Pharmacology

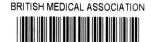

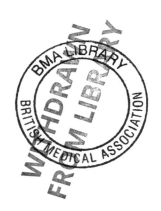

First and second edition authors:

Magali N F Taylor

Peter J W Reide

James S Dawson

Third edition author:

Gada Yassin

Fourth edition author:

Elisabetta Battista

5th Edition
CRASH COURSE

SERIES EDITORS

Philip Xiu
MA, MB BChir, MRCP
GP Registrar
Yorkshire Deanery
Leeds, UK

Shreelata Datta
MD, MRCOG, LLM, BSc (Hons), MBBS
Honorary Senior Lecturer
Imperial College London
Consultant Obstetrician and Gynaecologist
King's College Hospital
London, UK

FACULTY ADVISOR

Clive Page
OBE, PhD
Director, Sackler Institute of Pulmonary Pharmacology
Institute of Pharmaceutical Science
King's College London
London, UK

Pharmacology

Catrin Page
BSc, Mb, ChB
Core trainee
St. George's hospital
London, UK

ELSEVIER

ELSEVIER

Senior Content Strategist: Jeremy Bowes
Senior Content Development Specialist: Alex Mortimer
Project Manager: Andrew Riley
Page design: Christian bilbow
Illustration Manager: Karen Giacomucci
Illustrator: MPS North America LLC
Marketing Manager: Deborah Watkins

Notices

Practitioners and researchers must always rely on their own experience and knowledge in evaluating and using any information, methods, compounds or experiments described herein. Because of rapid advances in the medical sciences, in particular, independent verification of diagnoses and drug dosages should be made. To the fullest extent of the law, no responsibility is assumed by Elsevier, authors, editors or contributors for any injury and/or damage to persons or property as a matter of products liability, negligence or otherwise, or from any use or operation of any methods, products, instructions, or ideas contained in the material herein.

First edition 1998
Second edition 2002
Third edition 2008
Fourth edition 2013
Updated fourth edition 2015
Fifth edition 2019

ISBN: 978-0-7020-7344-1
eISBN: 978-0-7020-7345-8

The *Crash Course* series was conceived by Dr Dan Horton-Szar who as series editor presided over it for more than 15 years – from publication of the first edition in 1997, until publication of the fourth edition in 2011. His inspiration, knowledge and wisdom lives on in the pages of this book. As the new series editors, we are delighted to be able to continue developing each book for the twenty-first century undergraduate curriculum.

The flame of medicine never stands still, and keeping this all-new fifth series relevant for today's students is an ongoing process. Each title within this new fifth edition has been re-written to integrate basic medical science and clinical practice, after extensive deliberation and debate. We aim to build on the success of the previous titles by keeping the series up-to-date with current guidelines for best practice, and recent developments in medical research and pharmacology.

We always listen to feedback from our readers, through focus groups and student reviews of the *Crash Course* titles. For the fifth editions we have reviewed and re-written our self-assessment material to reflect today's 'single-best answer' and 'extended matching question' formats. The artwork and layout of the titles has also been largely re-worked and are now in colour, to make it easier on the eye during long sessions of revision. The new on-line materials supplement the learning process.

Despite fully revising the books with each edition, we hold fast to the principles on which we first developed the series. *Crash Course* will always bring you all the information you need to revise in compact, manageable volumes that still maintain the balance between clarity and conciseness, and provide sufficient depth for those aiming at distinction. The authors are junior doctors who have recent experience of the exams you are now facing, and the accuracy of the material is checked by a team of faculty editors from across the UK.

We wish you all the best for your future careers!

Philip Xiu and Shreelata Datta

Prefaces

Author

This book has been thoroughly updated to provide an accessible learning and revision aid for understanding the principles and applications of pharmacology.

The introductory chapter provides a comprehensive overview of the basic principles of pharmacology. The remaining chapters highlight the effect of drugs on different organ systems and include updates on the most recent pharmacological advance (e.g. novel anti coagulants and newer targeted therapies used in oncology). The self-assessment section has been updated to reflect the content contained within several undergraduate and post-graduate examinations. The self-assessment section includes questions focused on clinical pharmacology and drug –drug interactions and is in a 'Best of fives' format.

I hope you find the book informative and enjoyable, and wish you luck in learning the fascinating and essential subject of pharmacology.

Catrin Page

Faculty Advisor

This volume of *Crash Course: Pharmacology* has been thoroughly revised from the previous editions. Even more than ever it provides a comprehensive and approachable text for medical students and others interested in the study of pharmacology. As part of the *Crash Course* series, the overall style is user friendly, consisting of concise bulleted text with informative illustrations, many of which are new. The content provides a comprehensive overview of the core material needed to pass the pharmacology component of the undergraduate medical curriculum. At the end of the chapter, there is a self-assessment section consisting of multiple-choice questions, short-answer questions and extended-matching questions which test the reader's understanding of the topic.

In line with the new style of curriculum recommended by the General Medical Council, the pharmacology is organized logically into body systems and the clinical relevance of the pharmacology is stressed throughout.

I have no doubt that this volume will be a useful study and revision aid for students. It provides a refreshing means of bringing the medical student up to speed in pharmacology. I would like to formally acknowledge the hard work of Catrin Page and the highly professional way she has updated this volume, significantly improving the value of this book as a revision aid for students.

Clive Page

Acknowledgements

I would like to thank Professor Clive Page for his advice and encouragement throughout the process of updating this book. Further thanks to everyone involved with the book at Elsevier.

I also am grateful for the support given to me by family and for the opportunity to complete my medical degree and teaching fellow role at the University of Bristol, which has enabled me to hopefully update this book to be a relevant and practical source of revision for other students and doctors alike.

Catrin Page

FIGURE ACKNOWLEDGEMENTS

Figures 1.3–1.5, 1.11B, 2.1–2.4, 5.2, 5.4, 5.11, 5.18, 5.19, 6.1–6.5, 6.7, 6.11, 6.17, 7.1–7.5, 8.1, 10.8–10.10 and 10.13 redrawn with kind permission from *Integrated Pharmacology,* 3rd edn, edited by Professor C Page, Dr M Curtis, Professor M Walker and Professor B Hoffman, Mosby, 2006.

KEY TO ICONS

	Agonists		Closed voltage-gated ion channel
	Antagonist		Open voltage-gated ion channel
	Receptor		Active state of pump
	Active state of an enzyme		Energy-dependent carrier molecule
	Inactive state of an enzyme		

Series Editors' acknowledgements

We would like to thank the support of our colleagues who have helped in the preparation of this edition, namely the junior doctor contributors who helped write the manuscript as well as the faculty editors who check the veracity of the information.

We are extremely grateful for the support of our publisher, Elsevier, whose staffs' insight and persistence has maintained the quality that Dr Horton-Szar has setout since the first edition. Jeremy Bowes, our commissioning editor, has been a constant support. Alex Mortimer and Barbara Simmons our development editors has managed the day-to-day work on this edition with extreme patience and unflaggable determination to meet the ever looming deadlines, and we are ever grateful for Kim Benson's contribution to the online editions and additional online supplementary materials.

Philip Xiu and Shreelata Datta

Contents

Introduction to pharmacology

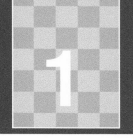

MOLECULAR BASIS OF PHARMACOLOGY

What is pharmacology?

Pharmacology is the study of the actions, mechanisms, uses and adverse effects of drugs.

A drug is any natural or synthetic substance that alters the physiological state of a living organism. Drugs can be divided into two groups.

- Medicinal drugs: substances used for the prevention, treatment and diagnosis of disease.
- Nonmedicinal (social) drugs: substances used for recreational purposes. These drugs include illegal substances such as cannabis, heroin and cocaine, as well as everyday substances such as caffeine, nicotine and alcohol (see Chapter 9).

Although drugs may have a selective action, there is always a risk of adverse effects associated with the use of any drug, and the prescriber should assess the balance of desired and adverse effects when deciding which drug to prescribe.

Drug names and classification

A single drug can have a variety of names and belong to many classes. Drugs are classified according to their:

- pharmacotherapeutic actions
- pharmacological actions
- molecular actions
- chemical nature

When a drug company's patent expires, the marketing of the drug is open to other manufacturers. Although the generic name is retained, the brand names can be changed.

How do drugs work?

Most drugs produce their effects by targeting specific cellular macromolecules, often proteins. The majority act as receptors in cell membranes, but they can also inhibit enzymes and transporter molecules. Some drugs directly interact with molecular targets found in pathogens. For example, β-lactam antibiotics are bactericidal, acting by interfering with bacterial cell wall synthesis.

Certain drugs do not have conventional targets. For example, succimer is a chelating drug that is used to treat heavy metal poisoning. It binds to metals, rendering them inactive and more readily excretable. Such drugs work by means of their physicochemical properties and are said to

have a nonspecific mechanism of action. For this reason, these drugs must be given in much higher doses than the more specific drugs. Another example would be antacids used to reduce the effect of excessive acid secretion in the stomach.

Transport systems

Ion channels

Ion channels are proteins that form pores in the cell membrane and allow selective transfer of ions (charged species) in and out of the cell. Opening or closing of these channels is known as *gating*; this occurs as a result of the ion channel undergoing a change in shape. Gating is controlled either by a neurotransmitter (receptor operated channels) or by the membrane potential (voltage-operated channels).

Some drugs modulate ion channel function directly by blocking the pore (e.g. the blocking action of local anaesthetics on sodium channels); others bind to a part of the ion channel protein to modify its action (e.g. anxiolytics acting on the γ-aminobutyric acid [GABA] channel). Other drugs interact with ion channels indirectly via a G-protein and other intermediates.

Carrier molecules

Carrier molecules located in the cell membrane facilitate the transfer of ions and molecules against their concentration gradients. There are two types of carrier molecule.

1. Energy-independent carriers: These are transporters (move one type of ion/molecule in one direction), symporters (move two or more ions/molecules) or antiporters (exchange one or more ions/molecules for one or more other ions/molecules).
2. Energy-dependent carriers: These are termed *pumps* (e.g. the Na^+/K^+ adenosine triphosphatase [ATPase] pump).

Enzymes

Enzymes are protein catalysts that increase the rate of specific chemical reactions without undergoing any net change themselves during the reaction. All enzymes are potential targets for drugs. Drugs either act as a false substrate for the enzyme or inhibit the enzyme's activity directly, usually by binding the catalytic site on the enzyme (Fig. 1.1).

Certain drugs may require enzymatic modification. This degradation converts a drug from its inactive form (prodrug) to its active form.

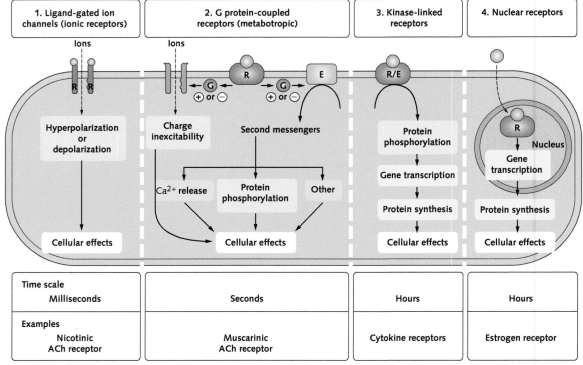

Fig. 1.1 How ion channel enzymes work. *ACh*, acetylcholine. (From Rang HP, Dale MM, Ritter JM, Moore PK. *Pharmacology*. 8th ed. Edinburgh: Churchill Livingstone, 2016.)

Receptors

Receptors are the means through which endogenous ligands produce their effects on cells. A receptor is a specific protein molecule usually located in the cell membrane, although intracellular receptors and intranuclear receptors also exist.

A ligand that binds and activates a receptor is an agonist. However, a ligand that binds to a receptor but does not activate the receptor and prevents an agonist from doing so is called an antagonist.

The following are naturally occurring ligands.

- Neurotransmitters: Chemicals released from nerve terminals that diffuse across the synaptic cleft, and bind to presynaptic or postsynaptic receptors.
- Hormones: Chemicals that, after being released locally, or into the bloodstream from specialized cells, can act at neighbouring or distant cells.

Each cell expresses only certain receptors, depending on the function of the cell. Receptor number and responsiveness to external ligands can be modulated.

In many cases, there is more than one receptor for each messenger so that the messenger often has different pharmacological specificity and different functions according to where it binds (e.g. adrenaline is able to produce different effects in different tissues because different adrenergic receptors are formed of different cell types).

There are four main types of receptor (Table 1.1).

Table 1.1 The four main types of receptor and their uses

Receptor type	Time for effect	Receptor example	Function example
Ion channel–linked	Milliseconds	Nicotinic acetylcholine receptor	Removing hand from hot water
G-protein–linked	Seconds	β-Adrenergic receptor	Airway smooth muscle relaxation
Tyrosine kinase–linked	Minutes	Insulin receptor	Glucose uptake into cells
DNA-linked	Hours to days	Steroid receptor	Cellular proliferation

1. Receptors directly linked to ion channels

Receptors that are directly linked to ion channels (Fig. 1.2) are mainly involved in fast synaptic neurotransmission. A classic example of a receptor linked directly to an ion channel is the nicotinic acetylcholine receptor (nicAChR).

The nicAChRs possess several characteristics:

- Acetylcholine (ACh) must bind to the N-terminal of both α subunits to activate the receptor.

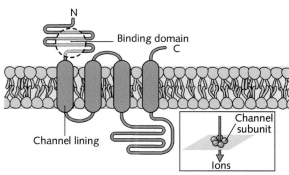

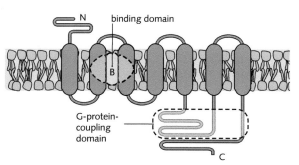

Fig. 1.2 General structure of the subunits of receptors directly linked to ion channels. *C*, C-terminal; *N*, N-terminal. (Modified from Page, C., Curtis, M. Walker, M, Hoffman, B. (eds) *Integrated Pharmacology*, 3rd edn. Mosby, 2006.)

Fig. 1.3 General structure of the subunits of receptors linked to G-proteins. *C*, C-terminal; *N*, N-terminal. (Modified from Page, C., Curtis, M. Walker, M, Hoffman, B. (eds) *Integrated Pharmacology*, 3rd edn. Mosby, 2006.)

- The receptor shows marked similarities with the two other receptors for fast transmission, namely the GABA$_A$ and glycine receptors.

2. G-protein–linked receptors

G-protein–linked receptors (Fig. 1.3) are involved in relatively fast transduction. G-protein–linked receptors are the predominant receptor type in the body; muscarinic, ACh, adrenergic, dopamine, serotonin and opiate receptors are all examples of G-protein–linked receptors.

Molecular structure of the receptor

Most of the G-protein–linked receptors consist of a single polypeptide chain of 400 to 500 residues and have seven transmembrane-spanning α helices. The third intracellular

loop of the receptor is larger than the other loops and interacts with the G-protein.

The ligand-binding domain is buried within the membrane on one or more of the α helical segments.

G-proteins

Fig. 1.4 illustrates the mechanism of G-protein–linked receptors.

- In resting state, the G-protein is unattached to the receptor and is a trimer consisting of α, β and γ subunits (see Fig. 1.4A).
- The occupation of the receptor by an agonist produces a conformational change, causing its affinity for the trimer to increase. Subsequent association of the trimer with the receptor results in the dissociation of bound guanosine diphosphate (GDP) from the α subunit.

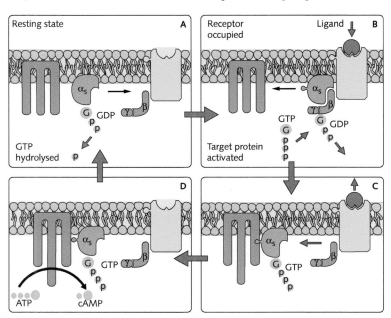

Fig. 1.4 Mechanism of action of G-protein–linked receptors. *α, β, γ*, subunits of G-protein; *ATP*, adenosine triphosphate; *cAMP*, cyclic adenosine monophosphate; *G*, guanosine; *GDP, GTP*, guanosine di- and triphosphate; *p*, phosphate. (Modified from Page, C., Curtis, M. Walker, M, Hoffman, B. (eds) *Integrated Pharmacology*, 3rd edn. Mosby, 2006).

Guanosine triphosphate (GTP) replaces GDP in the cleft thereby activating the G-protein and causing the α subunit to dissociate from the βγ dimer (see Fig. 1.4B).

- Alpha-GTP represents the active form of the G-protein (although this is not always the case: in the heart, potassium channels are activated by the βγ dimer and recent research has shown that the γ subunit alone may play a role in activation). This component diffuses in the plane of the membrane where it is free to interact with downstream effectors such as enzymes and ion channels. The βγ dimer remains associated with the membrane owing to its hydrophobicity (see Fig. 1.4C).
- The cycle is completed when the α subunit, which has enzymic activity, hydrolyses the bound GTP to GDP. The GDP-bound α subunit dissociates from the effector and recombines with the βγ dimer (see Fig. 1.4D).

This whole process results in an amplification effect because the binding of an agonist to the receptor can cause the activation of numerous G-proteins, which in turn can each, via their association with the effector, produce many other molecules intracellularly.

Many types of G-protein exist. This is probably attributable to the variability of the α subunit. G_s and G_i/G_o cause stimulation and inhibition, respectively, of the target enzyme adenylyl cyclase. This explains why muscarinic ACh receptors (G_i/G_o–linked) and β-adrenoreceptors (G_s-linked) located in the heart produce opposite effects. The bacterial toxins cholera and pertussis can be used to determine which G-protein is involved in a particular situation. Each has enzymic action on a conjugation reaction with the α subunit, such that:

- Cholera affects G_s causing continued activation of adenylyl cyclase. This explains why infection with cholera toxin results in uncontrolled fluid secretion from the gastrointestinal tract.
- Pertussis affects G_i and G_o causing continued inactivation of adenylyl cyclase. This explains why infection with *Bordetella pertussis* causes a "whooping" cough, characteristic of this infection, because the airways are constricted, and the larynx experiences muscular spasms.

Targets for G-proteins

G-proteins interact with either ion channels or secondary messengers. G-proteins may activate ion channels directly, for example, muscarinic receptors in the heart are linked to potassium channels which open directly on interaction with the G-protein, causing a slowing down of the heart rate. Secondary messengers are a family of mediating chemicals that transduces the receptor activation into a cellular response. These mediators can be targeted, and three main secondary messenger systems exist as targets of G-proteins (Fig. 1.5).

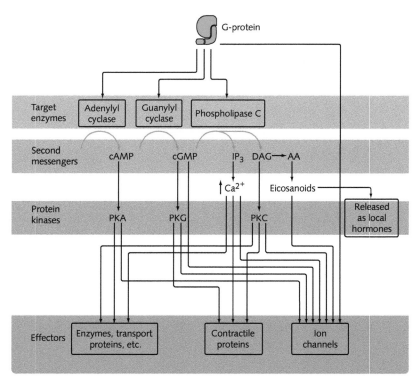

Fig. 1.5 Second-messenger targets of G-proteins and their effects. *AA*, arachidonic acid; *cAMP*, cyclic adenosine monophosphate; *cGMP*, cyclic guanosine monophosphate; *DAG*, diacylglycerol; IP_3, inositol (1,4,5) triphosphate; *PK*, protein kinase.

Adenylyl cyclase/cyclic adenosine monophosphate system—Adenylyl cyclase catalyses the conversion of ATP to cyclic adenosine monophosphate (cAMP) within cells. The cAMP produced causes activation of certain protein kinases, enzymes that phosphorylate serine and threonine amino acid residues in various proteins, thereby producing either activation or inactivation of these proteins. An example of this system can be observed in the activation of β_1-adrenergic receptors found in cardiac muscle. The activation of β_1-adrenergic receptors results in the activation of cAMP-dependent protein kinase A, which phosphorylates and opens voltage-operated calcium channels. This increases calcium levels in the cells and results in an increased rate and force of contraction. An inhibitory example of this system can be observed in activation of opioid receptors. The receptor linked to the "G_i" protein inhibits adenylyl cyclase and reduces cAMP production.

Phospholipase C/inositol phosphate system—Activation of M_1, M_3, 5-hydroxytryptamine (5-HT_2), peptide and α_1-adrenoreceptors, via G_q, cause activation of phospholipase C, a membrane-bound enzyme, which increases the rate of degradation of phosphatidylinositol (4,5) bisphosphate into diacylglycerol (DAG) and inositol (1,4,5) triphosphate (IP_3). DAG and IP_3 act as second messengers. IP_3 binds to the membrane of the endoplasmic reticulum, opening calcium channels and increasing the concentration of calcium within the cell. Increased calcium levels may result in smooth muscle contraction, increased secretion from exocrine glands, increased hormone or transmitter release, or increased force and rate of contraction of the heart. DAG, which remains associated with the membrane owing to its hydrophobicity, causes protein kinase C to move from the cytosol to the membrane where DAG can regulate the activity of the latter. There are at least six types of protein kinase C, with over 50 targets which can lead to:

- release of hormones and neurotransmitters
- smooth muscle contraction
- inflammation
- ion transport
- tumour promotion

Guanylyl cyclase system—Guanylyl cyclase catalyses the conversion of GTP to cyclic guanosine monophosphate (cGMP). This cGMP goes on to cause activation of protein kinase G which in turn phosphorylates contractile proteins and ion channels. Transmembrane guanylyl cyclase activity is exhibited by the atrial natriuretic peptide receptor upon the binding of atrial natriuretic peptide. Cytoplasmic guanylyl cyclase activity is exhibited when bradykinin activates receptors on the membrane of endothelial cells to generate nitric oxide, which then acts as a second messenger to activate guanylyl cyclase within the cell.

3. Tyrosine kinase-linked receptors

Tyrosine kinase-linked receptors are involved in the regulation of growth and differentiation, and responses to metabolic signals. The response time of enzyme-initiated transduction is slow (minutes). Examples include the receptors for insulin, platelet-derived growth factor and epidermal growth factor.

Activation of tyrosine kinase receptors results in autophosphorylation of tyrosine residues leading to the activation of pathways involving protein kinases. These receptors have become important targets for certain types of anticancer drugs (see Chapter 13).

4. Deoxyribonucleic acid–linked receptors

Deoxyribonucleic acid (DNA)–linked receptors are located intracellularly and so agonists must pass through the cell membrane to reach the receptor. The agonist binds to the receptor and this receptor–agonist complex is transported to the nucleus, aided by chaperone proteins. Once in the nucleus, the complex can bind to specific DNA sequences and so alter the expression of specific genes. As a result, transcription of this specific gene to messenger ribonucleic acid (mRNA) is increased or decreased and thus the amount of mRNA available, for translation into a protein, increases or decreases. The process is much slower than for other receptor–ligand interactions, and the effects usually last longer. Examples of molecules with DNA-linked receptors are corticosteroids, thyroid hormone, retinoic acid and vitamin D.

HINTS AND TIPS

Drugs, like naturally occurring chemical mediators, act on receptors located in the cell membrane, in the cytoplasm of the cell, or in the cell nucleus, to bring about a cellular, and eventually organ or tissue, response.

DRUG–RECEPTOR INTERACTIONS

Most drugs produce their effects by acting on specific protein molecules called receptors.

Receptors respond to endogenous chemicals in the body that are either synaptic transmitter substances (e.g. ACh, noradrenaline) or hormones (endocrine, e.g. insulin; or local mediators, e.g. histamine). These chemicals or drugs are classed in two ways.

- **Agonists**: Activate receptors and produce a subsequent response.
- **Antagonists**: Associate with receptors but do not cause activation. Antagonists reduce the chance of transmitters or agonists binding to the receptor and thereby oppose their action by effectively diluting or removing the receptors from the system.

Electrostatic forces initially attract a drug to a receptor. If the shape of the drug corresponds to that of the binding site of the receptor, then it will be held there temporarily by weak bonds or, in the case of irreversible antagonists, permanently by stronger covalent bonds. It is the number of bonds and goodness of fit between drug and receptor that determines the affinity of the drug for that receptor, such that the greater the number of bonds and the better the goodness of fit, the higher the affinity will be.

The affinity is defined by the dissociation constant, which is given the symbol K_d. The lower the K_d, the higher the affinity. K_d values in the nanomolar range represent drugs (D) with a high affinity for their receptor (R):

$$D + R \underset{k_{-1}}{\overset{k_{+1}}{\rightleftharpoons}} DR$$

The rate at which the forward reaction occurs depends on the drug concentration [D] and the receptor concentration [R]:

$$\text{Forward rate} = K_{+1}\left[D\right]\left[R\right]$$

The rate at which the backward reaction occurs mainly depends on the interaction between the drug and the receptor [DR]:

$$\text{Backward rate} = K_{-1}\left[DR\right]$$
$$K_d = K_{-1} / K_{+1}$$

K_a is the association constant and is used to quantify affinity. It can be defined as the concentration of drug that produces 50% of the maximum response at equilibrium, in the absence of receptor reserve:

$$K_a = 1 / K_d$$

Drugs with a high affinity stay bound to their receptor for a relatively long time and are said to have a slow off-rate. This means that at any time the probability that any given receptor will be occupied by the drug is high.

The ability of a drug to combine with one type of receptor is termed *specificity*. Although no drug is truly specific, most exhibit relatively selective action on one type of receptor.

Agonists

Agonist (A) binds to the receptor (R) and the chemical energy released on binding induces a conformational change that sets off a chain of biochemical events within the cell, leading to a response (AR*). The equation for this is:

$$A + R \xrightarrow{(1)} AR \xrightarrow{(2)} AR^*$$

where: (1) affinity; (2) efficacy.

Partial agonists cannot bring about the same maximum response as full agonists, even if their affinity for the receptor is the same (Fig. 1.6).

The ability of agonists, once bound, to activate receptors is termed *efficacy*, such that:

- Full agonists have high efficacy and are able to produce a maximum response while occupying only a small percentage of the receptors available.
- Partial agonists have low efficacy and are unable to elicit the maximum response even if they are occupying all the available receptors.

Antagonists

Antagonists bind to receptors but do not activate them; they do not induce a conformational change and thus have no intrinsic efficacy. However, because antagonists occupy the receptor, they prevent agonists from binding and therefore block their action.

Two types of antagonist exist: competitive and noncompetitive.

Competitive antagonists

Competitive antagonists bind to receptors reversibly, and effectively produce a dilution of the receptors such that:

- A parallel shift is produced to the right of the agonist dose–response curve (Fig. 1.7).
- The maximum response is not depressed. This reflects the fact that the antagonist's effect can be overcome by increasing the dose of agonist, that is, the block is surmountable. Increasing the concentration of agonist increases the probability of the agonist taking the place of an antagonist leaving the receptor.

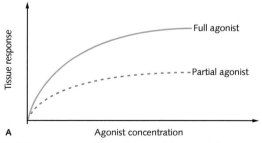

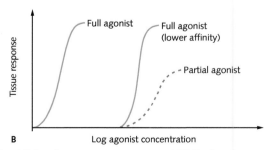

Fig. 1.6 Comparison of a partial agonist and a full agonist showing (A) the dose–response curve and (B) the log dose–response curve. (From Neal MJ. *Medical Pharmacology at a Glance,* 6th edition. Wiley-Blackwell, 2009.)

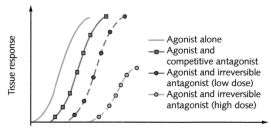

Fig. 1.7 Comparison of the log dose–response curves for competitive and noncompetitive (irreversible) antagonists. (From Neal MJ. *Medical Pharmacology at a Glance,* 6th edition. Wiley-Blackwell, 2009.)

- The size of the shift in the agonist dose–response curve produced by the antagonist reflects the affinity of the antagonist for the receptor. High-affinity antagonists stay bound to the receptor for a relatively long period of time allowing the agonist little chance to take the antagonist's place.

This concept can be quantified in terms of the dose ratio (known as a Schild plot). The dose ratio is the ratio of the concentration of agonist producing a given response in the presence and absence of a certain concentration of antagonist, for example, a dose ratio of 3 tells us that three times as much agonist was required to produce a given response in the presence of the antagonist than it did in its absence.

CLINICAL NOTE

A 22-year-old man is admitted to hospital with signs of respiratory depression, drowsiness, bradycardia and confusion. His girlfriend tells the medical team that he uses heroin and an overdose is therefore suspected. Heroin acts as an agonist, activating the opioid receptors. Naloxone is a competitive antagonist at those receptors and so is administered as treatment. Minutes later the man's condition improves, and his respiratory rate returns to normal. Careful titration of the naloxone dose should allow treatment of respiratory depression without provoking acute withdrawal signs.

Noncompetitive antagonists

Noncompetitive antagonists are also known as irreversible antagonists.

- Noncompetitive antagonists also produces a parallel shift to the right of the agonist dose–response curve (see Fig. 1.7).
- Their presence depresses the maximum response, reflecting the fact that the antagonist's effect cannot be

overcome by the addition of greater doses of agonist. At low concentrations, however, a parallel shift may occur without a reduced maximum response. This tells us that not all the receptors need to be occupied to elicit a maximum response because irreversible antagonists effectively remove receptors, there must be a number of spare receptors.

Receptor reserve

Although on a log scale the relation between the concentration of agonist and the response produces a symmetric sigmoid curve, rarely does a 50% response correspond to 50% receptor occupancy. This is because there are spare receptors.

This excess of receptors is known as receptor reserve and serves to sharpen the sensitivity of the cell to small changes in agonist concentration. The low efficacy of partial agonists can be overcome in tissues with a large receptor reserve and in these circumstances, partial agonists may act as full agonists.

Potency

Potency relates to the concentration of a drug needed to elicit a response. The EC_{50}, where EC stands for effective concentration, is a number used to quantify potency. EC_{50} is the concentration of drug required to produce 50% of the maximum response. Thus the lower the EC_{50}, the more potent the drug. For agonists, potency is related to both affinity and efficacy, but for antagonists, only affinity is considered because they have no efficacy (Table 1.2).

Other variables can affect the efficacy of a drug beyond its potency. For example, if a potent drug in vitro is metabolized in the stomach or affected by the pH in the stomach, less would be available to reach the target site. This means that, if given as a tablet, it would be less than the in vitro potency predicted.

- Thus the effectiveness of a drug (Pharmacodynamics: the biological effect of the drug on the body) is influenced by many factors which are covered by the term *pharmacokinetics*: the way the body affects the drug with time, that is, the factors that determine its absorption, distribution, metabolism and excretion.

Table 1.2 Key definitions

Definition	Explanation
Affinity	Number of bonds and goodness of fit between drug and receptor.
Agonist	A ligand that binds and activates a receptor.
Antagonist	A ligand that binds to but does not activate a receptor. Prevents an agonist from binding.
Efficacy	The ability of agonists, once bound, to activate receptors.
Potency	Concentration of a drug needed to elicit a response.

PHARMACOKINETICS

Pharmacology can be divided into two disciplines. These are: Pharmacokinetics and Pharmacodynamics

Administration

The drug can be administered by a variety of routes.

Topical

Topical drugs are applied where they are needed, giving them the advantage that they do not have to cross any barriers or membranes. This means a higher concentration of the drug in the target tissue, with less drug being absorbed into the systemic circulations and therefore less likelihood of unwanted side effects. Examples include skin ointments; ear, nose or eye drops; and aerosols inhaled in the treatment of asthma.

Enteral

Enteral administration means that the drug reaches its target via the gut. This is the least predictable route of administration, owing to potential metabolism by the liver following absorption into the hepatoportal circulation (so called *first pass metabolism*)(Fig. 1.8), chemical breakdown and possible binding to food within the gastrointestinal tract. Drugs must cross several barriers, which may or may not be a problem according to their physicochemical properties, such as charge and size.

- However, most drugs are administered orally unless the drug is unstable, or is rapidly inactivated in the gastrointestinal tract, or if the efficacy of absorption from the gastrointestinal tract is uncertain (e.g. vomiting or diarrhoea).
- In addition, absorption of drugs via the buccal or sublingual route avoids the hepatoportal circulation and is, therefore valuable when administering drugs subject to a high degree of first-pass metabolism (which is unavoidable if taken orally). It is also useful for potent drugs with a nondisagreeable taste, such as sublingual nitroglycerin given to relieve acute attacks of angina.
- Also, administration of drugs rectally, such as in the form of suppositories, means that there is less first-pass metabolism by the liver because the venous return from the lower gastrointestinal tract is less than that from the upper gastrointestinal tract. It has the disadvantage, however, of being inconsistent.

Parenteral

Parenteral administration means that the drug is administered in a manner that avoids the gut. The protein drug insulin, for example, is destroyed by the acidity of the stomach and the digestive enzymes within the gut and must, therefore be injected, usually subcutaneously.

Intravenous injection of drugs is sometimes used and has several advantages.

- It is the most direct route of administration. The drug enters the bloodstream directly and thus bypasses absorption barriers.
- A drug is distributed in a large volume and acts rapidly.

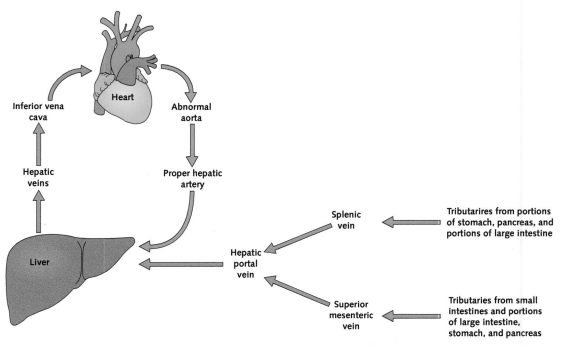

Fig. 1.8 The hepatoportal circulation and arterial supply and venous drainage of liver.

For drugs that must be given continuously by infusion, or for drugs that damage tissues, this is an important method of administration.

Alternative parenteral routes of administration include subcutaneous, intramuscular, epidural or intrathecal injections, as well as transdermal patches.

Binding the drug to a vehicle or coadministering a vasoconstrictor, such as adrenaline, to reduce blood flow to the site can decrease the rate of drug absorption from the site of the injection. This approach is commonly used in the administration of local anaesthetics and the presence of adrenaline in proportions of local anaesthetics has the added benefit of reducing bleeding by reducing blood flow when used in dental procedures or when carrying out skin biopsies.

Drug absorption

Bioavailability takes into account both absorption and metabolism and describes the proportion of the drug that passes into the systemic circulation. This will be 100% after an intravenous injection, but following oral administration, it will depend on the physiochemical characterizations of the drug, the individual and the circumstances under which the drug is given.

Drugs must cross membranes to enter cells or to transfer between body compartments; therefore drug absorption will be affected by both physiochemical and physiological factors.

Cell membranes

Cell membranes are composed of lipid bilayers and thus absorption is usually proportional to the lipid solubility of the drug. Unionized molecules (B) are far more soluble than those that are ionized (BH$^+$) and surrounded by a "shell" of water.

$$B + H^+ \rightleftharpoons BH^+$$

Size

Small molecular size is another factor that favours absorption. Most drugs are small molecules that are able to diffuse across membranes in their uncharged state.

pH—Because most drugs are either weak bases, weak acids or amphoteric, the pH of the environment in which they dissolve, as well as the pK$_a$ value of the drug, will be important in determining the fraction in the unionized form that is in solution and able to diffuse across cell membranes (see Fig. 1.9). The pK$_a$ of a drug is defined as the pH at which 50% of the molecules in solution are in the ionized form, and is characterized by the Henderson–Hasselbalch equation:

For acidic molecules:

$$HA \rightleftharpoons H^+ + A^-$$
$$pK_a = pH + \log [HA]/[A^-]$$

For basic molecules:

$$BH^+ \rightleftharpoons B + H^+$$
$$pK_a = pH + \log[BH^+]/[B]$$

Drugs will tend to exist in the ionized form when exposed to an environment with a pH opposite to their own state. Therefore acids become increasingly ionized with increasing pH (i.e. basic).

It is useful to consider three important body compartments to plasma (pH = 7.4), stomach (pH = 2) and urine (pH = 8). Examples include the following.

- Aspirin is a weak acid (pK$_a$= 3.5) and its absorption will therefore be favoured in the stomach, where it is uncharged, and not in the plasma or the urine, where it is highly charged; aspirin in high doses may even damage the stomach.
- Morphine is a weak base (pK$_a$ = 8.0) that is highly charged in the stomach, quite charged in the plasma, and half charged in the urine. Morphine can cross the blood–brain barrier but is poorly and erratically absorbed from the stomach and intestines, and metabolized by the liver; it must, therefore be given by injection or delayed-release capsules.
- Some drugs, such as quaternary ammonium compounds (e.g. suxamethonium, tubocurarine), are always charged and must, therefore be injected or inhaled (e.g. tiotropium bromide).

Drug distribution

Once drugs have reached the circulation, they are distributed around the body. Because most drugs have a very small molecular size, they can leave the circulation by capillary filtration to act on the tissues.

The half-life of a drug (t$_{1/2}$) is the time taken for the plasma concentration of that drug to fall to half of its original value. Bulk transfer in the blood is very quick.

- Drugs exist either dissolved in the blood or bound to plasma proteins such as albumin. Albumin is the most important circulating protein for binding many acidic drugs.
- Drugs that are basic tend to be bound to a globulin fraction that increases with age. A drug that is bound is confined to the vascular system and is unable to exert its actions; this becomes a problem if more than 80% of the drug is bound.
- Drugs can interact, and one drug may displace another. For example, aspirin can displace the benzodiazepine diazepam from albumin.

The apparent volume of distribution (V$_d$) is the calculated pharmacokinetic space in which a drug is distributed.

$$V_d = \frac{dose\ administered}{initial\ apparent\ plasma\ concentration}$$

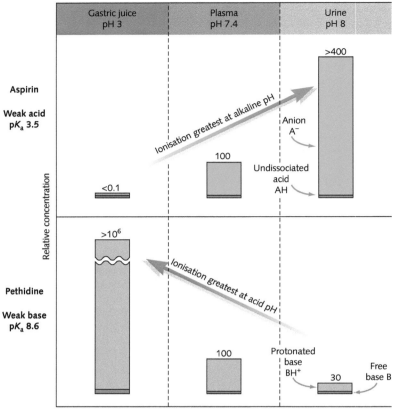

Fig. 1.9 Theoretic partition of a weak acid (aspirin) and a weak base (pethidine) between aqueous compartments (urine, plasma, and gastric juice) according to the pH difference between them. (From Rang HP, Dale MM, Ritter JM, Moore PK. *Pharmacology*. 8th ed. Edinburgh: Churchill Livingstone, 2016.)

- V_d values that amount to less than a certain body compartment volume indicate that the drug is contained within that compartment. For example, when the volume of distribution is less than 5 L, it is likely that the drug is restricted to the vasculature.
- V_d values less than 15 L implies that the drug is restricted to the extracellular fluid.
- V_d values greater than 15 L suggests distribution within the total body water. Some drugs (usually basic) have a volume of distribution that exceeds body weight, in which case tissue binding is occurring. These drugs tend to be contained outside the circulation and may accumulate in certain tissues. Very lipid-soluble substances, such as thiopental, can build up in fat. Mepacrine, an antimalarial drug, has a concentration in the liver 200 times that in the plasma because it binds to nucleic acids. Some drugs are even actively transported into certain organs, for example, iodine hormones accumulate in the thyroid.

CLINICAL NOTE

Anaesthetists need to consider the weight of their patient before administering thiopental given that it is a highly lipid soluble medication that will accumulate in the fat of obese patients and thus have a longer half-life than in a thinner patient.

Drug metabolism

Before being excreted from the body, most drugs are metabolized. A small number of drugs exist in their fully ionized form at physiological pH (7.4) and, owing to this highly polar nature, are metabolized to only a minor extent, if at all. The sequential metabolic reactions that occur have been categorized as phases 1 and 2.

Sites of metabolism

The liver is the major site of drug metabolism although most tissues can metabolize specific drugs. Other sites of metabolism include the kidney, the lung and the gastrointestinal tract. Diseases of these organs may therefore affect a drug's pharmacokinetics.

Orally administered drugs, which are usually absorbed in the small intestine, reach the liver via the portal circulation. At this stage, or within the small intestine, the drugs may be extensively metabolized; this is known as the first-pass metabolism and means that considerably less drug reaches the systemic circulation than enters the portal vein (see Fig. 1.10). This causes problems because it means that higher doses of the drug must be given and, owing to individual variation in the degree of the first-pass metabolism, the effects of the drug can be unpredictable. Drugs that are subject to a high degree of the first-pass metabolism, such as the local anaesthetic lidocaine, cannot be given orally and must be administered by some other route.

Phase 1 metabolic reactions

Phase 1 metabolic reactions include oxidation, reduction and hydrolysis. These reactions introduce a functional group, such as OH^- or NH_2, which increases the polarity of the drug molecule and provides a site for phase 2 reactions.

Oxidation

Oxidations are the most common type of reaction and are catalysed by an enzyme system known as the microsomal mixed function oxidase system, which is located on the smooth endoplasmic reticulum. The enzyme system forms small vesicles known as microsomes when the tissue is homogenized.

- Cytochrome P_{450} is the most important enzyme, although other enzymes are involved. This enzyme is a haemoprotein that requires the presence of oxygen, reduced nicotinamide adenine dinucleotide phosphate (NADPH) and NADPH cytochrome P_{450} reductase to function.

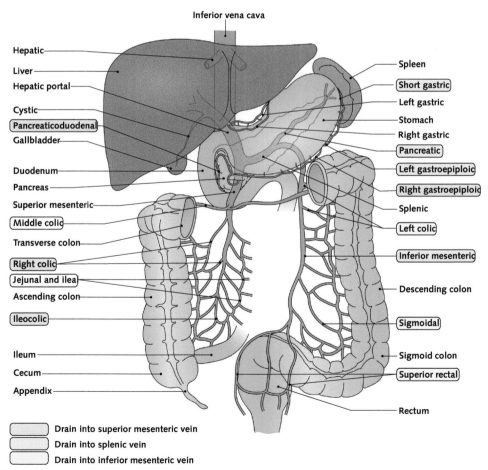

Inferior vena cava

Hepatic
Liver
Hepatic portal
Cystic
Pancreaticoduodenal
Gallbladder
Duodenum
Pancreas
Superior mesenteric
Middle colic
Transverse colon
Right colic
Jejunal and ilea
Ascending colon
Ileocolic
Ileum
Cecum
Appendix

Spleen
Short gastric
Left gastric
Stomach
Right gastric
Pancreatic
Left gastroepiploic
Right gastroepiploic
Splenic
Left colic
Inferior mesenteric
Descending colon
Sigmoidal
Sigmoid colon
Superior rectal
Rectum

Drain into superior mesenteric vein
Drain into splenic vein
Drain into inferior mesenteric vein

Fig 1.10 Portal venous system.

- It exists in several hundred isoforms, some of which are constitutive, whereas others are synthesized in response to specific signals. The substrate specificity of this enzyme depends on the isoform but tends to be low, meaning that a whole variety of drugs can be oxidized.

Although oxidative reactions usually result in inactivation of the drug, sometimes a metabolite is produced that is pharmacologically active and may have a duration of action exceeding that of the original drug. In these cases, the drug is known as a prodrug, for example, codeine that is demethylated to morphine.

Reduction

Reduction reactions also involve microsomal enzymes but are much less common than oxidation reactions. An example of a drug subject to reduction is prednisone, which is given as a prodrug and reduced to the active glucocorticoid prednisolone.

Hydrolysis

Hydrolysis is not restricted to the liver and occurs in a variety of tissues. Aspirin is spontaneously hydrolysed to salicylic acid in moisture.

Phase 2 metabolic reactions

Drug molecules possessing a suitable site that was either present before phase 1 or is the result of a phase 1 reaction, are susceptible to phase 2 reactions. Phase 2 reactions involve conjugation, the attachment of a large chemical group to a functional group of the drug molecule. Conjugation results in the drug being more hydrophilic and thus more easily excreted from the body.

- In conjugation it is mainly the liver that is involved, although conjugation can occur in a wide variety of tissues.
- Chemical groups involved are endogenous activated moieties such as glucuronic acid, sulphate, methyl, acetyl and glutathione.
- The conjugating enzymes exist in many isoforms and show relative substrate and metabolite specificity.

Unlike the products of phase 1 reactions, the conjugate is almost invariably inactive. An important exception is morphine, which is converted to morphine 6-glucuronide, which has an analgesic effect lasting longer than that of its parent molecule.

Factors affecting metabolism

Enzyme induction is the increased synthesis or decreased degradation of enzymes and occurs as a result of the presence of an exogenous substance. Examples include the following.

- Some drugs can increase the activity of certain isoenzyme forms of cytochrome P_{450} and thus increase their own metabolism, as well as that of other drugs.

- Smokers can show increased metabolism of certain drugs because of the induction of cytochrome P_{448} by a constituent in tobacco smoke.
- In contrast, some drugs inhibit microsomal enzyme activity and therefore increase their own activity as well as that of other drugs.

Table 1.3 gives some examples of enzyme-inducing agents, and the drugs whose metabolism is affected. Competition for a metabolic enzyme may occur between two drugs, in which case there is a decreased metabolism of one or both drugs. This is known as inhibition.

Enzymes that metabolize drugs are affected by many aspects of diet, such as the ratio of protein to carbohydrate, flavonoids contained in vegetables, and polycyclic aromatic hydrocarbons found in barbequed foods.

Overdose

Drugs that are taken at 2 to 1000 times their therapeutic dose can cause unwanted and toxic effects. Paracetamol can be lethal at high doses (2–3 times the maximum therapeutic dose), owing to the accumulation of its metabolites.

In phase 2 of the metabolic process, paracetamol is conjugated with glucuronic acid and sulphate. When high doses of paracetamol are ingested, these pathways become saturated and the drug is metabolized by the mixed

Table 1.3 Examples of drugs that induce or inhibit drug-metabolizing enzymes

Drugs modifying enzyme action	Drugs whose metabolism is affected
Enzyme induction	
Phenobarbital and other barbiturates	Warfarin
Rifampicin	Oral contraceptives
Phenytoin	Corticosteroids
Ethanol	Cyclosporine
Carbamazepine	
Enzyme inhibition	
Allopurinol	Azathioprine
Chloramphenicol	Phenytoin
Corticosteroids	Various drugs—TCA, cyclophosphamide
Cimetidine	Many drugs—amiodarone, phenytoin, pethidine
MAO inhibitors	Pethidine
Erythromycin	Cyclosporine
Ciprofloxacin	Theophylline

MAO, *monoamine oxidase*; TCA, *tricyclic antidepressant.*
Modified from Rang et al. 2012 Pharmacology, 7th edition, Churchill Livingstone.

function oxidases. This results in the formation of the toxic metabolite *N*-acetyl-*p*-benzoquinone which is inactivated by glutathione. However, when glutathione is depleted, this toxic metabolite reacts with nucleophilic constituents in the cell leading to necrosis in the liver and kidneys.

N-Acetylcysteine or methionine can be administered in cases of paracetamol overdose, because these increase liver glutathione formation and the conjugation reactions, respectively.

Drug excretion

Drugs are excreted from the body in a variety of different ways. Excretion predominantly occurs via the kidneys into urine or by the gastrointestinal tract into bile and faeces. Volatile drugs are predominantly exhaled by the lungs into the air. To a lesser extent, drugs may leave the body through breast milk and sweat.

The volume of plasma cleared of drug per unit time is known as the clearance.

Renal excretion

Glomerular filtration, tubular reabsorption (passive and active), and tubular secretion all determine the extent to which a drug will be excreted by the kidneys.

Glomerular capillaries allow the passage of molecules with a molecular weight less than 20 000. The glomerular filtrate thus contains most of the substances in plasma except proteins.

- In the glomerular capillaries the negative charge of the corpuscular membrane repels negatively charged molecules, including plasma proteins.
- In addition, drugs that bind to plasma proteins such as albumin will not be filtered.

Most of the drug in the blood does not pass into the glomerular filtrate but passes into the peritubular capillaries of the proximal tubule where, depending on its nature, one of two transport mechanisms will transport it into the lumen of the tubule. One transport mechanism deals with acidic molecules, the other with basic molecules.

- In the peritubular capillaries tubular secretion is responsible for most of the drug excretion carried out by the kidneys and, unlike glomerular filtration, allows the clearance of drugs bound to plasma proteins. Competition between drugs that share the same transport mechanism may occur, in which case the excretion of these drugs will be reduced.
- Reabsorption of a drug will depend upon the fraction of molecules in the ionized state, which is in turn dependent on the pH of the urine.
- Renal disease will affect the excretion of certain drugs. The extent to which excretion is impaired can be deduced by measuring 24-hour creatinine clearance.

Gastrointestinal excretion

Some drug conjugates are excreted into the bile and subsequently released into the intestines where they are hydrolysed back to the parent compound and reabsorbed. This "enterohepatic circulation" prolongs the effect of the drug.

> **HINTS AND TIPS**
>
> The liver is the main site of drug inactivation, and the kidneys and gastrointestinal tract the main sites for drug excretion. Disease of these organs will alter the pharmacokinetics of a drug.

Mathematic aspects of pharmacokinetics

Kinetic order

Two types of kinetics, related to the plasma concentration of a drug, describe the rate at which a drug leaves the body.

- Zero-order kinetics (Fig. 1.11A) describes a decrease in drug levels in the body that is independent of the plasma concentration, and the rate is held constant by a limiting factor, such as a cofactor of enzyme availability.

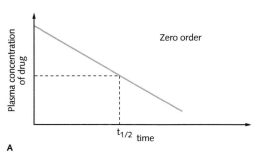 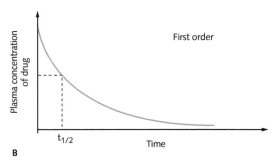

Fig. 1.11 Plasma drug concentration versus time plot. (A) For a drug displaying zero-order kinetics. (B) For a drug displaying first-order kinetics. *t* ½, half-life.

When the plasma concentration is plotted against time, the decrease is a straight line. Alcohol is an example of a drug that displays zero-order kinetics.

- First-order kinetics (Fig. 1.11B) is displayed by most drugs. It describes a decrease in drug levels in the body that is dependent on the plasma concentration because the concentration of the substrate (drug) is the rate-limiting factor. When the plasma concentration is plotted against time, the decrease is exponential.

One-compartment model

The one-compartment model usually gives an adequate clinical approximation of drug concentration by considering the body to be a single compartment. Within this single compartment, a drug is absorbed, immediately distributed, and subsequently eliminated by metabolism and excretion.

If the volume of the compartment is V_d and the dose administered D, then the initial drug concentration, C_o, will be:

$$C_o = D / V_d$$

The time taken for the plasma drug concentration to fall to half of its original value is the half-life of that drug. The decline in concentration may be exponential, but this situation expresses itself graphically as a straight line when the log plasma concentration is plotted against the time after intravenous dose (Fig. 1.12A).

Half-life is related to the elimination rate constant (K_{el}) by the following equation:

$$t_{1/2} \times K_{el} = \text{natural log } 2 (\ln 2)$$

Half-life is related to V_d, but does not determine the ability of the body to remove the drug from the circulation, because both V_d and half-life change in the same direction. The body's ability to remove a drug from the blood is termed *clearance* (Cl_p) and is constant for individual drugs.

$$Cl_p = V_d \times K_{el}$$

If the drug is not administered parenterally, plotting the log plasma drug concentration against time will require the consideration of both absorption and elimination from the compartment (Fig. 1.12B).

The one-compartment model is widely used to determine the dose of the drug to be administered. The two-compartment model expands on this model by considering the body as two compartments to allow some consideration of drug distribution.

Model-independent approach

For drugs displaying first-order kinetics, the level of the drug in the body increases until it is equal to the level excreted, at which point steady-state is reached (Fig. 1.13), such that:

- The time to reach steady-state is usually equal to four to five half-lives.
- The amount of drug in the body at steady-state will depend upon the frequency of drug administration: the greater the frequency, the greater the amount of drug and the less the variation between peak and trough plasma concentrations. If the frequency of administration is greater than the half-life, then an accumulation of the drug will occur.

The loading dose can be calculated according to the desired plasma concentration at steady-state (C_{ss}) and the volume of distribution (V_d) of the drug:

$$\text{Loading dose} (mg / kg) = V_d (L / kg) \times C_{ss} (mg / L)$$

Adherence

Lastly, despite not being a pharmacological property, it is important to consider adherence. For some drugs to be effective (e.g. antibiotics), they must be taken at regular intervals and for a certain period of time. Adherence can be an issue in paediatric and elderly patients. With children, parents must remember to give the medicine and follow directions

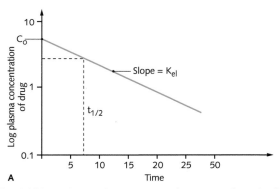

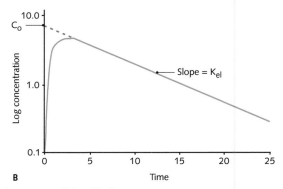

Fig. 1.12 Log plasma drug concentration versus time plot for a drug compatible with the one-compartment open pharmacokinetic model for drug disposition. (A) After a parenteral dose, assuming first-order kinetics. (B) After an oral dose. C_o, initial drug concentration; K_{el}, elimination rate constant. (modified from Page, C., Curtis, M. Walker, M, Hoffman, B. (eds) *Integrated Pharmacology*, 3rd edn. Mosby, 2006.)

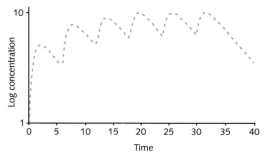

Fig. 1.13 Log plasma drug concentration versus time plot for a drug administered by mouth every 6 hours when its terminal disposition half-life is 6 hours.

accurately; the child must cooperate and not spit out or spill the medicine. Similarly, elderly patients' capacity to understand and remember to take their medicines must be ascertained, as well as their physical ability to carry out the task. For example, an elderly patient with arthritis may struggle to administer medicines unaided. Furthermore, adherence is limited if patients are required to take several medications.

Practical dosage forms are important in achieving adherence. Many tablets are now sugar coated, making them easier to take, and a large number of the drugs manufactured for children are in the form of elixirs or suspensions, which may be available in a variety of different flavours, making their administration less of a problem.

The route of administration of a drug may affect adherence. Taking a drug orally, for example, is simpler than injecting it. The wide variety of devices available to deliver inhaled drugs are often challenging because this may require good coordination to work properly, something the young, infirm and elderly find difficult.

The dosing schedule is also an important aspect of adherence. The easier this is to follow, and the less frequently a drug needs to be taken or administered, the more likely adherence will be achieved.

DRUG INTERACTIONS AND ADVERSE EFFECTS

Drug interactions

Drugs interact in a number of ways that may produce unwanted effects. Two types of interactions exist: pharmacodynamic and pharmacokinetic.

Pharmacodynamic interactions

Pharmacodynamic interactions involve a direct conflict between the effects of drugs. This conflict results in the effect of one of the two drugs being enhanced or reduced. Examples include the following.

- Propranolol, a β-adrenoceptor antagonist given for angina and hypertension, will reduce the effect of

salbutamol, a β_2-adrenoceptor agonist given for the treatment of asthma. The administration of beta-blockers to asthmatics should therefore be avoided, or undertaken with caution.
- Administration of monoamine oxidase inhibitors, which inhibit the metabolism of catecholamines, enhances the effects of drugs such as ephedrine. This enhancement causes the release of noradrenaline from stores in the nerve terminal and is known as potentiation.

Pharmacokinetic interactions

Absorption, distribution, metabolism and excretion all affect the pharmacokinetic properties of drugs. Thus any drug that interferes with these processes will be altering the effect of other drugs.

- If administered with diuretics, nonsteroidal antiinflammatory drugs (NSAIDs) will reduce the antihypertensive action of these drugs. NSAIDs bring about this effect by reducing prostaglandin synthesis in the kidney, thus impairing renal blood flow and consequently decreasing the excretion of waste and sodium. This results in an increased blood volume and a rise in blood pressure.
- Enzyme induction, which occurs as a result of the administration of certain drugs, can affect the metabolism of other drugs served by that enzyme (see Table 1.3).

In some cases, however, drugs are used together so that their interaction can bring about the desired effect.

- For example, carbidopa is a drug used in conjunction with levodopa (L-dopa) in the treatment of Parkinson disease. L-Dopa, which is converted to dopamine in the body, can cross the blood–brain barrier. Carbidopa prevents the conversion of L-dopa to dopamine; however, it cannot cross the blood–brain barrier and so acts to reduce the peripheral side effects while still allowing the desired effects of the drug.

CLINICAL NOTE

Mr Abbas is a 66-year-old man who takes metoprolol, a β-blocker, for his hypertension. He had a myocardial infarction 2 days ago and has now developed ventricular tachycardia (a type of cardiac arrhythmia). He was given amiodarone (a class III antiarrhythmic agent) to slow down his heart rate. Because amiodarone inhibits the cytochrome P_{450} enzymes responsible for breaking down metoprolol, there is a risk that the plasma concentration of metoprolol would be higher than expected. The prescribing doctor, therefore needs to monitor for an excessive slow beating of the heart and for heart block.

Adverse effects

As well as interacting with one another and with their target tissue, drugs will also interact with other tissues and organs and alter their function. No drug is without side effects, although the severity and frequency of these will vary from drug to drug and from person to person.

The liver and the kidneys are susceptible to the adverse effects of drugs, as these are the sites of drug metabolism and excretion. Some drugs cause hepatotoxicity or nephrotoxicity.

Some people are more prone to the adverse effects of drugs.

- Pregnant women must be careful about taking certain medications that are teratogenic, that is, cause foetal malformations (e.g. thalidomide taken in the 1960s for morning sickness).
- Breastfeeding women must also be careful about which drugs they take, because many drugs can be passed on in the breast milk to the developing infant.
- Patients with an underlying illness, such as liver or kidney disease. These illnesses will result in decreased metabolism and excretion of the drug and will produce the side effects of an increased dose of the same drug.
- Elderly people who tend to take a large number of drugs have an increased risk of drug interactions and the associated side effects. In addition, elderly patients have a reduced renal clearance and a nervous system that is more sensitive to drugs. The dose of drug initially given is usually 50% of the adult dose, and certain drugs are contraindicated.
- Children, like the elderly, are at an increased risk of toxicity because of immature clearance systems.
- Patients with genetic enzyme defects, such as glucose 6-phosphate dehydrogenase deficiency. The deficiency will result in haemolysis if an oxidant drug, such as aspirin, is taken.

Certain drugs are carcinogenic, that is, induce cancer. Allergic reactions to certain drugs are common, occurring in 2% to 25% of cases. Most of these are not serious, for example, skin reactions; however, rarely, reactions such as anaphylactic shock (type 1 hypersensitivity) occur that may be lethal, unless treated with intramuscular adrenaline. The most common allergic reaction is to penicillin, which produces an anaphylactic shock in approximately 1 in 50,000 people.

HINTS AND TIPS

Adverse reactions and allergy to a drug are different. Adverse reactions are usually minor irritations, whereas an allergic reaction can be life threatening.

DRUG HISTORY AND DRUG DEVELOPMENT

Drug history

A patient's drug history is a crucial component of the clerking process, because drug effects account for a significant proportion of hospital admissions, and potential drug interactions and adverse events are crucial to foresee.

A complete list of the names and doses of prescribed drugs taken by the patient (noting the proprietary and the generic name, for example, Viagra and sildenafil, respectively) and any other medications or supplements they may have bought themselves over the counter at a pharmacy should be documented. Women often forget the contraceptive pill and hormone replacement therapy and should be sensitively questioned about these. NSAIDs and paracetamol are often taken by patients with arthritis and should be specifically asked about. Make sure to note how often the drugs were taken, and at what times.

If presented with numerous bottles and packets of tablets, ensure they all belong to the patient, and not the partner of the patient, or to someone else. Always ask the patient if they are taking all their medicines as prescribed.

Occasionally, it is useful to know what drugs have been taken in the recent and distant past; for example, monoamine oxidase inhibitors should be stopped at least 3 weeks before starting a different antidepressant therapy.

Previous adverse reaction to drugs, and to nondrug products such as latex, is essential to ascertain. Explore what happened to the patient, and what was done about it. An upset stomach a day after taking penicillin is a common side effect, and is not grounds for choosing another antibiotics when treating a penicillin-sensitive infection in the future. A widespread cutaneous rash and difficulty breathing which required adrenaline and a hospital admission suggests an allergic drug reaction and therefore this, or any related drug should be clearly avoided in the future. Allergy to drugs should be clearly marked in the patient's notes and drug charts.

The family history of adverse drug reactions is usually confined to the anaesthetic history, where the concern is largely in relation to the muscle-relaxing drugs, particularly suxamethonium.

A history of recreational or illicit drug use is an important but sensitive issue to approach. One must use discretion when questioning the patient. A history of smoking should also be established.

Knowledge about any hepatic or renal disease and general health problems is important when it comes to management and prescribing, as are specific considerations, such as not prescribing aspirin in peptic ulcer disease, or oestrogen to patients with oestrogen-dependent cancers. These aspects are usually brought to light in the rest of the history taking.

The salient points of the drug history are:
- current and previous drugs and their doses
- adverse drug reactions and allergies
- family history of allergies
- recreational drug use
- existing renal or hepatic and general disease.

Drug development

Hundreds of thousands of substances have been produced by the pharmaceutical industry over the past 50 years, although very few ever get past preclinical screening, and fewer than 10% of these survive clinical assessment.

There are four stages a potential drug goes through from discovery to being approved (Table 1.4).

Phase 4 can be regarded as an ongoing phase, where drugs are monitored once licensed for general use. By this stage, the efficacy and dose–response relationship are known, although the side-effect profile is often incomplete, and information is gathered on these "adverse reactions" which are caused by, or likely caused by new drugs.

In the United Kingdom, this is known as the yellow card scheme. The British National Formulary (BNF) contains detachable yellow cards, which medical staff complete, documenting adverse drug reactions in their patients, which can then be forwarded to the Medicines Control Agency. The Medicines Control Agency collates these data and uses them for surveillance of common or severe adverse effects. The data are publicized in future copies of the BNF, or used in the reassessment of certain drug licences.

Table 1.4 The five stages of drug development and monitoring

Phase	Main aims/means of investigation	Subjects
Preclinical	Pharmacology	In vitro
	Toxicology	In laboratory animals
Phase 1	Clinical pharmacology and toxicology	Healthy individuals and/or patients
	Drug metabolism and bioavailability	
	Evaluate safety	
Phase 2	Initial treatment studies	Small numbers of patients
	Evaluate efficacy	
Phase 3	Large randomized controlled trials	Large numbers of patients
	Comparing new to old treatments	
	Evaluate safety and efficacy	
Phase 4	Postmarketing surveillance	All patients prescribed the drug
	Long-term safety and rare events	
	Yellow card scheme	

● Chapter Summary

- Drugs can produce their effects by targeting specific cellular macromolecules, often proteins. The majority act via receptors in cell membranes but they can also work on transporter molecules and enzymes.
- Interaction with ligand-gated ion channels (ionic receptors) results in hyperpolarization or depolarization. Interaction with G protein-coupled receptors (metabotropic) results in secondary messenger involvement and either calcium release or protein phosphorylation. Kinase-linked receptor activation results in protein phosphorylation which induces gene transcription and protein synthesis. Nuclear receptor activation results in gene transcription and protein synthesis.
- Drugs can be administered topically, enterally, or parenterally. Drug excretion, metabolism and dosage can be modelled by pharmacokinetics to relate to plasma concentration of a drug.
- Drugs can interact in unwanted ways, involving pharmacokinetics and pharmacodynamics. Adverse drug effects stem from the drug interacting with tissues and organs to alter their function. Adverse reactions are usually minor, whereas allergic reactions can be life-threatening.
- Drug development is divided into preclinical and then 4 subsequent phases involving ever larger trials. Phase 4 is postmarketing surveillance and is always ongoing once the drug is in the market.

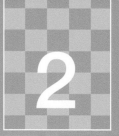
BASIC CONCEPTS

The nervous system consists of the peripheral nervous system (PNS), which consists of the nerves and ganglia outside of the brain and spinal cord (the central nervous system [CNS]). The PNS connects the CNS to the limbs and organs, providing a route of transmission between the brain and spinal cord and the rest of the body. The PNS is further divided into the somatic nervous system (SNS) and the autonomic nervous system (ANS). The SNS provides voluntary skeletal muscle control, whereas the ANS provides involuntary control of smooth muscle and glands. Afferent nerves are responsible for relaying sensation from the body to the CNS and efferent nerves are responsible for sending out commands from the CNS to the body, within the SNS. The hypothalamus regulates the ANS and is responsible for regulating heart rate, respiratory rate, digestion, pupillary response and urination as well as the fight-or-flight response.

NERVE CONDUCTION

Conduction of impulses through nerves occurs as an all-or-none event called the *action potential*. The action potential is caused by the voltage-dependent opening of sodium and potassium channels in the cell membrane.

All cells maintain a negative internal potential between $-30\,mV$ and $-80\,mV$. This arises because the permeability of the plasma membrane is different for sodium (Na^+) and potassium (K^+). The membrane is relatively impermeable to Na^+. Na^+ is also exchanged for K^+ via the Na^+/K^+ pump. The result is that the intracellular K^+ concentration is higher and the Na^+ lower than the respective extracellular concentrations. The sodium equilibrium potential (Eq Na^+) is $-60\,mV$ and the potassium equilibrium potential (Eq K^+) is $-90\,mV$. Because a resting nerve has 50 to 75 more potassium channels open than sodium channels, the resting membrane potential is $-70\,mV$.

Fig. 2.1 shows the concentrations of Na^+ and K^+ inside and outside a resting nerve. The Na^+/K^+ pump (Na^+/K^+ adenosine triphosphate [ATPase]) is an energy-dependent pump that functions to maintain the concentration gradient of these two ionic species across the membrane. Three sodium ions are pumped out of the cell for every two potassium ions pumped in, and thus the excitability of the cell is retained. Fig. 2.2 and Table 2.1 summarize the events that occur during a nerve action potential.

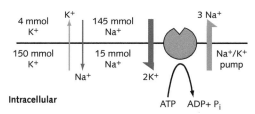

Fig. 2.1 Intracellular and extracellular sodium and potassium concentrations. The Na^+/K^+ pump maintains these concentration gradients across the cell membrane. *ADP*, Adenosine diphosphate; *ATP*, adenosine triphosphate.

- During a nerve action potential, the rate of sodium entry into the nerve axon becomes greater than the rate of potassium out of the axon, at which point the membrane becomes depolarised (the loss of an electrical gradient across the membrane).
- Depolarisation sets off a sodium-positive feedback whereby more voltage-gated sodium channels open and the membrane becomes more depolarized.
- A threshold, which is usually $15\,mV$ greater than the resting membrane potential, must be reached if an action potential is to be generated.
- The membrane repolarizes when the sodium channels become inactivated; a special set of potassium channels open and potassium leaves the axon.
- The sodium channels; eventually regain their resting excitable state and the Na^+/K^+ ATPase restores the membrane potential back to $-70\,mV$.

Fig. 2.3 shows the voltage-operated sodium channels in their inactivated, activated and resting states. Two types of gate exist within the channel; the m-gates and the h-gates. These gates are open or closed according to the state of the channel.

In the resting sodium channel, the m-gates are held closed by the strongly negative ($-70\,mV$) electrical gradient across the membrane. Once an action potential begins to propagate, the loss of the membrane potential causes the m-gates to open, allowing sodium into the cell, further propagating the action potential. After a very short time, a further conformational change causes the h-gates to close, inactivating the sodium channel. The membrane then repolarizes, and once at $-70\,mV$, the m-gates again close, and the h-gates open so the sodium channel is back in its resting state.

Sodium channel

The voltage-operated sodium channel is present in all excitable tissues. It is a transmembrane protein made up of four domains, each with six transmembrane regions. It is sensitive to membrane potential and selectively passes sodium ions.

Local anaesthetics block the sodium channel (see Chapter 10), and thus nerve conduction, by binding to the sixth transmembrane region of the fourth domain.

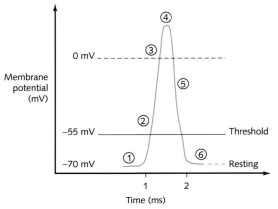

Fig. 2.2 Nerve action potential. For explanation of points 1 to 6, see Table 2.1.

Size of the nerve fibre

Small nerve fibres are preferentially blocked because of their high surface-area to volume ratio. This results in a differential block whereby the small nociceptive (pain) and autonomic fibres are blocked, but not the larger fibres responsible for the mediation of movement and touch.

SOMATIC NERVOUS SYSTEM

Neuromuscular junction

The neuromuscular junction is a chemical synapse formed by motor nerve axons and muscle fibres. It is the site where a motor neurone is able to transmit a signal to the muscle fibre, resulting in a muscle contraction.

Physiology of transduction

Skeletal (voluntary) muscle is innervated by motor neurones, the axons of which can propagate action potentials at high velocities. The area of muscle that lies below the axon terminal is known as the motor end plate, and the chemical synapse between the two is known as the neuromuscular junction (NMJ). The axon terminal incorporates membrane-bound vesicles containing the neurotransmitter acetylcholine (ACh). Depolarisation of the presynaptic terminal of the nerve by an action potential (generated

Table 2.1 State of sodium and potassium channels and membrane potential at different stages of the neuronal action potential

Sodium channels	Potassium channels	Membrane potential
1 Closed resting	Closed resting	Resting (−70 mV)
2 Open	Closed resting	Depolarisation (action potential upstroke)
3 More channels open	Closed resting	More depolarisation
4 Channels close (inactive)	Special set of channels start opening	Peak of action potential reached
5 All inactivated	More channels open	Repolarisation
6 Closed resting	Channels close	Resting membrane potential reestablished

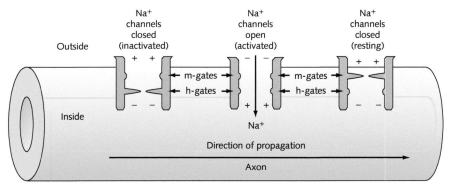

Fig. 2.3 Voltage-operated sodium channels in their inactivated, activated and resting states. The m-gates and h-gates open or close according to the state of the channel.

by sodium influx) causes voltage-sensitive calcium channels to open, allowing calcium ions into the terminal. Normally, the levels of calcium ions inside the nerves are very low and are much lower compared with the external concentration. This calcium influx results in the release of ACh by exocytosis from vesicles. ACh diffuses across to the muscle membrane where it binds to the nicotinic acetylcholine receptor (nicAChR) and/or is inactivated by the enzyme acetylcholinesterase (AChE) (Fig. 2.4). Several events then occur.

- During association, ACh binds to the nicAChR, which is an ion channel that allows cations into the muscle (mainly sodium, but also potassium to a lesser extent).
- During the conformational change, the pore of the ion channel is open for 1 ms, during which approximately 20,000 sodium ions enter the cell. The resulting depolarisation, called an end-plate potential (EPP), depolarizes the adjacent muscle fibre.
- If the cellular response is large enough, an action potential is generated in the rest of the muscle fibre

(sodium influx), resulting in the opening of voltage-operated calcium channels, but this time the calcium influx mediates contraction.
- ACh is rapidly inactivated by AChE, which hydrolyses ACh into the inactive metabolites choline and acetic acid.
- In the synthesis of ACh, the choline generated is taken up by the nerve terminal where another enzyme, choline acetyl transferase (ChAT), converts it back to ACh to be reused.

HINTS AND TIPS

Within the neuromuscular junction, an electrical impulse from the motor nerve is converted into a chemical signal that results in muscle fibre contraction. Several drugs act at the neuromuscular junction.

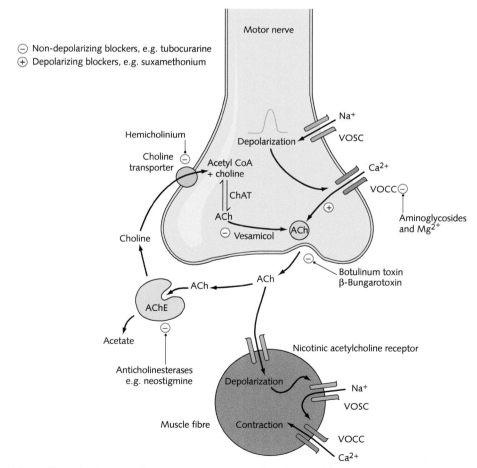

Fig. 2.4 Physiology of impulse transduction at the neuromuscular junction (NMJ) showing the site of action of drugs used in conjunction with the NMJ. *ACh*, Acetylcholine; *AChE*, acetylcholinesterase; *ChAT*, choline acetyltransferase; *Vesamicol*, an experimental drug; *VOCC*, voltage-operated calcium channel; *VOSC*, voltage-operated sodium channel.

Nicotinic acetylcholine receptor

The nicAChR is made up of five subunits (two α, one β, two γ) that traverse the membrane and surround a central pore. The binding site for ACh lies on the α subunits, therefore ACh must bind to both α subunits to open the channel.

Each subunit has four membrane-spanning regions (helices), that is, each receptor has a total of 20 regions. One of the transmembrane helices (M_2) from each subunit forms the lining of the channel pore.

Pharmacological targets

There are three major targets within the NMJ for clinically useful drugs (Table 2.2).

- Presynaptic release
- nicAChR
- Acetylcholinesterase.

Drugs affecting the neuromuscular junction

Presynaptic agents

Drugs can block neuromuscular transmission by acting presynaptically to inhibit Ach synthesis or release.

Drugs inhibiting acetylcholine synthesis—The rate-limiting step in the synthesis of ACh is the uptake of choline into the nerve terminal.

Hemicholinium is an analogue of choline that competitively blocks the choline transporter and causes a depletion of ACh stores. Because of the time taken for the stores to run down, the onset of this drug is slow. This, and the frequency-dependent nature of the block (depletion of stores is related to release of ACh), means that it is not useful clinically. The block is reversed by the addition of choline.

Drugs inhibiting vesicular packaging of acetylcholine—Vesamicol inhibits the active transport of ACh into storage vesicles and results in neuromuscular block. However, this drug is only an experimental tool and is not approved for clinical use.

Drugs inhibiting acetylcholine release—Calcium entry into the nerve terminal is necessary for the release of ACh; thus agents such as aminoglycoside antibiotics (e.g. streptomycin) that prevent this step will cause neuromuscular blockade. Muscle paralysis is occasionally a side effect of aminoglycoside antibiotics, but it can be reversed by the administration of calcium salts.

Botulinum toxin is a neurotoxin produced by the anaerobic bacillus *Clostridium botulinum*. The toxin is very potent, and it is believed to inhibit ACh release by inactivating actin, which is necessary for exocytosis. In botulism, a serious type of food poisoning caused by this toxin, patients experience progressive parasympathetic and motor paralysis. β-bungarotoxin contained in snake venom acts in a similar manner to botulinum toxin.

Botulinum toxin type A is sometimes used clinically in the treatment of excessive muscle contraction disorders (dystonias), spasticity and involuntary movements. Botulinum toxin is also given via a local injection for treatment of strabismus, urinary incontinence and hyperhidrosis. More often, however, it is used cosmetically to diminish the appearance of wrinkles.

CLINICAL NOTE

Lambert-Eaton myasthenic syndrome is caused by autoantibodies to the presynaptic voltage-gated calcium channels and is a rare autoimmune disorder associated with small cell lung cancer.

Postsynaptic agents

Drugs can also block neuromuscular blockade postsynaptically and the majority of anaesthetic medications are postsynaptic agents.

Nondepolarising blockers—These act as competitive antagonists by binding to the nicAChR, but they do not activate it. They produce motor paralysis and are often used as adjuncts to general anaesthesia. Approximately 80% to 90% of receptors must be blocked to prevent transmission, because the amount of ACh released by nerve terminal depolarisation usually greatly exceeds what is required to generate an action potential in the muscle. The drugs are all quaternary ammonium compounds and therefore do not cross the blood-brain barrier or the placenta. They are poorly absorbed orally and therefore must be administered via intravenous injection.

The main side effect is hypotension caused by the blocking of ganglionic transmission. Bronchospasm may also be a problem in certain individuals because of histamine release from mast cells.

Some of these drugs cause a "tetanic fade" (nonmaintained muscle tension during brief nerve stimulation). This is caused by the blocking of presynaptic autoreceptors,

Table 2.2 Targets for clinically useful drugs at the neuromuscular junction

Site	Action	Use
nicAChR	Block transmission	Neuromuscular blockers for surgery
AChE	Enhance transmission	Peripheral neuropathy, e.g. myasthenia gravis
Release	Block transmission	Spasms, e.g. squints, tics, tremors, etc.

AChE, Acetylcholinesterase; nicAChR, nicotinic acetylcholine receptor.

Table 2.3 Nondepolarising blockers of postsynaptic receptors at the neuromuscular junction

| Drug | Approximate duration (mins) | Side effects | | | Elimination |
		Ganglion block	Histamine release	Other	
Pancuronium	40–60	X	Minimal	Block of muscarinic receptors in the heart → tachycardia	Mainly renal
Gallamine	15	X	X	Block of muscarinic receptors in the heart → tachycardia	Mainly renal: avoid in patients with renal disease
Alcuronium	20	X	X	Dose dependency	Mainly hepatic
Vecuronium	20–30	X	X		Mainly hepatic
Atracurium	15–30	X	Sometimes		Degradation in plasma at body pH (Hofmann elimination)

which usually maintain the release of ACh during repeated stimulation. The block can be reversed by anticholinesterases and depolarising drugs.

The majority of anaesthetic drugs used clinically are nondepolarising blockers. Further details are given in Table 2.3.

Depolarising (noncompetitive) blockers—Depolarising blockers initially activate receptors, causing depolarisation, but in doing so block further activation.

Depolarising blockers act on the motor end plate in the same manner as ACh, that is, they increase the cation permeability of the end plate. However, unlike ACh, which is released in brief spurts and rapidly hydrolysed, depolarising blockers remain associated with the receptors long enough to cause a sustained depolarization and a resulting loss of electrical excitability (phase I).

Repeated or continuous administration of depolarising blockers leads to the block becoming more characteristic of nondepolarising drugs. This is known as phase II and is probably caused by receptor desensitisation, whereby the end plate becomes less sensitive to ACh. The block starts to show, and it is partly reversed by anticholinesterase drugs.

Suxamethonium is the only depolarising blocker used clinically because of its rapid onset time and short duration of action (approximately 4 mins). It must be given by intravenous injection. It is rapidly hydrolysed by plasma cholinesterase, although certain people with a genetic variant of this enzyme may experience a neuromuscular block that may last for hours. Of note, suxamethonium can cause malignant hyperthermia (intense muscle spasm and a dramatic rise in body temperature) in some patients with a rare inherited condition affecting calcium channels.

The side effects of depolarising blockers include the following.

- Initial spasms, which occur before paralysis, often resulting in postoperative muscle pain.

- Muscarinic receptor activation resulting in bradycardia. Bradycardia can be prevented by the administration of atropine.
- Potassium release from muscle resulting in elevated plasma potassium levels. This is usually a problem only in the case of trauma.

CLINICAL NOTE

Myasthenia gravis is a disorder of neuromuscular transmission resulting from autoantibodies binding to the postsynaptic acetylcholine receptors. This leads to muscle weakness with easy fatigability. In patients with myasthenia gravis, who have fewer niAChRs at the end plate, the blocking potency of depolarising blockers is reduced. Thus suxamethonium is likely to have no effect in these patients.

Anticholinesterases

Anticholinesterases inhibit AChE and thus increase the amount of ACh in the synaptic cleft and enhance cholinergical transmission. Most of the anticholinesterases used are quaternary ammonium compounds and, therefore, they do not penetrate the blood–brain barrier.

Short-acting anticholinesterases include edrophonium, which is selective for the NMJ. Edrophonium's duration of action is only 2 to 10 minutes because it binds by electrostatic forces (no covalent bonds) to the active site of the enzyme. Clinically, it is used in the diagnosis of myasthenia gravis.

Intermediate-acting anticholinesterases include neostigmine, pyridostigmine and physostigmine.

Neostigmine is used intravenously to reverse the effects of nondepolarising blockers. Its duration of action is 2 to

4 hours, and it is used orally in the treatment of myasthenia gravis. Although neostigmine shows some selectivity for the NMJ, atropine is sometimes coadministered to block the muscarinic effects of the drug.

Pyridostigmine has a duration of action of 3 to 6 hours, and it is also used orally in the treatment of myasthenia gravis. It has few parasympathetic actions.

Anticholinesterase inhibitors that cross the blood-brain barrier, such as physostigmine, have marked CNS effects because of its selectivity for the postganglionic parasympathetic junction. These include bradycardia, hypotension, excessive secretions and bronchoconstriction. A helpful effect is the reduction of intraocular pressure and therefore physostigmine is used in the form of eye drops to treat glaucoma.

Most of the long-lasting or irreversible anticholinesterases are organophosphorus compounds. For example, sarin and tabun were developed as nerve gases and can cause anticholinesterase poisoning. Parathion was developed as an insecticide and these drugs have many adverse effects, such as bradycardia, hypotension, breathing problems, depolarising neuromuscular block, central effects and possible death from peripheral nerve demyelination.

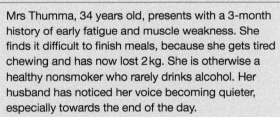

CLINICAL NOTE

Mrs Thumma, 34 years old, presents with a 3-month history of early fatigue and muscle weakness. She finds it difficult to finish meals, because she gets tired chewing and has now lost 2 kg. She is otherwise a healthy nonsmoker who rarely drinks alcohol. Her husband has noticed her voice becoming quieter, especially towards the end of the day.

On examination, she looks well. Power in all muscle groups is grossly normal but weakens after repeated testing. Tone, coordination, reflexes and sensation are normal. She is referred to a neurologist, who orders more investigations. Serum acetylcholine receptor antibodies test positive. A computed tomography scan of her thymus reveals an enlarged thymus gland.

She, therefore has a thymectomy, histopathological examination of which revealed benign hyperplasia. She is also given the anticholinesterase pyridostigmine to treat her myasthenia gravis.

AUTONOMIC NERVOUS SYSTEM

The autonomic nervous system comprises the sympathetic and parasympathetic systems, which generally have opposite effects on the body. It innervates all tissues, except skeletal muscle (Fig. 2.5). The axons of the autonomic nervous system arise from their cell body, located in the CNS, as preganglionic fibres. These synapse in the appropriate ganglion, and leave as postganglionic fibres, which reach the effector cells.

The neurotransmitter released by preganglionic fibres at autonomic ganglia is ACh. The receptors for ACh are located on postganglionic nicotinic fibres.

Autonomic ganglia

Table 2.4 summarizes the differences between ganglionic nicAChR and those found in skeletal muscle at the NMJ.

Ganglion-stimulating drugs

Nicotinic agonists
There are few agonists that act selectively on the nicAChR without affecting muscarinic receptors. Carbachol is the best example of a drug that shows preference for the nicotinic receptor, but still its action is not selective. Nicotine and lobeline both show a preference for ganglionic nicotinic receptors in comparison with the NMJ.

These drugs have no clinical use, because their range of effects is vast, affecting both sympathetic and parasympathetic transmission.

- Sympathetic effects include tachycardia and vasoconstriction leading to hypertension.
- Parasympathetic effects include increased gastrointestinal motility and glandular secretions.

Ganglion-blocking drugs
Autonomic ganglia can be blocked presynaptically by inhibiting ACh synthesis, vesicular packaging or release, or postsynaptically by blocking the nicotinic receptors.

Nondepolarising ganglion blockers
A few of these drugs act solely as competitive antagonists, blocking receptors without depolarising the ganglion. Most block the ion channel, as well as the associated receptor, and they produce their action through this former mechanism.

Ganglion-blocking drugs have a wide range of complex effects, although the sympathetic and parasympathetic systems tend to oppose one another. The effects of ganglion-blocking drugs include the following.

- Arteriolar vasodilatation leading to a marked reduction in blood pressure (block of sympathetic ganglia).
- Postural and postexercise hypotension (loss of cardiac reflexes).
- A slight reduction in cardiac output.
- Inhibition of gastrointestinal secretions and motility, leading to constipation, urinary retention, impotence and failure of ejaculation.

Despite having a broad pharmacological profile, rocuronium and vecuronium are the only widely used drugs of this class; they are used as muscle relaxants in surgical intubation.

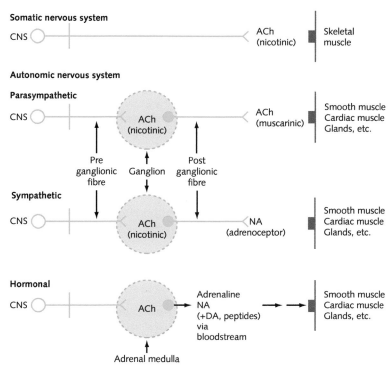

Fig. 2.5 Somatic and autonomic nervous systems: organisation and neurotransmitters. *ACh*, Acetylcholine; *CNS*, central nervous system; *DA*, dopamine; *NA*, noradrenaline.

Table 2.4 Distinguishing features of the ganglionic nicotinic acetylcholine receptors and those found in skeletal muscle at the neuromuscular junction

	Skeletal muscle	Neurones
Structure	2α	2α
	1β	3β
	1γ or ε	
	1δ	
Specific agonists	Suxamethonium	DMPP
Specific antagonists	Gallamine	Hexamethonium
	Tubocurarine	Mecamylamine
	α-Bungarotoxin	κ-Bungarotoxin
Function	End plate region depolarisation at NMJ	Neuronal depolarization in ganglia and CNS

CNS, Central nervous system; DMPP, dimethylphenylpiperazinium; NMJ, neuromuscular junction.

Sympathetic nervous system

The fibres of the sympathetic nervous system leave the CNS from the thoracolumbar regions of the spinal cord (T1–L3). They synapse in ganglia located close to the spinal cord.

These ganglia form a chain along each side of the spinal cord, which is known as the sympathetic trunk.

The major neurotransmitter is noradrenaline.

> **HINTS AND TIPS**
>
> Sympathetic transmission is enhanced under conditions of stress, known as the "fight-or-flight response".

Adrenal medulla

Some postganglionic neurones in the sympathetic arm do not have axons, but instead they release their transmitters directly into the bloodstream. These neurones are in the adrenal medulla.

On stimulation by preganglionic fibres, the adrenal medulla acts as an endocrine gland, releasing its hormones/transmitters into the systemic circulation and consist of ~80% adrenaline, ~20% noradrenaline, as well as small amounts of dopamine, neuropeptides and ATP.

Adrenoceptors

The two receptor subtypes are α and β.

- Potency at α receptors is noradrenaline > adrenaline > isoprenaline.
- Potency at β receptors is isoprenaline > adrenaline > noradrenaline.

Effects mediated by α-adrenoreceptors

α₁ Receptors

α_1 Receptors are located postsynaptically. Their activation causes smooth muscle contraction (except for the non-sphincter part of the gastrointestinal tract, where activation causes relaxation), glycogenolysis in the liver, and potassium release from the liver and salivary glands. Transduction is via G-proteins and an increase in the intracellular second messengers, inositol (1,4,5) triphosphate (IP_3) and diacylglycerol (DAG).

α₂ Receptors

α_2 Receptors are located mainly presynaptically, but also postsynaptically on liver cells, platelets and the smooth muscle of blood vessels. The activation of presynaptic α_2 receptors inhibits noradrenaline release and, therefore provides a means of end-product negative feedback. Activation of postsynaptic α_2 receptors causes blood vessel constriction and platelet aggregation. Transduction is via G-proteins and a decrease in the intracellular second messenger cyclic adenosine monophosphate (cAMP).

Some drugs, such as phenoxybenzamine and phentolamine, are nonselective α-adrenoceptor antagonists. Phenoxybenzamine is an irreversible antagonist as it forms covalent bonds with the receptor, whereas phentolamine binds reversibly and so has a much shorter duration of action. These drugs cause a fall in arterial blood pressure, caused by the block of α-receptor–mediated vasoconstriction.

CLINICAL NOTE

Mrs Pharasha, a 26-year-old librarian, presents to her doctor with episodes of anxiety, sweating, tremor and palpitations. These attacks had been increasing in frequency and are now occurring almost daily. The only change Mrs Pharasha can think of is the increased stress at work, which she now feels she is not handling well. She is a nonsmoker and seldom drinks alcohol. She is on no medication.

On examination, her heart rate is 106 beats per minute and her blood pressure is elevated. To treat her hypertension, she is prescribed propranolol, a β-blocker, which causes her blood pressure to increase by 30 mm Hg and her heart rate to reach 145 beats per minute. So, her condition worsens markedly. She is rushed to accident and emergency where the doctor suspects phaeochromocytoma.

Resting plasma catecholamines and urinary metanephrines (catecholamine metabolites) are raised, supporting the diagnosis. Imaging reveals a tumour in the adrenal medulla, which is resectable. Intravenous phentolamine is given to safely reduce her blood pressure. Following stabilisation of her blood pressure, she is put on phenoxybenzamine to achieve α blockade, with propranolol added later to achieve β blockade as well. She is maintained on this until complete α and β blockade is established and plasma volume has reexpanded. Surgery to remove the secreting tumour can then be performed, with an expert anaesthetist and surgeon, and readily available nitroprusside.

Effects mediated by β-adrenoceptors

β₁ Receptors

β_1 Receptors are mainly postsynaptic and located in the heart, platelets and nonsphincter part of the gastrointestinal tract. They can, however, be found presynaptically. Activation causes an increase in the rate and force of contraction of the heart, relaxation of the nonsphincter part of the gastrointestinal tract, aggregation of platelets, an increase in the release of noradrenaline, lipolysis in fat, and amylase secretion from the salivary glands. Presynaptically, their activation causes an increase in noradrenaline release. Transduction is via G-proteins and an increase in the intracellular second messenger cAMP.

β₂ Receptors

β_2 Receptors are located postsynaptically. Their activation causes smooth muscle relaxation, glycogenolysis in the liver, inhibition of histamine release from mast cells, and tremor in skeletal muscle. Transduction is via G-proteins and an increase in the second messenger cAMP.

Drugs acting on the sympathetic system

Fig. 2.6 summarizes the drugs acting on the sympathetic system.

Presynaptic agents

Noradrenaline synthesis—The precursor to noradrenaline is L-tyrosine, which is taken up by adrenergic neurones.

Drugs decreasing noradrenaline synthesis—The rate-limiting step is the conversion of tyrosine to dihydroxyphenylalanine (dopa), which is catalysed by tyrosine hydroxylase and inhibited by metyrosine. Noradrenaline provides a negative feedback upon this step. Carbidopa inhibits dopa decarboxylase and is used in Parkinson disease to increase dopamine levels. Because this is not the rate-limiting step in the synthesis of noradrenaline, drugs that inhibit dopa decarboxylase do not greatly affect noradrenaline synthesis. Administering α-methyldopa (used

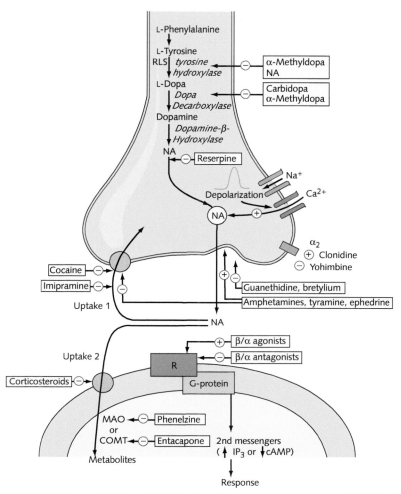

Fig. 2.6 Drugs affecting adrenergic transmission. *cAMP*, Cyclic adenosine monophosphate; *COMT*, catechol-*O*-methyltransferase; *IP₃*, inositol triphosphate; *MAO*, monoamine oxidase; *NA*, noradrenaline; *RLS*, rate-limiting step.

in hypertension) results in the formation of a false transmitter, α-methylnoradrenaline, decreasing noradrenaline synthesis.

Drugs increasing noradrenaline synthesis—Noradrenaline is stored in vesicles as a complex with ATP and a protein called chromogranin A.

Drugs inhibiting noradrenaline storage—Reserpine is a drug used in the treatment of hypertension and schizophrenia. It reduces stores of noradrenaline by preventing the accumulation of noradrenaline in vesicles. Its action is effectively irreversible because it has a very high affinity for the noradrenaline storage site. The displaced noradrenaline is immediately broken down by monoamine oxidase (MAO) and is therefore unable to exert sympathetic effects.

Drugs inhibiting the breakdown of leaked noradrenaline stores—MAO inhibitors (MAOIs) and catechol-*O*-methyltransferase (COMT) inhibitors prevent the breakdown of leaked catecholamines so that noradrenaline that leaves the vesicles is protected and eventually leaks out from the nerve ending.

Drugs inhibiting noradrenaline release—These include guanethidine and bretylium. These are adrenergic neurone-blocking drugs that prevent the exocytosis of noradrenaline from nerve terminals; they are used as hypotensive drugs. They are taken up by "uptake 1" and concentrated in nerve terminals where they have a local anaesthetic effect on impulse conduction. The tricyclic antidepressants, which inhibit uptake 1, prevent these drugs from exerting their effects. Clonidine is an α₂-receptor agonist and therefore inhibits noradrenaline release. It is used as the fourth line in treatment of hypertension.

Drugs promoting noradrenaline release—These include amphetamines, tyramine and ephedrine, which are sympathomimetic drugs that act indirectly. They are taken up by uptake 1 and displace noradrenaline from the vesicles. Because they also inhibit MAO, the displaced noradrenaline is not broken down and is able to exert sympathetic effects. These drugs act in part through a direct agonist effect on adrenoceptors. Yohimbine is an α₂ receptor antagonist that prevents noradrenaline from exerting a negative feedback effect on noradrenaline release.

Postsynaptic agents

Adrenoceptor agonists—These are termed *sympathomimetics*. They activate postsynaptic adrenoceptors, eliciting a response (Table 2.5).

Adrenoceptor antagonists—These are termed *sympatholytics*. They block postsynaptic adrenoceptors (Table 2.6).

Inactivation

Uptake 1—Noradrenaline can be taken up into presynaptic nerve terminals via active transports systems. One of these, termed uptake 1, is located on neuronal terminals and uptake of noradrenaline into nerve terminals is the main mechanism

for inactivation of this neurotransmitter. Uptake 1 has a high affinity for the uptake of noradrenaline ($K = 0.3$ mmol/L in the rat), but the maximum rate of uptake is low ($V_{max} = 1.2$ nmol/g per min in the rat). It has a specificity rank of noradrenaline > adrenaline > isoprenaline; it is blocked by cocaine, amphetamines and tricyclic antidepressants (e.g. imipramine), which therefore potentiate the actions of noradrenaline.

Uptake 2—Uptake 2 is located outside neurones (e.g. in smooth muscle, cardiac muscle and endothelium), and it is the main mechanism for the removal of circulating adrenaline from the bloodstream. It has a low affinity for the uptake of noradrenaline ($K = 250$ mmol/L in the rat) but a high maximum rate of uptake ($V_{max} = 100$ nmol/g per min in the rat). Uptake 2 has a specificity rank of adrenaline > noradrenaline > isoprenaline, and it is blocked by corticosteroids.

Table 2.5 Adrenoceptor agonists and their clinical uses

Drug	Receptor	Uses	Side effects	Pharmacokinetics
Noradrenaline	α/β	No use clinically	Hypertension, tachycardia, ventricular arrhythmias	Poor oral absorption, metabolized by MAO and COMT $t_{1/2}$ ~2 min
Adrenaline	α/β	Anaphylactic shock Cardiac resuscitation with local anaesthetics	Hypertension, tachycardia, ventricular arrhythmias	Poor oral absorption, metabolized by MAO and COMT $t_{1/2}$ ~2 min given intravenously or intramuscularly
Oxymetazoline	α	Nasal decongestant	Rebound congestion	Given intranasally
Phenylephrine	α₁	Hypotension Nasal decongestant	Hypertension Reflex bradycardia	Metabolized by MAO $t_{1/2}$ <1 min, given intramuscularly or intranasally
Clonidine	α₂	Hypertension Migraine	Drowsiness, hypotension	Good oral absorption $t_{1/2}$ ~12 hours
Isoprenaline	β	Asthma Cardiac resuscitation	Arrhythmias, tachycardia	Metabolized by COMT, given sublingually or as aerosol $t_{1/2}$ ~2 hours
Dobutamine	β₁	Heart failure	Tachycardia	
Salbutamol	β₂	Asthma Premature labour	Arrhythmias, tachycardia, vasodilatation	Given by aerosol $t_{1/2}$ ~4 hours

COMT, Catechol-O-methyltransferase; MAO, monoamine oxidase.

Table 2.6 Adrenoceptor antagonists and their clinical uses

Drug	Receptor	Uses	Side effects	Pharmacokinetics
Labetalol	α/β	Hypertension	Postural hypotension	Oral absorption $t_{1/2}$ ~4 hours
Phentolamine	α	No clinical use	Hypotension Tachycardia Nasal congestion	Metabolized by the liver, given intravenously $t_{1/2}$ ~4 hours
Prazosin	α₁	Hypertension	Hypotension Tachycardia Nasal congestion Drowsiness	Oral absorption, metabolized by the liver $t_{1/2}$ ~2 hours
Yohimbine	α₂	No clinical use	Hypertension Excitement	Oral absorption, metabolized by the liver $t_{1/2}$ ~4 hours
Propranolol	β	Hypertension Angina Arrhythmias	Bronchoconstriction Heart failure	Oral absorption, first-pass metabolism, 90% plasma-protein bound $t_{1/2}$ ~4 hours
Practolol	β₁	Hypertension Angina Arrhythmias	Bronchoconstriction Heart failure	Oral absorption $t_{1/2}$ ~4 hours

Metabolism of catecholamines by the enzyme mono-amine oxidase—MAO is found on the surface of mitochondria, principally within adrenergic nerve terminals but also in other cells, such as those of the liver and intestines. MAO metabolizes catecholamines into their corresponding aldehydes. It comprises two major forms: MAO_A and MAO_B. Noradrenaline is mainly broken down by MAO_A in nerve terminals. Inhibitors of MAO increase the releasable store of noradrenaline, but they do not greatly potentiate sympathetic transmission because catecholamines are mainly inactivated by reuptake. MAO_A has a substrate preference for 5HT (serotonin) and is the main target for antidepressants. These include phenelzine and tranylcypromine. MAO_B has a substrate preference for dopamine and is selectively inhibited by selegiline used in the treatment of Parkinson disease.

Note that interaction with other drugs and food is a serious issue with MAO inhibitors and includes the "cheese reaction" in which patients are at risk of severe hypertension following the ingestion of tyramine-containing foods. When tyramine is ingested, it is normally metabolized by MAO and little dietary tyramine reaches the systemic circulation. MAO inhibition allows tyramine to be absorbed and enhances the sympathomimetic effect resulting in acute hypertension.

Metabolism of catecholamines by catechol-O-methyltransferase—COMT is found in all tissues and breaks down most catecholamines and the byproducts of the actions of MAO. COMT metabolizes catecholamines to give a methoxy derivative. Entacapone, a COMT inhibitor, is a drug used clinically for parkinsonism.

Parasympathetic nervous system

The fibres of the parasympathetic nervous system leave the CNS from the sacral region (S3 and S4) of the spinal cord and via cranial nerves III, VII, IX and X. The fibres synapse in ganglia, which, unlike the sympathetic system, are located within the innervated organs themselves.

The major transmitter released by the postganglionic fibres at the junction with effector cells is ACh (Fig. 2.7).

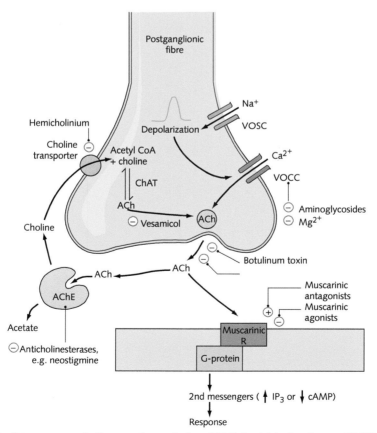

Fig. 2.7 Drugs acting on the parasympathetic nerve transmission. *AChE*, Acetylcholinesterase; *ChAT*, choline acetyl transferase; *VOCC*, voltage-operated calcium channel; *VOSC*, voltage-operated sodium channel.

Parasympathetic receptors

The ACh released by postganglionic nerve fibres acts on muscarinic (M) receptors, of which between three and five subtypes exist.

Neuroparietal M$_1$ receptors

M1 "neuroparietal" receptors are principally found in the CNS, peripheral neurones and gastric parietal cells. Their effects tend to be excitatory, depolarising membranes through a decrease in potassium conductance. Activation causes central excitation and gastric acid secretion, whereas transduction is via G-proteins and an increase in the second messengers IP$_3$ and DAG through stimulation of phospholipase C.

Neurocardiac M$_2$ receptors

M$_2$ "neurocardiac" receptors are found in the heart and on peripheral neurones. Their effects are inhibitory, increasing potassium conductance and inhibiting calcium channels. In the heart, their activation causes a decrease in the rate (via potassium) and force of contraction (via calcium). Transduction is via G-proteins and a decrease in the second messenger cAMP through inhibition of adenylyl cyclase.

Smooth muscle-glandular M$_3$ receptors

M$_3$ "smooth muscle-glandular" receptors are found in smooth muscle and glands. Their effects tend to be excitatory, increasing sodium conductance. Activation causes glandular secretions such as saliva and sweat, and smooth muscle contraction. Transduction is via G-proteins and an increase in the second messengers IP$_3$ and DAG. M$_3$ receptors are also located on vascular endothelium, activation of which causes vasodilatation, through the release of an endothelium-derived relaxing factor that is now known to be nitric oxide.

Eye M$_4$ receptors

M$_4$ "eye" receptors are believed to be exclusive to the eye. Their activation causes constriction of the pupil and accommodation for near vision. Transduction is via G-proteins and a decrease in the second messenger cAMP through inhibition of adenylyl cyclase.

Drugs acting on the parasympathetic system

Fig. 2.7 summarizes the drugs that act on the parasympathetic system.

Presynaptic agents

For information regarding presynaptic agents, see pp. 34.

Anticholinesterases

For information regarding anticholinesterases, see p. 31.

Postsynaptic agents

Muscarinic-receptor agonists—These are termed *parasympathomimetic* and such drugs activate postsynaptic receptors (Table 2.7).

Muscarinic-receptor antagonists—These are termed *parasympatholytic* and block postsynaptic receptors (Table 2.8).

Nonselective antagonists can be used as an adjunct to anaesthesia to prevent bronchial secretions and vagal slowing of heart rate.

Different tissues respond differently to muscarinic antagonists (Table 2.9). Salivary, sweat and bronchial glands are the most sensitive and can be blocked by very low doses of atropine. In contrast, the parietal cells are the most resistant, and the block of gastric acid secretion requires high doses

Table 2.8 Muscarinic antagonists and their clinical uses

Drug	Muscarinic receptor	Specific uses
Atropine	Nonselective	Reduces GI motility Cardiac arrest
Hyoscine	Nonselective	Motion sickness
Ipratropium	Nonselective	Bronchodilator
Cyclopentolate	M$_4$	Dilation of pupil
Tropicamide	M$_4$	Dilation of pupil
Pirenzepine	M$_1$	Reduces gastric acid secretion
Trihexyphenidyl (benzhexol)	M$_1$	Parkinson disease

GI, Gastrointestinal.

Table 2.7 Muscarinic agonists and their clinical uses

Drug	Muscarinic receptors	Nicotinic receptors	Uses
Carbachol	++	+	Gut and bladder stimulation postoperatively
Methacholine	+++	+	
Bethanechol	+++	−	Gut and bladder stimulation postoperatively
Muscarine	+++	−	
Pilocarpine	++	−	To decrease intraocular pressure in glaucoma

Table 2.9 Summary of the opposing effects of sympathetic and parasympathetic nerve stimulation on body tissues

Target tissue	Sympathetic		Parasympathetic		Overall effect
Nerve terminals	α_2	Decreased release	M_2	Decreased release	Decreased transmission
Smooth muscle					
Blood vessels	$\alpha_{1/2}$	Contraction	M_3	Relaxation (via EDRF)	Vasoconstriction
	β_2	Relaxation			Vasodilatation
Bronchi	β_2	Relaxation	M_3	Contraction	Bronchodilation
	α_1	Contraction	M_3	Secretion	Bronchoconstriction
					Bronchosecretion
GI tract: nonsphincter sphincter secretions	β/α_1	Relaxation	M_3	Contraction	Increased/decreased motility and tone GI secretions
		Contraction	M_3	Relaxation	
	α_1		M_3	Secretion	
Parietal cells			M_1	Contraction	Gastric acid secretion
Pancreas			M_3	Contraction	Increased secretions
Uterus	α_1	Contraction	M_3		
	β_2	Relaxation	M_3		
Bladder: detrusor sphincter	β_2	Relaxation	M_3	Contraction	Micturition
	α_1	Contraction	M_3	Relaxation	Urine retention
Seminal tract	α_1	Contraction			Ejaculation
	β_2	Relaxation			Ejaculation
Vas deferens	α_1				
Penis: venous sphincter	α_1	Contraction	M_3	Vasodilatation	Erection
Radial muscle (iris)	α_1	Contraction	M_4	Relaxation	Pupil relaxation/constriction
	β_2	Relaxation	M_4	Contraction	
Ciliary muscle			M_4	Contraction	Accommodation
Lacrimal gland					Tear secretion
Heart	β_1	Increased rate and force	M_2	Decreased rate and force	
Liver	α_1/β_2	Glycogenolysis			
Fat	β_1	Lipolysis			
Salivary glands	α_1/β_1	Secretion of thick saliva	M_3	Abundant secretion of watery saliva	
Platelets	α_2	Platelet aggregation			
Mast cells	β_2	Inhibition of histamine release			

EDRF, Endothelium-derived relaxing factor; GI, gastrointestinal.

of atropine. Muscarinic receptor antagonists such as glycopyrronium are also used to treat urinary incontinence (see Chapter 10) and motion sickness (hyoscine).

The side effects of muscarinic antagonists include:

- Dry mouth and skin, and increased body temperature (inhibition of salivary and sweat glands)
- Blurred vision and pupil no longer responsive to light (dilation of the pupil)

- Paralysis of accommodation: cycloplegia (relaxation of ciliary muscle)
- Urinary retention
- Central excitation: irritability and hyperactivity
- Sedation (hyoscine)

Certain Muscarinic antagonists can also be administered by inhalation (e.g. ipratropium bromide and tiotropium bromide) to treat airways obstruction associated with asthma and chronic obstructive pulmonary disease (see Chapter 3) where the side effects associated with systemically active drugs are much reduced.

NITRERGIC NERVOUS SYSTEM

Nitric oxide is now well recognized as a neurotransmitter and is generated by the action of the enzyme nitric oxide synthase (NOS) that converts the amino acid, L-arginine into nitric oxide.

Nitric oxide activates the guanylyl cyclase enzyme inside cells, which is responsible for generating the second messenger cyclic guanosine monophosphate (cGMP). In smooth muscle cells, the synthesis of cGMP in turn activates a protein kinase, which phosphorylates ion channels in the plasma membrane and causes hyperpolarization of the smooth muscle cell. Intracellular calcium ions are consequently sequestered into the endoplasmic reticulum, and further calcium influx into the cell inhibited by the closure of calcium channels. The overall effect of a fall in intracellular calcium is a relaxation of the smooth muscle.

The smooth muscle effects of nitric oxide in the peripheral nervous system are now recognized to be important in the gastrointestinal system, in vascular smooth muscle and in sexual arousal in both sexes, particularly in the male. For example, the therapeutic benefit of nitrovasodilator drugs such as nitroglycerin are now recognized as being through mimicking the action of nitric oxide in vascular smooth muscle to generate the second messenger cGMP. Furthermore, therapeutic manipulation of the nitrergic nervous system is confined to the male reproductive system at present, and the agents currently used in the management of erectile dysfunction (e.g. sildenafil). Such drugs inhibit phosphodiesterase 5 (PDE5) which normally breaks down cGMP in cells. Inhibition of PDE5 by sildenafil increases the intracellular levels of cGMP in the vascular smooth muscle cells of the corpus carvenosum leading to penile erection.

Chapter Summary

- The peripheral nervous system (PNS) consists of the nerves and ganglia outside of the brain and spinal cord.
- Conduction of nerve impulses through nerves occurs as an all-or-none event called the action potential (A). The AP is caused by the voltage-dependent opening of sodium and potassium channels in the cell membrane.
- Skeletal muscle is innervated by motor neurones via a chemical synapse at the neuromuscular junction (NMJ). The pre-synaptic axon terminal incorporates acetylcholine neurotransmitter which is released upon depolarisation. The ACh then causes a calcium influx at the post-synapse after binding to nicotinic acetylcholine receptors.
- Drugs can affect the NMJ such as hemicholiunium which depletes ACh stores, and vesamicol which inhibits the active transport of ACh, botulinum toxin also stops ACh release by inactivating actin.
- Nondepolarising blockers act as competitive antagonists and need 80-90% blockage of all receptors to prevent transmission, the vast majority of anaesthetic drugs act in this way. Depolarising blockers (e.g. suxamethonium) initially activate receptors and then blocks further activation.
- Anticholinesterases inhibit AChE and this increase the amount of ACh in the synaptic cleft. Examples include the short-acting edrophonium and intermediate-acting pyridostigmine.

Respiratory system

BASIC CONCEPTS

Respiration is the process of exchange of oxygen and carbon dioxide between an organism and its external environment. This principally involves the lungs, which possess the largest surface area in the body in contact with the external environment. The respiratory system (Fig. 3.1) has defence mechanisms, which can be divided into physical (such as coughing or the mucociliary escalator, to remove foreign agents) and immunologic (such as enzymes, pulmonary macrophages and lymphoid tissue, to "disarm" foreign agents). These defence mechanisms can be launched inappropriately or may be insufficient to deal with the triggering agent, and thus disease may occur.

OBSTRUCTIVE AIRWAYS DISEASES

Asthma

Asthma is a chronic inflammatory disease of the bronchiolar airways. It is characterized by recurrent reversible obstruction to airflow causing airflow limitation, airway hyperresponsiveness and inflammation of the bronchi. Asthma may be allergic (extrinsic) or nonallergic (intrinsic).

In asthma, smooth muscle that surrounds the bronchi is hyperresponsive to stimuli, and underlying inflammatory changes are present in the airways. Asthmatic stimuli

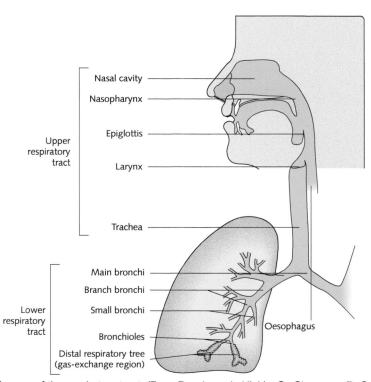

Nasal cavity
Nasopharynx
Epiglottis
Larynx
Trachea

Upper respiratory tract

Main bronchi
Branch bronchi
Small bronchi
Bronchioles
Distal respiratory tree (gas-exchange region)

Lower respiratory tract

Oesophagus

Fig. 3.1 A schematic diagram of the respiratory tract. (From Renshaw, J., Hickin, S., Chapman, R. *Crash Course: Respiratory System*, 4th edition. Mosby, London, 2013).

include inhaled allergens (e.g. pollen, animal dander), occupational allergens and drugs or nonspecific stimuli such as cold air, exercise, stress and pollution.

The stimuli cause asthmatic changes through several complex pathways (Fig. 3.2). The possible mechanisms of these pathways include the following.

- Immune reactions (type 1 hypersensitivity) and release of inflammatory mediators: the cross-linking of immunoglobulin E (IgE) by allergens causes mast cell degranulation, which releases histamine, eosinophilic and neutrophilic chemotactic factors. The eosinophils, neutrophils and other inflammatory

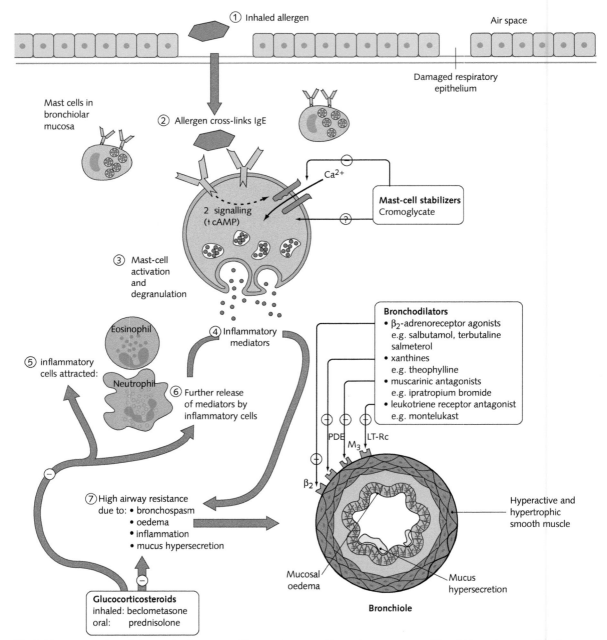

Fig. 3.2 Pathogenesis and drug action in asthma. Allergens interact with respiratory mucosa (1) and trigger immunoglobulin E–mediated mast cell response (2). Activation of mast cells causes them to degranulate (3) and release various proinflammatory mediators (4) which attract and recruit further inflammatory response cells (5). These cells also secrete mediators, which amplify the inflammatory response (6). The overall effect is narrowing of small airways (7) by bronchospasm, oedema and increased secretions. *cAMP*, Cyclic adenosine monophosphate; *LT-Rc*, Leukotriene receptor; *PDE*, phosphodiesterase.

cells release inflammatory mediators that cause a bronchial inflammatory reaction, tissue damage and an increase in airway hyperresponsiveness. Bronchial inflammatory mediators include leukotrienes, prostaglandins, thromboxane, platelet-activating factor and eosinophilic major basic protein.

- Physiologically, airway smooth muscle tone is controlled by the balance between contraction induced by release of acetylcholine (Ach) released from parasympathetic nerves (carried in the vagus) acting on muscarinic receptors and relaxation induced by release of nonadrenergic noncholinergic (NANC) nerves and circulating noradrenaline. There is also release of noradrenaline at parasympathetic ganglia to indirectly reduce airway smooth muscle tone.
- Abnormal calcium flux across cell membranes, increasing smooth muscle contraction and mast cell degranulation.
- Leaky tight junctions between bronchial epithelial cells allowing allergen access.

The aforementioned result in symptoms of wheezing, breathlessness and sometimes a cough. In many people, the asthmatic attack consists of two phases: an immediate-phase response and a late-phase response.

Immediate-phase response

An immediate-phase response occurs on exposure to the eliciting stimulus. The response consists mainly of bronchospasm. Bronchodilators are effective in this early phase.

Late-phase response

Several hours later, the late-phase response occurs. This consists of bronchospasm, vasodilatation, oedema and mucus secretion caused by inflammatory mediators released from eosinophils, platelets and other cells, and neuropeptides released by axon reflexes. This is associated with an influx of inflammatory cells into the airways, particularly eosinophils, which can be inhibited by treatment with glucocorticosteroids (see Fig. 3.2).

Chronic Obstructive Pulmonary Disease

Chronic Obstructive Pulmonary Disease (COPD) is a chronic and progressive disease with fixed or poorly reversible airflow obstruction. It encompasses several disease components, namely chronic bronchitis and bronchiolitis, consisting of inflammation and mucus hypersecretion and emphysema, involving the destruction of alveolar walls. Long-term smoking is the leading factor in the development of COPD. Cigarette smoke activates inflammatory cells (mainly macrophages and neutrophils), which can cause connective tissue damage in the lung parenchyma, resulting in emphysema and hypersecretion of mucus. α_1-Antitrypsin is an endogenous protease inhibitor, deficiency of which can result in decreased inhibition of proteases released by neutrophils, thus predisposing to the destruction of lung tissue leading to emphysema. Other factors, such as atmospheric pollution, can also have causal links.

Patients with COPD experience a cough productive of sputum, wheeze and breathlessness. Infective exacerbations can occur, giving purulent sputum. Current treatment of COPD is not very satisfactory and is aimed at improving the quality of life, minimising progressive lung destruction and treating acute exacerbations as they arise.

Management of obstructive airways disease

Antiasthmatic drugs include symptomatic bronchodilators and antiinflammatory agents, which are used for maintenance treatment. The stepwise management of asthma is summarized in Table 3.1; the stage-dependent treatment of COPD is shown in Fig. 3.3. Most patients with COPD get some symptom relief from bronchodilators and antiinflammatory agents in a fashion similar to people with asthma, yet the response of their airways to these drugs is much less marked, and there are no proven benefits for life expectancy. Long-term oxygen therapy does prolong survival in patients with COPD; however, this must be undertaken with care in patients with carbon dioxide retention because it will reduce their hypoxic drive to breathe.

Bronchodilators

β_2-Adrenoceptor agonists

Examples of β_2-adrenoceptor agonists include salbutamol (short acting) and salmeterol (long acting). Salbutamol has a half-life of 4 to 6 hours and salmeterol 12 hours. More recently indacaterol has been introduced as a once daily-inhaled drug.

Mechanism of action—Airway smooth muscle does not have a sympathetic nervous supply, but it does contain β_2-adrenoceptors that respond to circulating adrenaline. The stimulation of β_2-adrenoceptors leads to a rise in intracellular cyclic adenosine monophosphate (cAMP) levels and subsequent smooth muscle relaxation and bronchodilation.

- β_2-Adrenoceptor agonists may also help prevent the activation of mast cells, as a minor effect.
- Modern selective β_2-adrenoceptor agonists are potent bronchodilators and have very few β_1-stimulating properties at recommended doses (i.e. they do not affect the heart).

Route of administration—Inhaled.

Oral administration is reserved for children and people unable to use inhalers. In acute bronchoconstriction, salbutamol can be given as a nebulizer and may be given intravenously if life-threatening.

Indications—β_2-Adrenoceptor agonists are used to relieve bronchospasm; as such they are the principle bronchodilators used in the management of asthma and COPD. They may be used alone but are more commonly used in conjunction with other drugs, for example, corticosteroids.

Table 3.1 Management of chronic asthma in adults

Step 1 (Reliever therapy)	Inhaled short-acting β2 agonist (SABA)
Step 2 (Preventer therapy)	Inhaled SABA plus low dose inhaled corticosteroid
Step 3	Add in inhaled long-acting β2 agonist (LABA) to low-dose inhaled corticosteroid (usually combination inhaler)
Step 4	No response to LABA: stop LABA and consider increased dose of inhaled corticosteroid If benefit from LABA but control still inadequate: continue LABA and increase inhaled corticosteroid to moderate dose If benefit from LABA but control still inadequate: continue LABA and inhaled corticosteroid and consider trial of other therapy (theophylline or long-acting muscarinic antagonist
Step 5	Consider trials of: Increasing inhaled corticosteroid to high dose Addition of fourth drug Refer to specialist care
Step 6	Use daily steroid tablet in the lowest dose to provide adequate control Maintain high dose inhaled corticosteroid Refer to specialist care
Stepping down. If control is achieved, stepwise reduction in therapy may be possible	

Therapy should be started at step 1 and worked upwards until control of symptoms is achieved. Once symptoms have been controlled it may be possible to step down Adapted from British Thoracic Society Guidance September 2016.
Modified from British Thoracic Society Guidance 2016

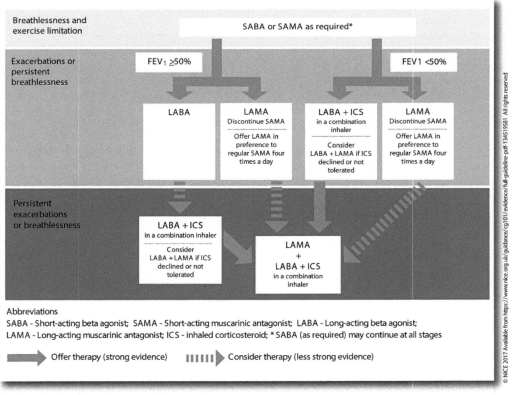

Abbreviations
SABA - Short-acting beta agonist; SAMA - Short-acting muscarinic antagonist; LABA - Long-acting beta agonist; LAMA - Long-acting muscarinic antagonist; ICS - inhaled corticosteroid; * SABA (as required) may continue at all stages

Offer therapy (strong evidence)   Consider therapy (less strong evidence)

Fig. 3.3 Inhaled therapy algorithm. *FEV1*, Forced expiratory volume during the first second. (From NICE guidance 2010 and updated with GOLD 2016 guidelines. Found in Primary Care Respiratory Society UK https://pcrs-uk.org/sites/pcrs-uk.org/files/COPDQuickGuide2016Academy.pdf).

Contraindications—Caution in hyperthyroidism, cardiovascular disease, arrhythmias.

Adverse effects—Fine tremor, tachycardia, hypokalaemia after high doses.

Therapeutic notes—β_2-Adrenoceptor agonists treat the symptoms of asthma but not the underlying disease process or inflammation. If a short-acting β2-adrenoreceptor agonist is used more frequently, it is often an indication of poorly controlled asthma or impending acute exacerbation. Salmeterol is a long-acting drug that can be administered twice daily. It is not suitable for relief of an acute attack.

Anticholinergics (Muscarinic receptor antagonists)

Ipratropium bromide (short acting) and tiotropium (long acting) are examples of anticholinergic (antimuscarinic) drugs.

Mechanism of action—Parasympathetic vagal fibres provide a bronchoconstrictor tone to the smooth muscle of the airways. They are activated by reflex on stimulation of sensory (irritant) receptors in the airway walls.

Muscarinic antagonists act by blocking muscarinic receptors, especially the M_3 subtype, which responds to this parasympathetic bronchoconstrictor tone.

Route of administration—Inhaled.

Indications—Anticholinergics are used as adjuncts to β_2-adrenoceptor agonists in the treatment of obstructive airway diseases.

Contraindications—Glaucoma, prostatic hypertrophy, pregnancy.

Adverse effects—Dry mouth may occur. Systemic anticholinergic effects are rare.

Therapeutic notes—Anticholinergics have a synergistic effect when administered with β_2-adrenoreceptor agonists in obstructive airway diseases.

Xanthines

Theophylline is an example of a xanthine.

Mechanism of action—The xanthines appear to increase cAMP levels in the bronchial smooth muscle cells by inhibiting phosphodiesterase, an enzyme which catalyses the hydrolysis of cAMP to AMP. Increased cAMP relaxes smooth muscle, causing bronchodilation.

Route of administration—Oral.

Aminophylline is the intravenous xanthine used in severe asthma attacks.

Indications—Xanthines are used in children with asthma who are unable to use inhalers and adults with predominantly nocturnal symptoms. They are administered intravenously in status asthmaticus.

Contraindications—Cardiac disease, hypertension, hepatic impairment.

Adverse effects—Nausea, vomiting, tremor, insomnia, tachycardia.

Therapeutic notes—Oral xanthines are formulated as sustained-release preparations and are useful in preventing attacks for up to 12 hours. However, they often cause adverse effects, having a narrow therapeutic window. Small increases above the therapeutic dose can be toxic and even fatal.

DRUG INTERACTION

In poorly controlled asthma, oral theophylline is sometimes prescribed. Caution should be taken when prescribing macrolide antibiotics (e.g. erythromycin) used in the treatment of respiratory infections. This is because erythromycin occupies the enzymes involved in theophylline breakdown, thus increasing the plasma concentration of theophylline. Small increases above the therapeutic dose of theophylline can be toxic and even fatal.

Leukotriene receptor antagonists

Montelukast and zafirlukast are examples of leukotriene receptor antagonists.

Mechanism of action—The leukotriene receptor antagonists are believed to act at leukotriene receptors in the bronchiolar muscle, antagonising endogenous leukotrienes, thus causing bronchodilation.

Leukotrienes are thought to be partly responsible for airway narrowing which is sometimes observed with the use of nonsteroidal antiinflammatory drugs (NSAIDs; see Chapter 10) in people with asthma.

Route of administration—Oral.

Indications—Prophylaxis of asthma.

Contraindications—Elderly, pregnancy, Churg–Strauss syndrome.

Adverse effects—Gastrointestinal disturbance, dry mouth, headache.

Therapeutic notes—Leukotriene receptor antagonists are used for children with asthma and can be prescribed for allergic rhinitis. 5-Lipoxygenase inhibitors, for example Zileuton, also inhibit the synthesis of leukotrienes and can be used in the management of asthma.

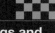

DRUG INTERACTION

Nonsteroidal antiinflammatory drugs and asthma

NSAIDs inhibit cyclooxygenase, and divert arachidonic acid breakdown via the lipoxygenase pathway, liberating leukotrienes among other mediators. Leukotrienes are thought to cause narrowing of bronchi in some asthmatics. Therefore caution should be exercised when prescribing ibuprofen (and other NSAIDs) in patients with asthma.

Magnesium sulphate

Intravenous magnesium sulphate is sometimes given in severe acute asthma when there has been a limited response to inhaled bronchodilator therapy. It is thought to relax smooth muscle and has bronchodilation properties when given intravenously.

HINTS AND TIPS

In an asthmatic emergency do not forget oxygen as well as salbutamol, ipratropium bromide and a glucocorticosteroid. You may also need to consider whether an antibiotic is needed to cover an infective component of the exacerbation.

Prophylactic and antiinflammatory drugs

Mast-cell stabilizers

Sodium cromoglycate and nedocromil sodium are examples of mast-cell stabilizers.

Mechanism of action—The exact modes of action of mast-cell stabilizers are unclear. These drugs appear to stabilize antigen-sensitized mast cells by reducing calcium influx and subsequent release of inflammatory mediators.

Route of administration—Inhaled.

Indications—Mast-cell stabilizers are useful in young patients (< 20 years old) with marked allergic disease and moderate asthma.

Adverse effects—Cough, transient bronchospasm, throat irritation.

Therapeutic notes—Mast-cell stabilizers have a prophylactic action; they must be taken regularly for several weeks before any beneficial effects are noted. These drugs are therefore not of use in acute asthma attacks.

Glucocorticoids

Antiinflammatory glucocorticoids include beclomethasone dipropionate, fluticasone propionate, fluticasone furoate, budesonide, mometasone and prednisolone.

Mechanism of action—Corticosteroids depress the inflammatory response in bronchial mucosa and so diminish bronchial hyperresponsiveness. The specific effects include the following.

- Reduced mucosal oedema and mucus production
- Decreased local generation of inflammatory mediators (prostaglandins and leukotrienes) and cytokines
- β_2-Adrenoceptor upregulation
- Long-term reduced T-cell cytokine production, and reduced eosinophil and mast-cell infiltration of bronchial mucosa.

For the intracellular events involved in corticosteroid action see Chapter 7.

Route of administration—Corticosteroids are usually delivered by metered-dose inhaler. Oral and intravenous administration is reserved for severe chronic asthma and status asthmaticus.

Indications—Corticosteroids are used in patients with more than minimal symptoms, often in combination with β_2-agonists or drugs that block allergies (see Table 3.1).

Inhaled corticosteroids are indicated in patients with severe COPD who suffer from frequent exacerbations, although there are growing concerns about an increased risk of pneumonia in patients with COPD regularly treated with corticosteroids.

Contraindications—Caution in growing children and in those with systemic and local respiratory/ear, nose and throat (ENT) infections.

Adverse effects—Dysphonia, oral thrush and with higher doses of inhaled corticosteroids, there can be some systemic absorption with the potential for suppression of the hypothalamic-pituitary-adrenal axis. If given orally, hypertension, diabetes and cushingoid effects may occur (Chapter 7).

Therapeutic notes—The initial treatment of severe or refractory asthma and COPD may require oral corticosteroids. If possible, maintenance should be achieved with inhaled corticosteroids via a metered dose to minimize side effects. Inhaled corticosteroids are usually effective in 3 to 7 days but must be taken regularly. Regular inhaled steroids improve airway irritability and reduce the number of exacerbations. However, acute exacerbations may require oral courses of corticosteroids.

CLINICAL NOTE

Mrs Connors is a 62-year-old woman who has been smoking approximately 15 cigarettes a day for the past 40 years. She presents with intermittent breathlessness and a 3-month history of a cough, which is productive of sputum. A diagnosis of COPD is made based on her history, examination and lung function tests. She is commenced on a short-acting β2 agonist (SABA) to relax the airways and increase the flow of air. Over winter, she has several exacerbations and a long-acting β2 agonist (LABA) is added. If her forced expiratory volume during the first second (FEV1) falls to < 50%, a combination inhaler consisting of a LABA and inhaled corticosteroid should be considered. In addition to her inhaled therapy, she should be advised to stop smoking, attend pulmonary rehabilitation and have her pneumococcal and annual influenza vaccine. In the future, she may require long-term oxygen therapy at home and short courses of oral steroids for exacerbations.

Use of inhalers, nebulizers and oxygen

In the treatment of asthma, inhalers and nebulizers are used to deliver drugs directly to the airways. This allows higher drug concentrations to be achieved locally while minimizing systemic effects. Whatever device is used, less than 15% of the dose is deposited on the bronchial mucosa.

Inhalers

There are several types of inhaler: metered dose, breath-activated spray, breath-activated powder. They vary in cost, delivery efficiency and ease of use.

A number of fixed-dose combination inhalers are now available for patients with mild to moderate asthma. These include fluticasone propionate and salmeterol and the combination of budesonide and formoterol, which can be administered twice daily. These fixed dose combinations increase adherence to taking the medication.

Inhaled long-acting muscarinic receptor antagonists (LAMA), tiotropium bromide that is administered once daily by inhalation is commonly used in the treatment of patients with COPD. However, increasingly LAMAs are administered in fixed-dose combination inhalers with a LABA for "dual bronchodilation", which appears to provide improved lung function when compared with the use of a single class of bronchodilator (e.g. tiotropium and formoterol) (see Fig. 3.3).

Spacer devices, used in conjunction with inhalers, improve drug delivery and are easy to use. Spacers are particularly effective in children and acute attacks.

Nebulizers

Nebulizers convert a solution of a drug into an aerosol for inhalation. Air or oxygen is driven through a solution of the drug which results in a mist, inhaled via a mask. They are more efficient than inhalers and are used to deliver higher doses of a drug. They are useful in the acute hospital treatment of severe asthma.

The long-term use of nebulizers is limited by cost, convenience and the danger of patient over reliance.

HINTS AND TIPS

The choice of medication in chronic asthma may be approached in stages, with the patient starting at the appropriate level and moving up or down according to the response to treatment. However, it is essential to check inhaler technique and compliance with medication before altering any medication and/or dose. Educating patients about avoiding triggers, using the medications in the correct situation (e.g. salbutamol as a reliever, inhaled steroid as a preventer) and being able to identify symptoms is critical to the management of asthma.

Oxygen

High-flow oxygen should be given to any patient in respiratory distress unless they have COPD and a hypoxic drive. In this situation, oxygen can be administered, but at a lower concentration. In very severe COPD (FEV1 <30% or <50% with chronic respiratory failure), long-term oxygen therapy may be required.

Oxygen increases alveolar oxygen tension and decreases the work of breathing necessary to maintain arterial oxygen tension.

Phosphodiesterase 4 inhibitors

Mechanism of action

Roflumilast inhibits phosphodiesterase 4 in inflammatory cells and, by exhibiting an antiinflammatory effect, improves lung function and reduces exacerbations of COPD.

Route of administration

Oral.

Indications

Added to existing therapy in severe patients with frequent exacerbations of their COPD in whom long-acting bronchodilators have limited control.

Adjunct to bronchodilators for severe COPD with frequent exacerbations

Contraindications

Severe immunologic disease, heart failure or depression.

Adverse effects

Narrow therapeutic window and can produce significant gastrointestinal side effects in a proportion of patients. It can also cause unexplained weight loss when used chronically in some patients as well as insomnia and suicidal ideation.

Therapeutic notes—Phosphodiesterase 4 inhibitor, roflumilast, has been shown to improve lung function and reduce the likelihood of exacerbations in COPD. However, it has little impact on quality of life or symptoms.

Biologics/monoclonal antibodies

Novel medications for the treatment of asthma have recently been developed for use by specialist respiratory physicians. Monoclonal antibodies are administered by injection for patients with severe asthma. They are administered every 2 to 3 weeks because antibodies have a long half-life. An IgE monoclonal antibody, omalizumab, has been shown to reduce the need for steroids and need for hospitalisation in severe asthmatics. More recently, an interleukin 5 monoclonal antibody, mepilumozab, has been introduced for treatment of severe asthma exacerbations by specialists.

ANTITUSSIVES AND MUCOLYTICS

Antitussives

Antitussives are drugs that inhibit the cough reflex.

A cough is usually a valuable protective reflex mechanism for clearing foreign material and secretions from the airways. In some conditions, however, such as inflammation or neoplasia, the cough reflex may become inappropriately stimulated and, in such cases, antitussive drugs may be used.

Antitussives either reduce sensory receptor activation or work by an ill-defined mechanism, depressing a "cough centre" in the brainstem.

Drugs that reduce receptor activation

Menthol vapour and topical local anaesthetics

Benzocaine is an example of a topical local anaesthetic.

Mechanism of action—Menthol vapour and topical local anaesthetics reduce the sensitivity of peripheral sensory "cough receptors" in the pharynx and larynx to irritation.

Route of administration—Topical as a spray, lozenge or vapour.

Indications—Menthol vapour and topical local anaesthetics are used for an unwanted cough.

Drugs that reduce the sensitivity of the 'cough centre'

Opioids

Opioids (see Chapter 10) reduce the sensitivity of the cough centre. Examples of these drugs include codeine and pholcodine.

Mechanism of action—Although not clearly understood, opioids seem to work via agonist action on opiate receptors, depressing a cough centre in the brainstem.

Route of administration—Oral.

Indications—Opioids are used for inappropriate coughing.

Adverse effects—There are generally few side effects of opioids at antitussive doses. Unlike pholcodine, codeine can cause constipation and inhibition of mucociliary clearance.

Mucolytics

N-acetylcysteine, carbocisteine and mecysteine hydrochloride

Mucolytics are used when excess bronchial secretions need to be cleared.

Mechanism of action—Carbocisteine and mecysteine hydrochloride reduce the viscosity of bronchial secretions by cleaving disulphide bonds cross-linking mucus glycoprotein molecules, loosening sputum and facilitating expectoration from the bronchial tree.

Route of administration—Oral.

Indications—Carbocisteine and mecysteine hydrochloride may be of benefit in some chronic obstructive airways disease, although there is no evidence supporting their use. N-acetylcysteine have successfully been used to reduce exacerbations of COPD.

Therapeutic notes—A novel drug with "mucolytic" properties is dornase alfa, a genetically engineered enzyme which cleaves extracellular deoxyribonucleic acid, and is used in cystic fibrosis, being administered by inhalation.

Mannitol is also a mucolytic, which when administered by inhalation, improves mucus clearance and has been used as add-on therapy for adults with cystic fibrosis. In the future, some patients with cystic fibrosis may be treated with cystic fibrosis transmembrane conductance regulator modulators (e.g. ivacaftor).

Allergic rhinitis

Rhinitis means an inflammatory response of the membrane lining the nose. *Allergic rhinitis* means that the inflammatory response is caused by specific allergens causing a type 1 hypersensitivity reaction. Based on symptoms, it may be further classified as seasonal or perennial (throughout the year). The inflammation can cause swelling, blockages to airflow and overactivity of the mucous membrane glands, causing excessive mucus production. Allergic rhinitis is treated with antihistamine drugs (H1 antagonists such as cetirizine and loratadine) or local corticosteroid sprays such as fluticasone propionate. Decongestants such as pseudoephedrine can sometimes be helpful by causing vasoconstriction of the nasal mucosa.

Decongestants

Nasal decongestion can occur acutely or be a chronic disorder.

Decongestion relies on administration of agents which ultimately have sympathomimetic effects. This results in vasoconstriction of the mucosal blood vessels of the nose, and a reduction in oedema and secretions.

Ephedrine

This drug is the most commonly used decongestant.

Mechanism of action—Ephedrine's sympathomimetic activity results in vasoconstriction of nasal blood vessels, limiting oedema and nasal secretions.

Route of administration—Topical or oral.

Indications—Nasal congestion.

Contraindications—Caution in children.

Adverse effects—Local irritation, nausea, headache. Rebound nasal congestion on withdrawal.

Therapeutic notes—Oral preparations are less effective than topical and are contraindicated in diabetes, hypertension and hyperthyroidism.

Histamine 1 receptor antagonists

There are two types of histamine 1 (H1) receptor antagonists.

- "Old" sedative types, for example, chlorphenamine and promethazine
- "New" nonsedative types, for example, cetirizine and loratadine

They are widely used in the treatment of allergic rhinitis because they antagonize H1 receptors and in the periphery can inhibit allergic reactions where histamine is the main mediator involved (see Chapter 6).

Topical glucocorticosteroids (see Chapter 7) are widely used to treat rhinitis and are commonly administered via nasal spray or drops. They help to reduce inflammation and swelling. Side effects include nasal dryness, irritation and nosebleeds.

RESPIRATORY STIMULANTS AND PULMONARY SURFACTANTS

Respiratory stimulants

Respiratory stimulants, or analeptic drugs, have a very limited place in the treatment of ventilatory failure in patients with chronic obstructive airways disease. They have largely been replaced by the use of ventilatory support. Example drugs are naloxone, flumazenil and doxapram.

Doxapram

Mechanism of action—Doxapram is used to improve both rate and depth of breathing. Doxapram is a central stimulant drug that acts on both carotid chemoreceptors and the respiratory centre in the brainstem to increase respiration.

Route of administration—Intravenous.

Indications—Acute respiratory failure.

Adverse effects—Perineal warmth, dizziness, sweating, increase in blood pressure and heart rate.

Pulmonary surfactants

Pulmonary surfactants are used in the management of respiratory distress syndrome, which is most common amongst premature babies. Pulmonary surfactants act to decrease the surface tension of the alveoli and allow ventilation to occur more easily. They are usually administered via endotracheal tubes directly into the pulmonary tree.

● Chapter Summary

- Asthma is characterized by recurrent reversible obstruction and inflammation of the bronchi
- Chronic obstructive pulmonary disease is a chronic and progressive disease with fixed or poorly reversible airflow obstruction
- Current management of obstructive airways disease requires ß-blockers, anticholinergics, xanthines and leukotriene receptor antagonists
- Allergic rhinitis is caused by a type 1 hypersensitivity reaction
- Allergic rhinitis is treated with antihistamine, H1 antagonists.

Cardiovascular system

4

THE HEART

Basic concepts

The heart is a pump, which together with the vascular system supplies the tissues with blood containing oxygen and nutrients and removes waste products.

The flow of blood around the body is as follows (Fig. 4.1).

- Deoxygenated blood from body tissues reaches the right atrium through the systemic veins (the superior and inferior venae cavae).
- Blood flows into the right ventricle, which then pumps the deoxygenated blood via the pulmonary artery to the lungs, where the blood becomes oxygenated before reaching the left atrium via the pulmonary vein.
- Blood flows from the left atrium into the left ventricle. From here, it is pumped into the systemic circulation via the aorta, to supply the tissues of the body.

Cardiac rate and rhythm

The sinoatrial node (SAN) and the atrioventricular node (AVN) govern the rate and timing of the cardiac action potential. The SAN is located in the superior part of the right atrium near the entrance of the superior vena cava; the AVN is located at the base of the right atrium. The SAN discharges at a frequency of 80 impulses per minute; it is the pacemaker for the heart and as such, determines the heart rate. The action potential generated by the SAN spreads throughout both atria, reaching the AVN. The AVN delays the action potential arising from the SAN to encourage the complete emptying of the atria before the ventricles contract.

The secondary action potential generated by the AVN descends into the interventricular septum via the bundle of His. The bundle of His splits into left and right branches making contact with the Purkinje fibres, which conduct the impulse throughout the ventricles, causing them to contract (Fig. 4.2).

The orderly pattern of sinus rhythm can be disrupted either by heart disease or by the action of drugs or circulating hormones. Therapeutically, drugs can be used to restore a normal cardiac rhythm where it has become disturbed (e.g. atrial fibrillation [AF] where the heart chambers stop contracting in a coordinated fashion because the rhythm is replaced by chaotic electrical activity).

Cardiac action potential

The shape of the action potential is characteristic of the location of its origin (i.e. whether from nodal tissue, the atria or the ventricles) (see Fig. 4.2).

Nonnodal cells

The resting membrane potential across the ventricular cell membrane is approximately -85 mV; this is because the resting membrane is more permeable to potassium than to other ions. Four phases occurring at the ventricular cell membrane are (Fig. 4.3).

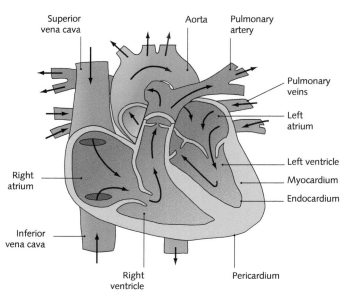

Fig. 4.1 . Blood flow through the heart chambers. (Modified from Page, C., Curtis, M. Walker, M, Hoffman, B. (eds) *Integrated Pharmacology*, 3rd edn. Mosby, 2006.)

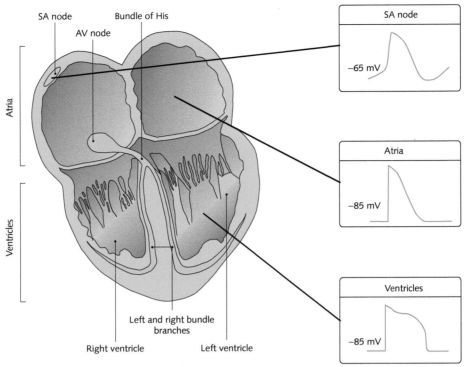

Fig. 4.2 . Regional variation in action potential configuration throughout the heart. *AV*, Atrioventricular; *SA*, sinoatrial. (Modified from Page, C., Curtis, M. Walker, M, Hoffman, B. (eds) *Integrated Pharmacology*, 3rd edn. Mosby, 2006.)

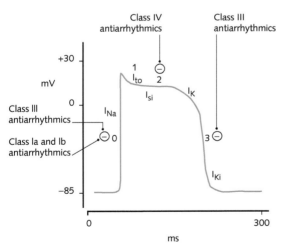

Fig. 4.3 . Configuration of a typical ventricular action potential showing the ionic currents, the phases and where class I, III and IV antiarrhythmic drugs act. *0, 1, 2* and *3*, Phases of the action potential; I_{Na}, fast inward Na^+ current; I_{si}, slow inward Ca^{2+} current; I_{to}, transient outward K^+ current; I_K, delayed rectifier K^+ current; I_{Ki}, inward rectifier K^+ current. (Modified from Page, C., Curtis, M. Walker, M, Hoffman, B. (eds) *Integrated Pharmacology*, 3rd edn. Mosby, 2006.)

- Phase 0 or depolarisation: Occurs when the membrane potential reaches a critical value of -60 mV. The upstroke of the action potential is caused by the transient opening of voltage-gated sodium channels, allowing sodium ions into the cell. In addition, potassium conductance falls to very low levels.
- Phase 1 (partial repolarisation): Occurs as a result of the inactivation of the sodium current, and a transient outward potassium current.
- Phase 2 (plateau phase): The membrane remains depolarized at a plateau of approximately 0 mV. This is caused by the activation of a voltage-dependent slow inward calcium current (conducting positive charge into the cell) and a delayed rectifier potassium current conducting positive charge out of the cell.
- Phase 3 (repolarisation): Repolarisation is caused by the inactivation of the calcium current and an increase in potassium conductance.

Nodal cells

The resting membrane potential of nodal cells is approximately -60 mV.

In nodal cells, there is no fast sodium current. Instead, the action potential is initiated by an inward calcium current, and, because calcium spikes conduct slowly, there is a delay of approximately 0.1 seconds between atrial and ventricular contraction.

Nodal cells have a phase known as phase 4 (the pacemaker potential). This phase involves a gradual depolarisation that

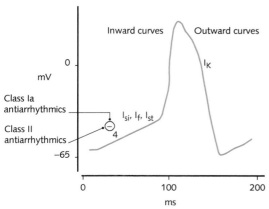

Fig. 4.4 . Configuration of a typical sinoatrial node action potential showing the ionic currents, the phases and where class Ia and II antiarrhythmic drugs act. *4*, Phase of the action potential; I_{si}, an inward current carried by Ca^{2+} ions; I_f, a 'funny' current carried by Na^+ and Ca^{2+} ions; I_{st}, the sustained inward Na^+ current; I_K, the delayed rectifier current which is an outward K^+ current. (Modified from Page et al. 2006.)

occurs during diastole and is known as the f current (I_f funny). The f current is activated by hyperpolarisation at -45 mV and consists of sodium and calcium ions entering the cell (Fig. 4.4).

CLINICAL NOTE

When a patient presents with chest pain or palpitations (sensation of feeling their heart beat), check their electrolytes (sodium and potassium), as well as calcium and magnesium levels, because the patient can be at risk of an arrhythmia if these are abnormal. In addition, many medications (e.g. digoxin) can affect intracellular potassium levels so a thorough drug history must be elicited.

Autonomic control of the heart

Both the parasympathetic and sympathetic nervous systems influence the heart, although parasympathetic activity predominates. This explains why the heart rate is lower than the inherent firing frequency of the SAN.

The sympathetic nervous system mediates its effects through the cardiac nerve and activation of β_1-adrenoceptors. These are linked to adenylyl cyclase and their activation causes increased levels of cyclic adenosine monophosphate (cAMP) and a subsequent increase in intracellular calcium levels.

The parasympathetic nervous system mediates its effects through the vagus nerve and activation of M_2 receptors by acetylcholine (ACh). These are also linked to adenylyl cyclase, but their activation causes decreased levels of cAMP and a subsequent decrease in intracellular calcium levels.

Table 4.1 Effects of the sympathetic and parasympathetic nervous systems on the heart

	Sympathetic	Parasympathetic
Heart rate	Increased	Decreased
Force of contraction	Increased	Decreased
Automaticity	Increased	Decreased
AV node conduction	Facilitated	Inhibited
Cardiac efficiency	Decreased	Increased
Effects mediated by	Cardiac nerve	Vagus nerve
Receptors activated	β_1-adrenoceptors	M_2 receptors
Effects on cAMP and intracellular calcium	Increased	Decreased

AV, Atrioventricular; cAMP, cyclic adenosine monophosphate.

The effects of the sympathetic and parasympathetic nervous systems on the heart are summarized in Table 4.1.

Cardiac contractility

Myocardial contraction is the result of calcium entry through L-type channels, giving rise to an increase in cytosolic calcium in the myocytes (Fig. 4.5).

The calcium is derived from two sources.

- The sarcoplasmic reticulum within the cell
- The extracellular medium

Extracellular calcium enters the cell, triggering larger amounts of calcium to be released from the sarcoplasmic reticulum, a process known as calcium-induced–calcium release.

During contraction, the intracellular levels of calcium increase to levels 10,000 times greater than those at rest. Calcium binds to troponin C, thereby modifying the position of actin and myosin filaments, and allowing the cell to contract. Contraction ceases only once calcium has been removed from the cytoplasm. This occurs through two mechanisms.

- Calcium is pumped out of the cell via the electrogenic Na^+/Ca^{2+} exchanger, which pumps one calcium ion out for every three sodium ions in.
- Calcium is resequestered into sarcoplasmic reticulum stores by a Ca^{2+} adenosine triphosphatase (ATPase) pump.

Cardiac output is the product of heart rate and mean left ventricular stroke volume (i.e. the volume of blood ejected from the ventricle with each heartbeat). Stroke volume is determined by both intrinsic factors (calcium and ATP) and extrinsic factors (elasticity and contractility of arteries and volume of blood). Drugs that influence these factors are essential in the treatment of cardiac dysfunction. Starling's Law is an important concept to understand—the stroke

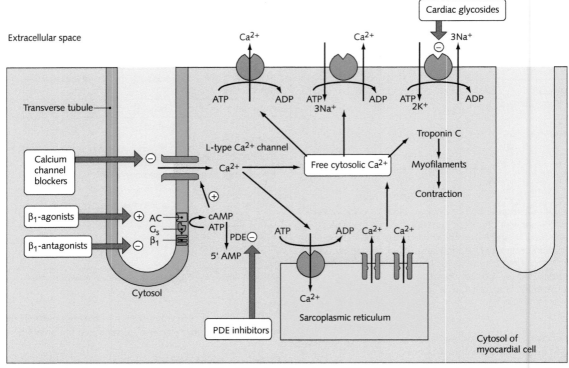

Fig. 4.5 . Effects of drugs on cardiac contractility. *AC*, Adenylyl cyclase; *ADP*, adenosine diphosphate; *AMP*, adenosine monophosphate; *ATP*, adenosine triphosphate; β_1, β_1-adrenoceptor; *cAMP*, cyclic adenosine monophosphate; G_s, stimulatory G-protein; *PDE*, phosphodiesterase.

volume of the heart increases in response to an increase in the volume of blood filling the heart (the end- diastolic volume). The increased volume of blood stretches the ventricular wall, causing cardiac muscles to contract more forcefully.

Cardiac dysfunction and treatment

Congestive cardiac failure

Congestive cardiac failure (CCF) is the combined failure of both the left and right sides of the heart. Around 900,000 people have chronic heart failure in the United Kingdom and the incidence is increasing with age. CCF occurs when the cardiac output does not meet the needs of the tissues. This is thought to be caused by defective excitation–contraction coupling, with progressive systolic and diastolic ventricular dysfunction. Some of the causes, symptoms and signs of acute and chronic cardiac failure are given in Table 4.2. The characteristics of left and right ventricular failure are listed in Table 4.3.

The body attempts to compensate for the effects of CCF by two processes: extrinsic and intrinsic.

Extrinsic cardiac compensation

Extrinsic cardiac compensation mechanisms aim to maintain cardiac output and blood pressure. The reflex pathway is as follows: hypotension → activation of baroreceptors (receptors responding to changes in pressure) → increased sympathetic activity → increased heart rate and

Table 4.2 Causes and symptoms/signs of acute and chronic cardiac failure

Causes		Symptoms/signs	
Acute CF	**Chronic CF**	**Acute CF**	**Chronic CF**
Myocardial infarction	Systemic hypertension	Tachycardia	Exertional dyspnoea
Acute valvular lesion	Myocardial infarction	Hypotension	Systemic oedema
	Valvular lesions	Dyspnoea	Cardiomegaly
	Cardiomyopathies	Pulmonary oedema	Fatigue
		Systemic oedema	Orthopnoea

CF, Chronic cardiac failure.

Table 4.3 Characteristics of right and left ventricular failure

Right Ventricular Failure (Cor pulmonale)	Left Ventricular Failure (Pink puffers)
Reduced cardiac output	Reduced cardiac output
Hypotension	Hypotension
Peripheral oedema	Pulmonary congestion
	= cough, crackles, wheeze, tachypnoea
	= pulmonary oedema
Raised JVP	Fatigue
Hepatomegaly/ splenomegaly	Paroxysmal nocturnal dyspnoea
Ascites	Orthopnoea
	Dyspnoea
Anorexia and GI disturbances	Confusion
Weight gain	

GI, Gastrointestinal; JVP, jugular venous pressure.

Positive inotropes and congestive cardiac failure (CCF)

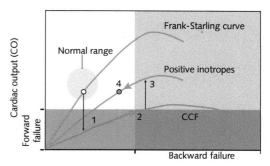

Left ventricular end-diastolic pressure

— Left ventricular end-diastolic pressure vs CO
▨ Low output symptoms: fatigue (forward failure)
▨ Congestive symptoms: dyspnoea, oedema (backward failure)
▨ Forward and backward failure
○ Normal set point
◉ New set point

Fig. 4.6 . Normal cardiac output is determined by the pressure in the left ventricle at end-diastole. In congestive cardiac failure, the set point for cardiac output is reduced and cardiac output falls (1). Compensatory neurohumoral responses become activated which increase end-diastolic pressure and improve cardiac output; however, this can give rise to backward failure (2). Positive inotropic agents increase cardiac output (3). The improved cardiac output reduces the drive for a high end-diastolic pressure, and decompensation occurs to a new set point (4).

vasoconstriction → increased cardiac contractility and vascular tone → increased arterial pressure.

However, the greater the resistance (arterial pressure) against which the heart must pump, the greater the reduction in both the ejection fraction (the volume of blood ejected by the ventricle relative to its end diastolic volume) and the perfusion of the tissues.

The reduced perfusion of the kidneys activates the renin–angiotensin system (RAS), leading to renin secretion and subsequent elevation of plasma angiotensin II and aldosterone levels (see Fig. 4.8). Angiotensin II causes peripheral vasoconstriction and aldosterone increases sodium retention, leading to increased water retention, oedema and an increased preload.

Intrinsic cardiac compensation
The increased cardiac preload leads to incomplete emptying of the ventricles and an increase in end-diastolic pressure. The heart eventually fails, owing to the massive increase in myocardial energy requirements.

Drugs used in heart failure

Introduction
The effects of medications are not independent of each other. A drug affecting the electrical properties of the myocardial cell membrane is likely to influence both the cardiac rhythm and myocardial contraction.

Cardiac glycosides
Digoxin is a commonly used cardiac glycoside. The drugs in this class shift the Frank–Starling ventricular function curve to a more favourable position (Fig. 4.6).

The chemical structure of these drugs consists of three components: a sugar moiety, a steroid and a lactone. The lactone ring is responsible for cardiotonic activity and the sugar moiety affects the potency and pharmacokinetic distribution of the drug. The steroid nucleus is responsible for the positive inotropic effect of these drugs. Positive inotropic actions of cardiac glycosides improve the symptoms of CCF, but there is no evidence they have a beneficial effect on the long-term prognosis of patients with CCF.

Mechanism of action—Cardiac glycosides act by inhibiting the membrane Na^+/K^+ ATPase pump (see Fig. 4.5). This increases intracellular Na^+ concentration, thus reducing the sodium gradient across the membrane and decreasing the amount of calcium pumped out of the cell by the Na^+/Ca^{2+} exchanger during diastole. Consequently, the intracellular calcium concentration rises, thus increasing the force of cardiac contraction and maintaining normal blood pressure.

In addition, cardiac glycosides alter the electrical activity of the heart, both directly and indirectly. At therapeutic doses, they indirectly decrease the heart rate, slow atrioventricular (AV) conductance and shorten the atrial action potential by stimulating vagal activity. This is useful in AF because when the ventricular rate is excessively high, the time available for diastolic filling is inadequate, so slowing the heart rate increases stroke volume and cardiac efficiency.

At toxic doses, they indirectly increase the sympathetic activity of the heart and cause arrhythmias, including heart block. The direct effects are mainly caused by loss of intracellular potassium and are most pronounced at high doses. The resting membrane potential is reduced, causing enhanced automaticity slowed cardiac conduction, and increased AVN refractory period.

The increased cytosolic calcium concentration may reach toxic levels thereby saturating the sarcoplasmic reticulum sequestration mechanism and causing oscillations in calcium owing to calcium-induced calcium release. This results in oscillatory after-potentials and subsequent arrhythmias.

In addition, cardiac glycosides have a direct effect on α-adrenoceptors, causing vasoconstriction and a consequent increase in peripheral vascular resistance, which is further enhanced by a centrally mediated increase in sympathetic tone.

Route of administration—Oral.

Indications—To slow the heart rate in AF and treatment of heart failure in patients who remain symptomatic despite optimal use of diuretics.

Contraindications—Heart block, hypokalaemia (the lack of competition from potassium potentiates the effects of cardiac glycosides on the Na^+/K^+ ATPase pump).

Adverse effects—Arrhythmias, anorexia, nausea and vomiting, visual disturbances, abdominal pain and diarrhoea.

Therapeutic notes—The cardiac glycosides have a very narrow therapeutic window, and toxicity is therefore relatively common. Effects of cardiac glycosides are increased if plasma potassium decreases, because of reduced competition at the K+ binding side on the Na^+/K^+ ATPase. This is clinically important because many diuretics, which are often used to treat heart failure, decrease plasma potassium thereby increasing the risk of glycoside-induced dysrhythmias. If this occurs, the drug should be withdrawn and, if necessary, potassium supplements and antiarrhythmic drugs administered. For severe intoxication, antibodies specific to cardiac glycosides are available.

CLINICAL NOTE

Digoxin is excreted via the kidney; therefore elderly patients and those with overt renal failure require a reduced dose of digoxin to avoid toxicity. Checking the plasma digoxin concentration in the blood is useful if toxicity is suspected.

Phosphodiesterase inhibitors

Examples of phosphodiesterase (PDE) 3 inhibitors include enoximone and milrinone. These have been developed as a result of the many adverse effects and problems associated with cardiac glycosides. There is no evidence that these improve the mortality rate.

Mechanism of action—The type 3 PDE isoenzyme is found in myocardial and vascular smooth muscle.

PDE is responsible for the degradation of cAMP; thus inhibiting this enzyme raises cAMP levels and causes an increase in myocardial contractility and vasodilatation (see Fig. 4.5). Cardiac output is increased, and pulmonary wedge pressure and total peripheral resistance are reduced, without much change in heart rate or blood pressure.

Route of administration—Intravenous.

Indications—PDE 3 inhibitors are given for severe acute heart failure that is resistant to other drugs.

Adverse effects—Nausea and vomiting, arrhythmias, liver dysfunction, abdominal pain, hypersensitivity.

β-Adrenoceptor and dopamine receptor agonists

Examples of β-adrenoceptor agonists include dobutamine and dopamine. They are used intravenously in CCF emergencies (see Fig. 4.5).

HINTS AND TIPS

Drugs with proven mortality benefits in cardiac failure should be remembered. They are β-adrenoceptor antagonists, angiotensin-converting enzyme (ACE) inhibitors, nitrates with hydralazine and spironolactone.

Diuretics

The main diuretic drug classes are:

* thiazides
* loop diuretics
* potassium-sparing diuretics

Diuretics inhibit sodium and water retention by the kidneys, and so reduce oedema because of heart failure. Venous pressure and thus cardiac preload are reduced, increasing the efficiency of the heart as a pump. Potassium-sparing diuretics (e.g. spironolactone) appears to have a beneficial effect in cardiac failure at doses lower than it would be expected to function as a diuretic (see Chapter 5)

Angiotensin-converting-enzyme inhibitors

For details of ACE inhibitors see p. 79.

Nitrates

See antianginal drugs (p. 76).

Vasodilating drugs

Hydralazine is discussed on p. 81.

Arrhythmias

The most common cause of sudden death in developed countries is arrhythmia and it usually results from underlying cardiovascular pathology such as atherosclerosis.

Myocardial ischaemia is one of the most important causes of arrhythmias and occurs when a coronary artery becomes occluded, thus preventing sufficient blood from reaching the myocardium. Accumulation of endogenous biological mediators, including potassium, cAMP, thromboxane A_2 and free radicals, is believed to initiate arrhythmias.

Reperfusion after coronary occlusion is necessary for tissue recovery and prevention of myocardial necrosis, but the spontaneous resumption of coronary flow is often itself a cause of the arrhythmia.

Arrhythmias have been defined according to their appearance on the electrocardiogram (ECG) by the Lambeth Conventions. These include the following.

- Ventricular: premature beats, tachycardia, fibrillation and torsades de pointes.
- Atrial: premature beats, tachycardia, flutter and fibrillation.

The two main mechanisms by which cardiac rhythm becomes dysfunctional are abnormal impulse generation (automatic or triggered) and abnormal impulse conduction.

Abnormal impulse generation

Automatic—Automatic abnormal impulse generation is likely to cause sinus and atrial tachycardia, and ventricular premature beats. It can be enhanced or abnormal.

- Enhanced: pathological conditions, such as ischaemia, may affect nodal and conducting tissue so their inherent pacemaker frequency is greater than that of the SAN (see Fig. 4.2). The automaticity of the slow pacemakers (AVN, Purkinje fibres, the bundle of His) is enhanced because ischaemia causes partial depolarisation of tissues (owing to a decrease in the activity of the electrogenic sodium pump and catecholamine release). This gives rise to an ectopic focus triggering the development of a premature beat.
- Abnormal: A premature beat may also develop in atrial or ventricular tissue, which is not normally automatic.

Triggered—Forms of triggered abnormal impulse generation are:

Early after-depolarisations: These are triggered during repolarisation, that is, phase 2 or 3, of a previously normal impulse (see Fig. 4.3). There is a decrease in the delayed K+ current that results in an abnormally long action potential. They are therefore more likely to occur during bradycardia and when taking class III antiarrhythmic drug treatment. It can cause torsades de pointes and reperfusion-induced arrhythmias.

Delayed after-depolarizations (DADs): DADs are triggered once the action potential has ended, that is, during phase 4, of a previously normal impulse. DADs usually result from cellular calcium overload, associated with ischaemia, reperfusion and cardiac glycoside intoxication.

Abnormal impulse conduction

Heart block—Heart block results from damage to nodal tissue, most commonly the AVN (e.g. after a myocardial infarction) and can cause ventricular premature beats. AV block may be first, second or third degree, manifesting itself from slowed conduction to complete block of conduction, where the atria and ventricles beat independently.

Reentry—Reentry is likely to cause ventricular and atrial tachycardia and fibrillation, atrial flutter and Wolff-Parkinson-White syndrome (a congenital abnormality that results in a supraventricular tachycardia that uses an AV accessory tract). Reentry is of two types, circus movement and reflection.

- Circus movement: An impulse reexcites an area of the myocardium recently excited and after the refractory period has ended. This usually occurs in a ring of tissue in which a unidirectional block is present, preventing anterograde conduction of the impulse, but allowing retrograde conduction of the same impulse. This results in its continuous circulation termed circus movement. The time taken for the impulse to propagate around the ring must exceed the refractory period; thus administration of drugs that prolong the refractory period will interrupt the circuit and terminate reentry.
- Reflection: Occurs in nonbranching bundles within which electrical dissociation has taken place. Owing to this electrical dissociation, an impulse can return over the same bundle.

CLINICAL NOTE

Mrs Fibbs, presented with palpitations and dyspnoea. She is known to have mitral stenosis. On examination, she had an irregularly irregular pulse, diagnostic of Atrial Fibrillation (AF). This was confirmed on ECG by absent P waves and irregular QRS complexes. Digoxin was given to slow the heart rate. Her management also included anticoagulation, because she is over 65 years of age and her AF puts her at increased risk of embolic stroke.

Antiarrhythmic drugs

Antiarrhythmic drugs are classified according to a system devized by Vaughan Williams in 1970 and later modified by Harrison. A summary of the effects of the different classes of drug is given in Table 4.4.

Table 4.4 Effects of antiarrhythmic drugs

Class	Example	Myocardial contractility	AV conduction	AP duration	Effective refractory period
Ia	Procainamide	↓	↓	↑	↑
Ib	Lidocaine	–	–	↓	↑↑
Ic	Flecainide	↓↓	↓↓	–	–
II	Propranolol	↓↓	–/↓	–	–
III	Amiodarone	–	↑	↑↑↑	↑↑↑
IV	Verapamil	↓↓↓	↓↓	↓↓	–

The number of arrows indicates the degree of the effect caused.
AP, Action potential; AV, atrioventricular.

Class I

All class I drugs block the voltage-dependent sodium channels in a dose-dependent manner. Their action resembles that of local anaesthetics (see Chapter 10).

All class I drugs have the following effects.

- They prolong the effective refractory period (terminate reentry).
- They convert unidirectional block to bidirectional block (prevent reentry).

Class Ia

Examples of class Ia drugs include quinidine, procainamide and disopyramide.

Class Ia drugs affect atrial muscle, ventricular muscle, the bundle of His, the Purkinje fibres and the AVN.

Mechanism of action—Class Ia drugs block voltage-dependent sodium channels in their open (activated) or refractory (inactivated) state (see Figs. 4.3 and 4.4). Their effects are to slow phase 0 (increasing the effective refractory period) and phase 4 (reducing automaticity) and to prolong action potential duration.

Route of administration—Oral, intravenous.

Indications—Ventricular, supraventricular arrhythmias.

Contraindications—Heart block, sinus node dysfunction, cardiogenic shock, severe uncompensated heart failure. Procainamide should not be given to patients with systemic lupus erythematosus.

Adverse effects—Arrhythmias, nausea and vomiting, hypersensitivity, thrombocytopenia and agranulocytosis. Procainamide can cause a lupus-like syndrome, and disopyramide causes hypotension.

Class Ib

Examples of class Ib drugs include lidocaine, mexiletine and phenytoin.

Mechanism of action—Class Ib drugs exert their effects in several ways (see Fig. 4.3). These include the following.

- Blocking voltage-dependent sodium channels in their refractory (inactivated) state, that is, when depolarized, as occurs in ischaemia.

- Binding to open channels during phase 0, and dissociating by the next beat, if the rhythm is normal, but abolishing premature beats.
- Decreasing action potential duration.
- Increasing the effective refractory period.

Route of administration—Lidocaine is administered intravenously, and mexiletine and phenytoin either orally or intravenously.

Indications—Ventricular arrhythmias following acute myocardial infarction. Phenytoin is used in epilepsy (see Chapter 8).

Contraindications—Class Ib drugs should not be given to patients with SAN disorders, AV block and porphyria.

Adverse effects—Hypotension, bradycardia, drowsiness and confusion, convulsions and paraesthesia (pins and needles).

Lidocaine may cause dizziness and respiratory depression; mexiletine may cause nausea and vomiting, constipation, arrhythmias and hepatitis; and phenytoin may cause nausea and vomiting and peripheral neuropathy.

Class Ic

Flecainide is the only drug used from class Ic.

Mechanism of action—Flecainide blocks sodium channels in a fashion similar to the class Ia and Ib drugs but shows no preference for refractory channels. This results in a general reduction in the excitability of the myocardium. They markedly inhibit conduction through the His Purkinje fibres.

Route of administration—Oral, intravenous.

Indications—Ventricular tachyarrhythmias, tachycardia associated with accessory pathways (e.g. Wolff-Parkinson-White syndrome), AF without left ventricular dysfunction.

Contraindications—Structural heart disease, heart failure, history of myocardial infarction.

Adverse effects—Dizziness, visual disturbances, arrhythmias.

Class II

Examples of class II drugs include propranolol, atenolol and metoprolol (see Figs. 4.4 and 4.5).

Class II drugs are β-adrenoceptor antagonists (atenolol is $β_1$ selective). Ventricular dysrhythmias following myocardial infarction are partly the result of increased sympathetic activity. β-adrenoceptor antagonists increase the refractory period of the AVN and therefore prevent recurrent attacks of supraventricular tachycardia and AF where there is sympathetic activation. Propranolol has some class I action in addition.

Class III

Examples of class III drugs include amiodarone, dronedarone, sotalol and ibutilide.

Mechanism of action—All class III drugs used clinically are potassium-channel blockers. They prolong cardiac action potential duration (increased QT interval on the ECG) and prolong the effective refractory period (see Fig. 4.3).

Amiodarone also blocks sodium and calcium channels, that is, slows phases 0 and 3, and blocks α and β-adrenoceptors. Sotalol is a β-adrenoceptor antagonist with class III activity (it prolongs the cardiac action potential and QT interval by delaying the slow outward K+ current).

Route of administration—Amiodarone and sotalol are administered orally or intravenously.

Indications—Class III drugs are given for ventricular and supraventricular arrhythmias.

Contraindications—Amiodarone should not be given to those with AV block, sinus bradycardia or thyroid dysfunction.

For contraindications regarding sotalol, see under β-blockers (p. 76).

Adverse effects—Class III drugs can cause arrhythmias, especially torsades de pointes. Amiodarone may cause thyroid dysfunction, liver damage, pulmonary disorders, photosensitivity and neuropathy as well as grey slate discolouration of the skin and irreversible corneal deposits.

For adverse effects regarding sotalol see under β-blockers (p. 76).

Class IV

Examples of class IV drugs include verapamil and diltiazem (see Figs. 4.3 and 4.5).

Class IV drugs are calcium antagonists that shorten phase 2 of the action potential, thus decreasing action potential duration. They are particularly effective in nodal cells, where calcium spikes initiate conduction. However, verapamil is contraindicated in patients with ventricular dysrhythmias and Wolff-Parkinson-White syndrome.

Details of the drugs are given in the section on antianginal drugs (p. 76).

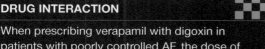

DRUG INTERACTION

When prescribing verapamil with digoxin in patients with poorly controlled AF, the dose of digoxin should be reduced and levels checked. Verapamil both displaces digoxin from tissue binding sites and reduces its renal excretion. There is a risk of digoxin accumulation and toxicity.

Other antiarrhythmics

The cardiac glycosides (e.g. digoxin) and adenosine are agents used in arrhythmias, but which do not fit into the four classes described.

Adenosine

Adenosine is produced endogenously and acts upon many tissues, including the lungs, afferent nerves and platelets.

Mechanism of action—Adenosine acts at A_1 receptors in cardiac conducting tissue and causes myocyte hyperpolarisation. This acts to slow the rate of the action potential rising and brings about delay in conduction.

Route of administration—Intravenous.

Indications—Paroxysmal supraventricular tachycardia. Aids diagnosis of broad and narrow-complex supraventricular tachycardia.

Contraindications—Second-degree or third-degree heart block, sick sinus syndrome.

Adverse effects—Transient facial flushing, chest pain, dyspnoea, bronchospasm. Side effects are very short lived, often lasting less than 30 seconds.

Angina pectoris

Angina is associated with acute myocardial ischaemia and results from underlying cardiovascular pathology, where the coronary flow does not meet the metabolic needs of the heart. It results in a radiating chest pain.

Stable or classic angina is caused by fixed stenosis of the coronary arteries and is brought on by exercise and stress. Unstable angina (crescendo angina) can occur suddenly at rest, and becomes progressively worse, with an increase in the number and severity of attacks. The following conditions can all cause unstable angina.

- Coronary atherosclerosis
- Coronary artery spasm
- Transient platelet aggregation and coronary thrombosis
- Endothelial injury causing the accumulation of vasoconstrictor substances
- Coronary vasoconstriction following adrenergic stimulation

Variant angina (Prinzmetal angina) occurs at rest, at the same time each day and is usually caused by coronary artery spasm. It is characterized by an elevated ST segment on the ECG during chest pain and may be accompanied by ventricular arrhythmias.

HINTS AND TIPS

The drugs used in stable angina pectoris are β-adrenoceptor antagonists, nitrates, calcium antagonists, antiplatelets and potassium-channel activators.

Antianginal drugs

Treatment of angina aims to dilate coronary arteries to allow maximal myocardial perfusion, decrease the heart rate to minimize oxygen demands of the myocardium, lengthen diastole when cardiac perfusion occurs and to prevent platelets from aggregating and forming platelet plugs. In addition to this, reversible risk factors need to be addressed to limit the progression of the disease.

Acute attacks of angina are treated with sublingual nitrates.

In the hospital setting, acute anginal pain is treated with an opiate (Chapter 10).

Stable angina is treated with the following.

- Long-acting nitrates
- β-Adrenoceptor antagonists
- Calcium antagonists
- Antiplatelet agents (e.g. aspirin)
- Potassium-channel activators

Unstable angina is a medical emergency and requires hospital admission. Unstable angina is treated with the following.

- Antiplatelets: aspirin, clopidogrel and dipyridamole (adenosine diphosphate [ADP] antagonists) and the glycoprotein IIb/IIIa inhibitors (p. 89).
- Heparin/low-molecular-weight heparin (LMWH) (p. 89).
- Standard antianginal drug regimen

Organic nitrates

The organic nitrates, glyceryl trinitrate (GTN), isosorbide mononitrate and isosorbide dinitrate, can relieve angina within minutes.

Mechanism of action—Most nitrates are prodrugs, decomposing to form nitric oxide (NO), which activates guanylyl cyclase, thereby increasing the levels of cyclic guanosine monophosphate (cGMP). Protein kinase G is activated, and contractile proteins are phosphorylated. Dilatation of the systemic veins decreases preload and thus the oxygen demand of the heart, whereas dilatation of the coronary arteries increases blood flow and oxygen delivery to the myocardium.

Route of administration—Sublingual, oral (modified release), transcutaneous patches. GTN can be given by intravenous infusion.

Indications—Organic nitrates are given for the prophylaxis and treatment of angina, myocardial infarction and in left ventricular failure.

Contraindications—Organic nitrates should not be given to patients with hypersensitivity to nitrates, or those with hypotension and hypovolaemia.

Adverse effects—Postural hypotension, tachycardia, headache, flushing and dizziness.

Therapeutic notes—To avoid nitrate tolerance, a drug-free period of approximately 8 hours is needed.

β-Adrenoceptor antagonists (β-blockers)

Examples of β-blockers include propranolol, atenolol, bisoprolol and metoprolol.

β-Adrenoceptors are found in many tissues, although the β_1-adrenoceptor is found predominantly in the heart, and the β_2-adrenoceptor is found mainly in the smooth muscle of the vasculature. Some overlap does exist.

Different β-blockers have different affinity for the two types of adrenoceptor. Propranolol is nonselective, having equal affinity for both the β_1-adrenoceptors and β_2-adrenoceptors. Atenolol, bisoprolol and metoprolol have a greater affinity for the β_1-adrenoceptor and are therefore more "cardiac-specific". Some β-blockers even appear to have partial agonist effects at β-adrenoceptors, as well as antagonistic effects.

Mechanism of action—The aim of using β-adrenoceptor antagonists in cardiac disease is to block β-adrenoceptors in the heart. This has the effect of causing a fall in heart rate (slowing of phase 4; see Fig. 4.4), in systolic blood pressure, in cardiac contractile activity and in myocardial oxygen demand.

Route of administration—Oral, intravenous.

Indications—Angina, postmyocardial infarction (reduce the risk of death), arrhythmias, hypertension, thyrotoxicosis, glaucoma and anxiety.

Contraindications—Nonselective β-blockers (e.g. propranolol) must not be given to asthmatic patients. At high doses, β_1-adrenoceptor antagonists lose their selectivity and should be used with caution in those with asthma. Other contraindications for β-blockers include bradycardia, hypotension and AV block.

Adverse effects—Bronchospasm (therefore are contraindicated in patients with asthma), fatigue and insomnia, dizziness, cold extremities (β_2-adrenoceptor effect), bradycardia, heart block, hypotension and decreased glucose tolerance in diabetic patients.

Calcium-channel blockers

There are two types of calcium-channel blocker (CCBs).

- Rate-limiting CCBs (verapamil)
- Dihydropyridine CCBs (short-acting nifedipine or long-acting felodipine)

Mechanism of action—Rate-limiting CCBs block L-type calcium channels found in the heart and in the vascular smooth muscle, thereby reducing calcium entry into cardiac and vascular cells (see Figs. 4.3, 4.5 and Fig. 4.7). This decrease in intracellular calcium reduces cardiac contractility and causes vasodilatation, which results in several effects: reduced preload caused by the reduced venous pressure; reduced afterload caused by the reduced arteriolar pressure; increased coronary blood flow; reduced cardiac contractility and thus reduced myocardial oxygen consumption; and a decreased heart rate. High doses of these drugs affect AVN conduction.

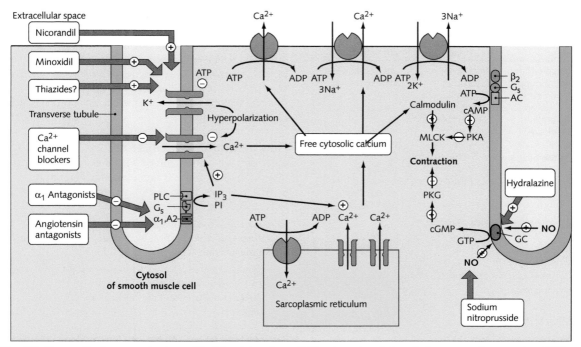

Fig. 4.7 . Drugs affecting vascular tone. *AC*, Adenylyl cyclase; *ADP*, adenosine diphosphate; α_1, α_1-adrenoceptor; *AMP*, adenosine monophosphate; *A2*, angiotensin II; *ATP*, adenosine triphosphate; β_2, β_2-adrenoceptor; *cAMP*; cyclic adenosine monophosphate; *cGMP*, cyclic guanosine monophosphate; *GC*, guanylyl cyclase; G_S, stimulatory G-protein; IP_3, inositol triphosphate; *MLCK*, myosin light-chain kinase; *NO*, nitric oxide; *PLC*, phospholipase C; *PI*, phosphatidylinositol; *PKA*, protein kinase A; *PKG*, protein kinase G.

Dihydropyridines block L-type calcium channels in vascular cells. They do not affect cardiac contractility or AVN conduction, and the beneficial effects are caused by increased coronary flow and peripheral vasodilatation.

Route of administration—Oral.

Indications—Prophylaxis and treatment of angina and hypertension. Dihydropyridines are especially useful in angina associated with coronary vasospasm (as they dilate coronary arteries), with the long-acting dihydropyridines being particularly useful for hypertension management. Verapamil and diltiazem are given for supraventricular arrhythmias and nifedipine for Raynaud syndrome (peripheral vasoconstriction).

Contraindications—CCBs should not be given to patients in cardiogenic shock.

Dihydropyridines are contraindicated in advanced aortic stenosis. Verapamil and diltiazem should not be given to patients with severe heart failure (owing to their negative inotropic action), to those taking β-blockers (risk of AV block and impaired cardiac output), and those with severe bradycardia.

Adverse effects—Verapamil and diltiazem may cause hypotension, rash, bradycardia, CCF, heart block and constipation.

Dihydropyridines may cause hypotension, rash, tachycardia, peripheral oedema, and flushing and dizziness.

HINTS AND TIPS

There are three classes of CCBs. Two of them act mostly on the heart (verapamil and diltiazem) and the other acts mostly on peripheral vascular tone (nifedipine). Concurrent use of a β-adrenoceptor antagonist and a nondihydropyridine CCB could result in profound bradycardia.

Potassium-channel activators

Nicorandil is the only licensed drug in this class.

Mechanism of action—Nicorandil acts to activate the potassium channels of the vascular smooth muscle. Once activated, potassium flows out of the cells, causing hyperpolarisation of the cell membrane. The hyperpolarized membrane inhibits the influx of calcium, and therefore inhibits contraction; the overall effect is the relaxation of the smooth muscle and vasodilatation (see Fig. 4.7).

Route of administration—Oral.

Indications—Angina prophylaxis.

Contraindications—Cardiogenic shock, left ventricular failure, hypotension.

Table 4.5 Classes of drugs used to treat angina, cardiac failure and arrhythmias

Angina	Heart failure	Arrhythmias
Organic nitrates	Cardiac	Na^+-channel
β_1-Adrenoceptor	glycosides	blockers (class I)
antagonists	Phosphodiesterase	β_1-Adrenoceptor
Ca^{2+} antagonists	inhibitors	antagonists (class
Antiplatelets	β_1-Adrenoceptor	II)
Potassium-	agonists	K^+-channel
channel	Diuretics	blockers (class III)
activators	ACE inhibitors	Ca^{2+} antagonists
	Nitrates	(Class IV)
	Vasodilating drugs	Cardiac
		glycosides
		Adenosine

ACE, Angiotensin-converting enzyme.

Adverse effects—Headache, cutaneous vasodilatation, nausea and vomiting.

See Table 4.5 for a summary of the drug classes used in cardiac dysfunction.

Ivabradine and Ranolazine

Ivabradine is used as an antianginal medication in patients with normal sinus rhythm. It can also be used in mild to severe chronic heart failure. Ivabradine slows the heart rate by inhibiting the sinus node current. The heart rate needs to be monitored to ensure that the patient does not become bradycardic.

Ranolazine has recently been introduced as an adjunct to current antianginal medication. It indirectly reduces intracellular calcium and the force of contraction, without affecting the heart rate.

CIRCULATION

Control of vascular tone

α-Adrenoceptor activation

α-Adrenoceptor activation (see Fig. 4.7) causes contraction of vascular smooth muscle through the activation of phospholipase C (PLC). The resulting increased levels of inositol triphosphate cause the release of calcium from the endoplasmic reticulum, thus increasing calcium levels. Calcium then binds to calmodulin, thus activating myosin light-chain kinase (MLCK) and allowing contraction.

β₂-Adrenoceptor activation

β₂-Adrenoceptor activation (see Fig. 4.7) causes relaxation of vascular smooth muscle through the activation of adenylyl cyclase. The resulting increased levels of cAMP activate protein kinase A, which phosphorylates and inactivates MLCK.

M₃-receptor activation

M₃-receptor activation causes relaxation of vascular smooth muscle through the release of endothelium-derived relaxing factor, which is believed to be nitric oxide (NO) (see Fig. 4.7). Guanylyl cyclase is activated by NO, thus increasing the levels of cGMP and activating protein kinase G. Protein kinase G inhibits contraction by phosphorylating contractile proteins.

Renin–angiotensin system

A decrease in plasma volume results in the activation of the RAS (Chapter 5), which is summarized in Fig. 4.8.

ACE catalyses the production of angiotensin II. The effects of angiotensin II are as follows.

- Potent direct vasoconstriction
- Indirect vasoconstriction by releasing noradrenaline
- Stimulates the secretion of aldosterone

ACE also catalyses the inactivation of bradykinin, which is an endogenous vasodilator.

Aldosterone is a steroid that induces the synthesis of sodium channels and Na^+/K^+ ATPase pumps in the luminal membrane of the cortical collecting ducts. This results in a greater amount of sodium and consequently water being reabsorbed, thus increasing the blood volume and pressure.

Certain renal diseases and renal artery occlusion will cause activation of the RAS and result in the development of hypertension.

Hypertension

Normal blood pressure is generally regarded as 120/80 mm Hg (systolic pressure/diastolic pressure). Hypertension is defined as a diastolic arterial pressure greater than 90 mm Hg, or a systolic arterial pressure greater than 140 mm Hg. The condition can be fatal if left untreated because it greatly increases the risk of thrombosis, stroke and renal failure.

Three factors determine blood pressure.

- Cardiac output
- Peripheral vascular resistance

"Primary" or "essential" hypertension accounts for 90% to 95% of all cases of hypertension. This has no known cause but is associated with the following.

- Age ($\geq$ 40 years)
- Obesity
- Physical inactivity
- Smoking and alcohol consumption
- Genetic predisposition

"Secondary hypertension" accounts for the remaining 5% to 10% of cases of hypertension. The cause is usually one of the following.

- Renal disease, which activates the RAS
- Endocrine disease, for example, phaeochromocytoma, a steroid-secreting tumour of the adrenal cortex or an adrenaline-secreting tumour of the adrenal medulla.

Table 4.6 Advantages and disadvantages of drugs used in hypertension with respect to associated conditions

	Diuretics	β-Blocker	ACE inhibitor/angiotensin II receptor antagonist	Calcium-channel blockers	α-Blocker
Diabetes	Care[a]	Care[a]	Yes	Yes	Yes
Gout	No	Yes	Yes	Yes	Yes
Dyslipidaemia	Care[b]	Care[b]	Yes	Yes	Yes
Ischaemic heart disease	Yes	Yes	Yes	Yes	Yes
Heart failure	Yes	Care[c]	Yes	Care[d]	Yes
Asthma	Yes	No	Yes	Yes	Yes
Peripheral vascular disease	Yes	Care	Care[e]	Yes	Yes
Renal artery stenosis	Yes	Care	No	Yes	Yes
Pregnancy	Caution	Not in late pregnancy	No	No	Caution

ACE, Angiotensin-converting enzyme.
[a] Diuretics may aggravate diabetes; β-blockers worsen glucose intolerance and mask symptoms of hypoglycaemia.
[b] Both diuretics and β-blockers disturb the lipid profile.
[c] There is some evidence for beneficial effects of some β-blockers when used cautiously in heart failure.
[d] Verapamil and diltiazem may exacerbate heart failure, although amlodipine appears to be safe.
[e] Patients with peripheral vascular disease may also have renal artery stenosis; therefore ACE inhibitors should be used cautiously.
From Kumar and Clark, Clinical Medicine, 4th edn. WB Saunders 1998.

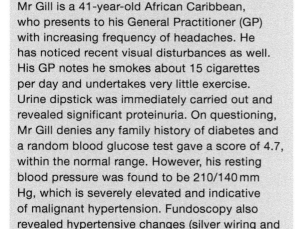

CLINICAL NOTE

Mr Gill is a 41-year-old African Caribbean, who presents to his General Practitioner (GP) with increasing frequency of headaches. He has noticed recent visual disturbances as well. His GP notes he smokes about 15 cigarettes per day and undertakes very little exercise. Urine dipstick was immediately carried out and revealed significant proteinuria. On questioning, Mr Gill denies any family history of diabetes and a random blood glucose test gave a score of 4.7, within the normal range. However, his resting blood pressure was found to be 210/140 mm Hg, which is severely elevated and indicative of malignant hypertension. Fundoscopy also revealed hypertensive changes (silver wiring and cotton wool spots). He is admitted for immediate treatment.

He was given the long-acting calcium-channel blocker, amlodipine. Two days later, bendroflumethiazide (a thiazide diuretic) was also added to his management. These two drug classes have been shown to be particularly effective in African Caribbeans with hypertension because of their effect on salt sensitivity and volume expansion. He is also advised to stop smoking, eat a healthier salt-restricted diet and do more exercise.

Treatment of hypertension

When prescribing, the choice of drug is usually influenced by age (over or under 55 years) and ethnicity. People aged under 55 years are usually commenced on an ACE inhibitor or angiotensin II receptor blockers (ARB). People aged over 55 years or who are of African or Caribbean origin are started on a CCB in the first instance (refer to NICE guidance on management of hypertension for more detail). Advantages and disadvantages of the different anti hypertensives are shown in Table 4.6.

Vasodilators

Angiotensin-converting enzyme inhibitors

Captopril, enalapril, lisinopril and ramipril are examples of ACE inhibitors.

Mechanism of action—ACE inhibitors cause inhibition of ACE with consequent reduced angiotensin II and aldosterone levels (see Fig. 4.8), and increased bradykinin levels. This, therefore causes vasodilatation with a consequent reduction in peripheral resistance, little change in heart rate and cardiac output and reduced sodium retention.

Route of administration—Oral.

Indications—Hypertension, heart failure and renal dysfunction (especially in diabetic patients to slow progression of diabetic or reduced renal functional nephropathy).

Contraindications—Pregnancy, renovascular disease, aortic stenosis.

Adverse effects—Characteristic cough (caused by increased bradykinin levels), angioedema, hypotension, dizziness and headache, diarrhoea, muscle cramps and hyperkalaemia.

Therapeutic notes—First-dose hypotension is relatively common and should ideally be given just before bed.

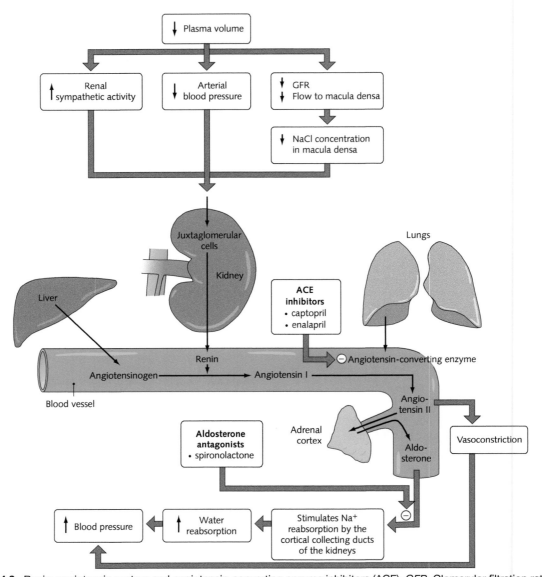

Fig. 4.8 . Renin–angiotensin system and angiotensin-converting enzyme inhibitors (ACE). *GFR*, Glomerular filtration rate.

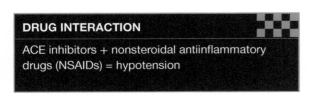

DRUG INTERACTION

ACE inhibitors + nonsteroidal antiinflammatory drugs (NSAIDs) = hypotension

Angiotensin-II receptor antagonists

Losartan and valsartan are examples of angiotensin-II receptor antagonists.

Mechanism of action—Angiotensin-II receptor antagonists cause inhibition at the angiotensin-II receptor (see Fig. 4.7), resulting in vasodilatation with a consequent reduction in peripheral resistance.

Route of administration—Oral.

Indications—Hypertension.

Contraindications—Pregnancy, breastfeeding. Caution in renal artery stenosis and aortic stenosis.

Adverse effects—Cough (less common than with ACE inhibitors), orthostatic hypotension, dizziness, headache and fatigue, hyperkalaemia and rash.

Calcium antagonists

Nifedipine has more effect upon vascular tone than diltiazem or verapamil, which are more cardioselective (see Fig. 4.7).

α₁-Adrenoceptor antagonists

Prazosin and doxazosin are examples of α_1-adrenoceptor antagonists.

Mechanism of action—α_1-Adrenoceptor antagonists cause inhibition of α_1-adrenoceptor-mediated vasoconstriction, thus reducing peripheral resistance and venous pressure (see Fig. 4.7). They also lower plasma low-density lipoprotein (LDL) cholesterol levels, very-low-density lipoprotein (VLDL) levels and triglyceride levels, and increase high-density lipoprotein (HDL) cholesterol levels, thus reducing the risk of coronary artery disease.

Route of administration—Oral.

Indications—Hypertension (especially in patients with CCF), prostate hyperplasia (reduced bladder and prostate resistance), coronary artery disease.

Contraindications—Prazosin should not be given to people with CCF because of aortic stenosis.

Adverse effects—Postural hypotension, dizziness, headache and fatigue, weakness, palpitations, nausea.

Hydralazine

Hydralazine is a second-line or third-line drug for the treatment of mild to moderate hypertension.

Mechanism of action—Hydralazine effects are unclear, although it appears to interfere with the action of inositol triphosphate in vascular smooth muscle, thereby reducing peripheral resistance and blood pressure (see Fig. 4.7).

Route of administration—Oral, intravenous.

Indications—Moderate to severe hypertension. Also used in conjunction with β-blockers and thiazides in hypertensive emergencies and in hypertensive pregnant women.

Contraindications—Idiopathic systemic lupus erythematosus, severe tachycardia.

Adverse effects—Tachycardia, fluid retention, nausea and vomiting, headache.

Minoxidil

Owing to its adverse effects, minoxidil is the drug of last resort in the long-term treatment of hypertension.

Mechanism of action—Minoxidil activates vascular smooth muscle ATP-sensitive potassium channels, resulting in hyperpolarisation of the cell membrane and consequently reduces calcium entry through L-type channels (see Fig. 4.7). The overall effect is inhibition of smooth muscle contraction, and subsequent vasodilatation.

Route of administration—Oral for hypertension; topical cream for baldness.

Indications—Severe hypertension, baldness.

Contraindications—Phaeochromocytoma, porphyria.

Adverse effects—Hirsutism (limits use in women), sodium and water retention, tachycardia, cardiotoxicity.

Sodium nitroprusside

Mechanism of action—Sodium nitroprusside is a prodrug that spontaneously decomposes into NO inside smooth muscle cells. NO activates guanylyl cyclase, thus increasing intracellular cGMP levels, and causing vasodilatation (see Fig. 4.7).

Route of administration—Intravenous.

Indications—Sodium nitroprusside is given in hypertensive crises, and for controlled hypotension in surgery, and in heart failure.

Contraindications—Sodium nitroprusside should not be given to patients with severe hepatic impairment, vitamin B_{12} deficiency or Leber's optic atrophy.

Adverse effects—Headache and dizziness, nausea, abdominal pain, palpitations, retrosternal discomfort.

Therapeutic notes—Sodium nitroprusside is broken down in the body to thiocyanate, which has a half-life of only a few minutes, although prolonged exposure to nitroprusside and thiocyanate can result in thiocyanate toxicity (weakness, nausea and inhibition of thyroid function).

HINTS AND TIPS

The more common adverse effects of the vasodilating drugs are hypotension and headache, both of which result directly from reducing peripheral vascular resistance.

Diuretic drugs

The main diuretics drug classes used in hypertension are:

- thiazides
- loop diuretics
- potassium-sparing diuretics

See Chapter 5 for details of each of these drugs.

Mechanism of action

The antihypertensive action of diuretic drugs does not seem to correlate with their diuretic activity; loop diuretics are powerful diuretics but only moderate antihypertensives whereas thiazides are moderate diuretics but powerful antihypertensives.

It has recently been suggested that the antihypertensive effects of diuretics (especially the thiazides) are not necessarily because of their diuretic effect but rather may be caused by activation of ATP-regulated potassium channels in resistance arterioles, with a mechanism of action similar to that of nicorandil (p. 77) and minoxidil. This causes hyperpolarisation, and thus inhibition of calcium entry into vascular smooth muscle cells with consequent vasodilatation and reduced peripheral vascular resistance (see Fig. 4.7).

Centrally acting antihypertensive drugs

Clonidine, methyldopa and moxonidine are examples of centrally acting antihypertensive drugs. These agents are second-line or third-line drugs in the treatment of hypertension.

Mechanism of action—Centrally acting antihypertensive drugs are α_2-adrenoceptor agonists. The activation of presynaptic α_2-adrenoceptors causes inhibition of noradrenaline release and consequent vasodilatation. The activation of postsynaptic α_2-adrenoceptors causes vasoconstriction, although presynaptic effects dominate.

Centrally acting antihypertensive drugs reduce the activity of the vasomotor centre in the brain, causing reduced sympathetic activity and subsequent vasodilatation. They also reduce heart rate and cardiac output.

Route of administration—Oral. Clonidine can be given by intravenous infusion.

Indications—Hypertensive patients when first-line antihypertensive agents are ineffective or contraindicated. Methyldopa is safe for hypertension in pregnancy, asthmatic patients and those with heart failure.

Contraindications—Methyldopa should not be given to people with depression, liver disease or phaeochromocytoma.

Adverse effects—Dry mouth, sedation, orthostatic hypotension, male sexual dysfunction, and galactorrhoea. Methyldopa can cause diffuse parenchymal liver injury, fever and, rarely, haemolytic anaemia. Clonidine can cause a withdrawal hypertensive crisis on stopping treatment.

Phaeochromocytoma

Phaeochromocytoma is a rare endocrine tumour, most commonly of the adrenal gland. These tumours can secrete adrenaline and various intermediates in its biosynthesis. These vasoactive compounds result in the clinical signs and symptoms of phaeochromocytomas, which include facial flushing, sweating, breathlessness, anxiety, tachycardia and paroxysmal hypertension.

Medical management of phaeochromocytoma-induced hypertension relies on the powerful α-adrenoceptor antagonist, phenoxybenzamine. α-Adrenoceptor blockade reduces peripheral vascular resistance and lowers blood pressure. The use of β-adrenoceptor antagonists is dangerous because tumour-secreted sympathomimetics act unopposed on α-adrenoceptors, increasing both peripheral vascular resistance and blood pressure.

Phenoxybenzamine

Mechanism of action—Phenoxybenzamine antagonizes α-adrenoceptors in the vascular smooth muscles, resulting in vasodilatation.

Route of administration—Oral, intravenous.

Indications—Hypertensive episodes in phaeochromocytoma.

Contraindications—History of cerebrovascular events, postmyocardial infarction.

Adverse effects—Postural hypotension, tachycardia, nasal congestion.

Therapeutic notes—Phentolamine is another powerful α-adrenoceptor antagonist which can be used in phaeochromocytoma, although it has a much shorter half-life and is commonly used before and during surgery to excise the tumour.

Vasoconstrictors and the management of shock

Shock

Shock is a state of circulatory collapse, characterized by an arterial blood pressure unable to maintain adequate tissue perfusion and oxygen delivery. Shock is a life-threatening condition.

The body responds inappropriately to shock, releasing mediators such as histamine, prostaglandins, bradykinin and serotonin, which cause capillary dilatation and increased capillary permeability. This further reduces blood pressure and cardiac output.

Signs of shock include:

- very low arterial blood pressure
- a weak, rapid pulse
- cold, pale, sweaty skin
- rapid breathing
- dry mouth
- reduced urine output
- confusion

Causes of shock include:

- haemorrhage
- burns
- dehydration
- severe vomiting or diarrhoea
- bacterial septicaemia
- myocardial infarction
- pulmonary embolism

Types of shock include the following.

- Hypovolemic: caused by a reduction in the circulating blood volume.
- Cardiogenic: reduced cardiac output caused by "pump failure".
- Septic: caused by massive vasodilatation.
- Anaphylactic: a severe allergic reaction, in which there is a massive generalized release of vasodilating mediators, particularly histamine.
- Spinal: disruption of neuronal control of vascular tone and cardiac output.

Management of shock

The medical management of shock ultimately depends upon its underlying cause, for example, if a child is shocked because of chronic diarrhoea and vomiting, fluid and electrolyte replacement is the most appropriate management. If an adult has had significant blood loss, management of their hypovolemic shock may require several blood transfusions. In addition, in septic shock, urgent antibiotics and fluid replacement are required.

The following drugs are useful in restoring blood pressure and tissue perfusion, but, on the whole, do not address the underlying cause of the different types of shock.

Sympathomimetic amines

Examples include adrenaline, noradrenaline, phenylephrine and ephedrine.

Sympathomimetic amines raise blood pressure at the expense of vital organs such as the kidneys, and raise peripheral resistance, which is already high in patients with shock.

Mechanism of action—Adrenaline and noradrenaline are agonists at both α- adrenoceptors and β-adrenoceptors, and phenylephrine is an α_1-adrenoceptor agonist. Ephedrine is a β-adrenoceptor agonist and causes noradrenaline release. These drugs work either by activating α-adrenoceptors which then activate PLC, causing vasoconstriction and a consequent increase in arterial blood pressure or by activating β-adrenoceptors which then activate adenylyl cyclase, causing an increased heart rate, increased cardiac contractility and vasodilatation.

Route of administration—Parenterally, commonly intravenously.

Indications—Shock, acute hypotension and reversal of hypotension caused by spinal or epidural anaesthesia. Adrenaline is used in cardiac arrest and anaphylaxis.

Contraindications—Sympathomimetic amines should not be given during pregnancy or in people who have hypertension.

Adverse effects—Tachycardia, anxiety, insomnia, arrhythmias, dry mouth, cold extremities.

Therapeutic notes—In a cardiac arrest, adrenaline is used at a concentration of 1 mg per 10 mL (1:10,000) intravenously, whereas, in anaphylaxis, adrenaline is used at a concentration of 1 mg per 1 mL (1:1000) intramuscularly.

Dopamine and dobutamine

Mechanism of action—Dopamine is a precursor of noradrenaline. It activates dopamine receptors and α-adrenoceptors and β-adrenoceptors. When administered by intravenous infusion, dopamine acts on the following.

- Dopamine receptors, causing vasodilatation in the kidneys at low doses.
- α_1-Adrenoceptors, causing vasoconstriction in other vasculature.
- β_1-Adrenoceptors, causing positive inotropic and chronotropic effects.

Dobutamine has no effect on dopaminergic receptors but does activate β_1-adrenoceptors.

If renal perfusion is not impaired, dobutamine and dopamine are a more appropriate means of treating shock than α-adrenoceptor agonists. This form of treatment maintains renal perfusion and inhibits the activation of the RAS.

Route of administration—Intravenous.

Indications—CCF (emergencies only), cardiogenic shock, septic shock, hypovolaemic shock, cardiomyopathy, cardiac surgery.

Contraindications—Tachyarrhythmias. Dopamine is contraindicated in people with phaeochromocytoma.

Adverse effects—Tachycardia and hypertension; dopamine causes nausea and vomiting and hypotension.

Therapeutic notes—Although low doses of dopamine cause vasodilatation, high doses cause vasoconstriction and may exacerbate heart failure.

Vasopressin and desmopressin

Vasopressin (antidiuretic hormone; ADH), and desmopressin are examples of antidiuretic peptides.

Vasopressin is short acting ($t_{1/2}$ = 10 minutes) whereas desmopressin is longer acting ($t_{1/2}$ = 75 minutes).

Mechanism of action—Antidiuretic peptides activate V_1 receptors on smooth muscle cells, which stimulate PLC, causing contraction. They also activate V_2 receptors on the tubular cells of the kidneys, which stimulate adenylyl cyclase and thereby increase the permeability of these cells to water and reduce sodium and water excretion. Vasopressin has a much greater affinity for V_2 receptors than V_1 receptors whereas desmopressin is selective for V_1 receptors.

Route of administration—Oral, intravenous, intranasal.

Indications—Pituitary diabetes insipidus. The antidiuretic peptides are no longer used in the management of shock, although their pharmacology is both academically interesting and a potential target for future drugs.

Contraindications—Vascular disease, chronic nephritis.

Adverse effects—Fluid retention, nausea, pallor, abdominal cramps, belching. They may induce anginal attacks (caused by coronary vasoconstriction).

Corticosteroids

The use of corticosteroids in septic shock remains controversial, although they are also given by intravenous injection in the treatment of anaphylactic shock as an adjunct to adrenaline (Chapter 7).

CLINICAL NOTE

It is possible to distinguish between the types of shock clinically.

- Hypovolaemic: low jugular venous pressure (JVP), cool, clammy peripheries, confusion/restlessness.
- Cardiogenic: raised JVP, cool, clammy peripheries, anxiousness/agitation.
- Septic: warm, sweaty peripheries, pyrexia, nausea.
- Anaphylactic: warm peripheries, urticaria, swollen face/mouth.
- Spinal: history of trauma or spinal anaesthesia.

Lipoprotein circulation and atherosclerosis

Lipoproteins provide a means of transporting lipids (cholesterol, triglycerides and phospholipids), which are insoluble in the blood, around the body.

Four classes of lipoproteins exist. These differ in size, density, constituent lipids and type of surface protein (apoprotein). These lipoproteins are as follow.

- HDL
- LDL
- VLDL
- Chylomicrons

Lipid transport in the blood is via two pathways, exogenous and endogenous, which are summarized in Fig. 4.9.

In the exogenous pathway (numbers refer to those in Fig. 4.9):

1. Diet-derived lipid breakdown leads to the formation of chylomicrons.
2. Lipoprotein lipase (LPL), found in the endothelium of extrahepatic tissues, hydrolyses the triglycerides in chylomicrons to glycerol and free fatty acids (FFAs), for use by the tissues.
3. The liver takes up the chylomicron remnant.
4. The liver secretes cholesterol and bile acids into the gut, creating an enterohepatic circulation.

In the endogenous pathway (numbers refer to those in Fig. 4.9):

1. The liver secretes VLDLs, the components of which may be derived either endogenously or from the diet.
2. LPL found in the endothelium of extrahepatic tissues, hydrolyses triglycerides in the VLDLs to glycerol and FFAs, for use by the tissues, and leaves LDL.

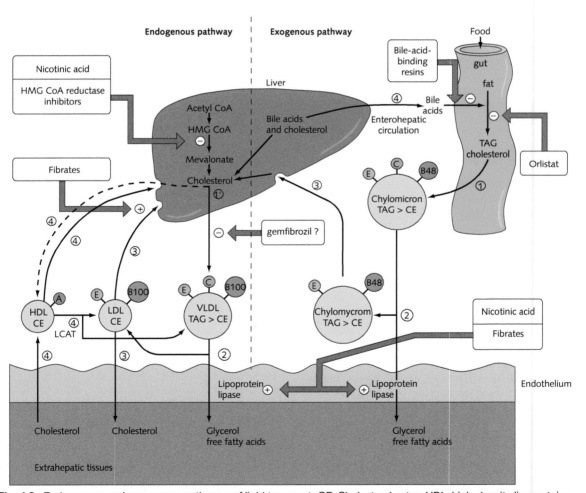

Fig. 4.9 . Endogenous and exogenous pathways of lipid transport. *CE*, Cholesterol ester; *HDL*, high-density lipoprotein; *HMG CoA*, 3-hydroxy-3-methylglutaryl coenzyme A; *LCAT*, lecithin cholesterol acyltransferase; *TAG*, triacylglycerol; *VLDL*, very-low-density lipoproteins; numbers refer to steps in pathways.

3. LDL is then taken up by the liver and extrahepatic tissues.
4. HDL is secreted by the liver into the plasma, where it is modified by lecithin-cholesterol acyltransferase (LCAT) and uptake of cholesterol from the tissues. LCAT transfers cholesterol esters to LDLs and VLDLs.

Hyperlipidaemias

Hyperlipidaemias are characterized by markedly elevated plasma triglycerides, cholesterol and lipoprotein concentrations.

Cholesterol is deposited in various tissues.

- Deposition in arterial plaques results in atherosclerosis, which leads to heart attacks, strokes and peripheral vascular disease.
- Deposition in tendons and skin results in xanthomas.

Primary

Primary hyperlipidaemias are genetic, and numerous types exist.

Secondary

Secondary hyperlipidaemias are the consequences of other conditions such as:

- diabetes
- liver disease
- nephrotic syndrome
- renal failure
- alcoholism
- hypothyroidism
- oestrogen administration.

Treatment (lipid-lowering drugs)

Changing a patient's diet alone can lower serum cholesterol and should be the first-line treatment option in mild to moderate hyperlipidaemia. The following drug classes, however, provide pharmacological control of a patient's cholesterol level, inhibiting its synthesis and its uptake from the intestine.

3-Hydroxy-3-methylglutaryl coenzyme A reductase inhibitors (statins)

Atorvastatin, pravastatin and simvastatin are examples of 3-hydroxy-3-methylglutaryl coenzyme A (HMG-CoA) reductase inhibitors. These drugs have been shown to reduce blood cholesterol by up to 35% in some patients. HMG-CoA reductase inhibitors can reduce the risk of dying from a coronary event by up to nearly one-half.

Mechanism of action—Statins reversibly inhibit the enzyme HMG-CoA reductase, which catalyses the rate-limiting step in the synthesis of cholesterol. The decrease in cholesterol synthesis also increases the number of LDL receptors, thus decreasing LDL levels.

Route of administration—Oral.

Indications—Hyperlipidaemia resistant to dietary control, as primary and secondary prevention in patients with serum cholesterol greater than 5.5 mmol/L (this value will vary depending upon local policy). Treatment of familial hypercholesterolaemia.

Contraindications—Pregnancy, breastfeeding, liver disease.

Adverse effects—Reversible myositis (rare), constipation or diarrhoea, abdominal pain and flatulence, nausea and headache, fatigue, insomnia, rash.

Therapeutics—They are typically prescribed at night to reduce peak cholesterol synthesis in the early morning.

DRUG INTERACTION

Simvastatin + Clarithromycin = myositis
Simvastatin is metabolized by the enzyme CYP3A4 and concomitant use of medications that inhibit this enzyme (e.g. the antibiotic clarithromycin) can lead to myositis.

Ezetimibe

Cholesterol absorption inhibitor, used as an adjunct to diet and statins in hypercholesterolaemia.

Mechanism of action—Inhibits absorption of cholesterol from the duodenum by blocking a transport protein in the brush border of enterocytes, without affecting the absorption of fat soluble vitamins, triglycerides or bile acids.

Route of administration—Oral

Indications—Hypercholesterolaemia

Contraindications—Breastfeeding

Adverse effects—In general, well tolerated. Diarrhoea, abdominal pain, headache.

Fibrates

Fibrates include bezafibrate, ciprofibrate and gemfibrozil. Used in the management of mixed dyslipidaemia (raised serum triglycerides and raised cholesterol).

Mechanism of action—Fibrates work in several ways (see Fig. 4.9).

- Stimulation of lipoprotein lipase, thus reducing the triglyceride content of VLDLs and chylomicrons.
- Stimulation of hepatic LDL clearance, by increasing hepatic LDL uptake (see Fig. 4.9).
- Reduction of plasma triglyceride, LDL and VLDL concentrations.

Increase of HDL-cholesterol concentration (except bezafibrate). Gemfibrozil decreases lipolysis and may decrease VLDL secretion.

Route of administration—Oral.

Indications—Hyperlipidaemia unresponsive to dietary control.

Contraindications—Gallbladder disease, severe renal or hepatic impairment, hypoalbuminaemia, pregnancy, breastfeeding.

Adverse effects—Myositis-like syndrome (especially if renal function is impaired), gastrointestinal disturbances, dermatitis, pruritus, rash and urticaria, impotence, headache, dizziness, blurred vision.

Nicotinic acid

The side effects of nicotinic acid limit its use in the treatment of hyperlipidaemias. Nicotinic acid has been shown to reduce the incidence of coronary artery disease.

Mechanism of action—Nicotinic acid has the following effects (see Fig. 4.9).

- It inhibits cholesterol synthesis thereby decreasing VLDL and thus LDL production.
- It stimulates lipoprotein lipase thus reducing the triglyceride content of VLDLs and chylomicrons.
- It increases HDL-cholesterol.
- It increases the levels of tissue plasminogen activator (p. 90)
- It decreases the levels of plasma fibrinogen.

Route of administration—Oral.

Indications—Hyperlipidaemias unresponsive to other measures.

Contraindications—Pregnancy, breastfeeding.

Adverse effects—Flushing, dizziness, headache, palpitations, nausea and vomiting, pruritus.

Bile acid binding resins

Colestyramine and colestipol have been shown to decrease the rate of mortality from coronary artery disease.

Mechanism of action—Basic anion exchange resins act by binding bile acids in the intestine (see Fig. 4.9), thus preventing their reabsorption and promoting hepatic conversion of cholesterol into bile acids. This increases hepatic LDL-receptor activity, thus increasing the breakdown of LDL-cholesterol. Plasma LDL-cholesterol is therefore lowered.

Route of administration—Oral.

Indications—When significantly elevated cholesterol is caused by a high LDL concentration.

Colestyramine also relieves pruritus associated with partial biliary obstruction and primary biliary cirrhosis.

Contraindications—Complete biliary obstruction.

Adverse effects—Bile acid binding resins are not absorbed and therefore have very few systemic side effects. Side effects include nausea and vomiting, constipation, heartburn, abdominal pain and flatulence and aggravation of hypertriglyceridaemia. They may interfere with the absorption of fat-soluble vitamins and certain drugs.

Therapeutic notes—To avoid interference with their absorption, other drugs should not be taken within 1 hour before or 3 to 4 hours after colestyramine or colestipol administration.

Other lipid-lowering drugs

Fish oils rich in omega-3 marine triglycerides can be useful in the treatment of severe hypertriglyceridaemia, although may sometimes worsen hypercholesterolaemia. Their role in clinical practice remains to be thoroughly ascertained.

Ispaghula husk is taken orally, and is presumed to act by binding bile acids, preventing their reabsorption, and is potentially useful in patients with hypercholesterolaemia but not hypertriglyceridaemia.

Note that a new class of cholesterol-lowering medications has been developed, two of which are licensed for use in the United Kingdom. These are proprotein convertase subtilisin/kexin type 9 (PCSK9) inhibitors (e.g. Evolocumab and Alirocumab). They target the PCSK protein, making it less effective at breaking down LDL receptors. The result is more working receptors on the surface of liver cells, and more cholesterol can then be removed from the blood.

HAEMOSTASIS AND THROMBOSIS

Haemostasis

Haemostasis is the cessation of bleeding from damaged blood vessels. If haemostasis is defective or unable to cope with blood loss from larger vessels, blood may accumulate in the tissues. This accumulated blood is called a haematoma.

Three stages are involved in haemostasis.

- Blood vessel constriction
- Formation of a platelet plug
- Formation of a clot

Blood vessel constriction

The first response to a severed blood vessel is the contraction of the smooth muscle of the vessel. This is mediated by the release of thromboxane A_2 and other substances from platelets.

Blood vessel constriction slows the flow of blood through the vessel, thus reducing the pressure, and pushes opposing surfaces of the vessel together. In very small vessels, this results in permanent closure of the vessel, but in most cases, blood vessel constriction is insufficient for this to occur.

Platelet plug formation

Exposure to the collagen underlying the vessel endothelium, as occurs during vessel injury, allows platelets to adhere to the collagen by binding to von Willebrand factor. This factor, secreted by the platelets and endothelium, binds to the exposed collagen; platelets then bind to this complex.

The release of adenosine diphosphate (ADP), serotonin, thromboxane A_2 and other substances by the platelets causes the platelets to aggregate. Fibrin binds them together. The synthesis and release of prostacyclin by the intact endothelium inhibits platelet aggregation limiting the extent of the platelet plug.

Intact endothelial cells also produce NO, a potent vasodilator and inhibitor of platelet aggregation.

Clot formation

Blood coagulation is the conversion of liquid blood into a solid gel, known as a clot.

- A clot consists of a meshwork of fibrin within which blood cells are trapped.
- It functions to reinforce the platelet plug.

Fibrin is formed from its precursor fibrinogen, through the action of an enzyme called thrombin. The formation of thrombin occurs via two distinct pathways, the intrinsic and the extrinsic pathways, which together are known as the coagulation cascade. Both pathways involve the conversion of inactive factors into active enzymes, which then go on to catalyse the conversion of other factors into enzymes (see Fig. 4.9). The liver is important in coagulation because it is the site at which many of the clotting factors are produced. It also produces bile salts necessary for the absorption of vitamin K, which is needed by the liver to produce prothrombin and clotting factors VII, IX and X.

The extrinsic pathway is thus termed because the component needed for its initiation is contained outside the blood. Tissue factor binds factor VII on exposure of blood to subendothelial cells and converts it to its active form, VIIa. This enzyme then catalyses the activation of factors X and IX.

The intrinsic pathway is thus termed because its components are contained in the blood. It merges with the extrinsic pathway at the step before thrombin activation.

The thrombin formed stimulates the activation of factors XI, VIII and V, and thus acts as a form of positive feedback.

Listed are three naturally occurring anticoagulants, which limit the extent of clot formation.

- Tissue factor pathway inhibitor, which binds to the tissue factor–VIIa complex and inhibits its actions.
- Protein C, which is activated by thrombin, and inactivates factors VII and V.
- Antithrombin III, which is activated by heparin, and inactivates thrombin and other factors.

Fibrinolysis

The fibrinolytic or thrombolytic system functions to dissolve a clot once repair of the vessel is under way.

Plasmin digests fibrin. It is formed from plasminogen through the action of plasminogen activators, the best example of which is tissue-plasminogen activator (tPA).

Thrombosis

Thrombosis is the pathological formation of a clot known as a thrombus, which may cause occlusion within blood vessels or the heart, and result in death.

- Thrombosis causes arterial occlusion, which may lead to myocardial infarction, stroke and peripheral ischaemia; or
- Venous occlusion, which may lead to deep venous thrombosis and pulmonary embolism.

COMMUNICATION

Mr Patel, a 50-year-old male with a body mass index of 31, presented to A&E with central crushing chest pain, shortness of breath and sweating. He is a longstanding smoker with a 60-pack a year history and his younger brother recently died from a stroke associated with significant vascular disease. ECG showed ST segment elevation which, combined with the history, is highly suggestive of myocardial infarction.

He was given oxygen, aspirin (antithrombotic agent) to prevent further platelet aggregation, morphine for pain relief and the antiischaemic vasodilating spray (glyceryl trinitrate). To prevent irreversible ischaemic damage following this episode of coronary thrombosis, opening the occluded artery promptly with a combination of ticagrelor (antiplatelet) and fondaparinux (LMWH) is essential to his management. He is then taken directly to the cardiac catheter laboratory for primary percutaneous intervention. He is later discharged home with secondary prevention medications including a ß-adrenoceptor antagonist, statin, ACE inhibitor and an antiplatelet agent.

Arterial thrombi form because of endothelial injury, which is, in turn, the result of underlying arterial wall pathology such as atherosclerosis. Venous and atrial thrombi tend to form as a result of blood stasis, allowing the build up of platelets and fibrin. People with hypercoagulability, caused by a lack of one or more of the naturally occurring anticoagulants, are particularly susceptible.

Arterial thrombi consist mainly of platelets, whereas venous thrombi consist mainly of fibrin.

TREATMENT OF THROMBOSIS

Anticoagulants

Vitamin K antagonists

Warfarin and phenindione are vitamin K antagonists.

Mechanism of action—Vitamin K antagonists block the reduction of vitamin K epoxide, which is necessary for its action as a cofactor in the synthesis of factors II, VII, IX and X (Figs. 4.10 and 4.11). The onset of action of vitamin K antagonists takes several hours, owing to the time needed for the degradation of factors that have already been carboxylated ($t_{1/2}$: VII = 6 hours, IX = 24 hours, X = 40 hours, II = 60 hours).

Route of administration—Oral.

Indications—Prophylaxis and treatment of deep vein thrombosis and pulmonary embolism, the prophylaxis of

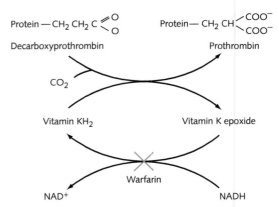

Fig. 4.11 . Role of vitamin K in prothrombin formation. Warfarin inhibits the reduction of vitamin K epoxide. *NAD*, Nicotinamide adenine dinucleotide.

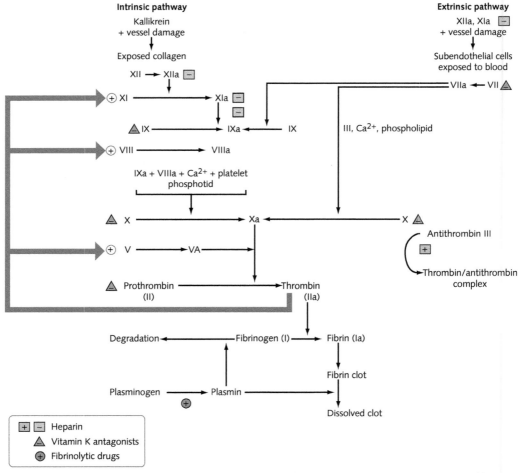

Fig. 4.10 . Effects of heparin, vitamin K and fibrinolytic drugs on the coagulation cascade. Factor III, factor/tissue thromboplastin.

embolisation in AF and rheumatic disease, and in patients with prosthetic heart valves.

Contraindications—Cerebral thrombosis, peripheral arterial occlusion, peptic ulcers, hypertension, pregnancy.

Adverse effects—Haemorrhage.

Therapeutic notes—Warfarin can be a therapeutic challenge; under dosing can increase the risk of a thrombus whereas overdosing can result in haemorrhage. Therefore vitamin K antagonists require frequent blood tests to individualize the dose and are consequently inconvenient as well as having a low margin of safety. In addition, many medications (and some foods) potentiate or lessen the effect of warfarin.

DRUG INTERACTION

Patients on warfarin who are concomitantly prescribed an antibiotic (e.g. ciprofloxacin or metronidazole) are at an increased risk of bleeding. This is because the antibiotics inhibit hepatic drug metabolism and the effects of warfarin are potentiated. Similarly, patients given NSAIDs (which inhibit platelet function) while on warfarin are also at risk of bleeding.

Direct Oral Anticoagulants

Recently emerged, these medications may come to replace warfarin. They can be used to prevent venous thromboembolism following hip or knee replacement. They are licensed in patients with AF as prophylaxis against stroke.

Dabigatran
Direct thrombin inhibitor, taken orally.

Rivaroxaban and Apixaban
Direct inhibitor of factor Xa, taken orally.

These drugs require no monitoring. Bleeding is the most common adverse effect.

Unfractionated heparin and the low-molecular-weight heparins

Mechanism of action—Unfractionated heparin activates antithrombin III, which limits blood clotting by inactivating thrombin and factor Xa. LMWHs (e.g. enoxaparin, dalteparin, fondaparinux) are simply fragments of unfractionated heparin, which exhibit very similar activity to heparin, but they only increase the action of antithrombin III on factor Xa and not its action on thrombin. LMWH are longer acting and used more frequently because their dosing is more predictable and thus requires no monitoring.

Route of administration—LMWHs are given subcutaneously (once daily).

Unfractionated heparin is given 12-hourly by the subcutaneous route or via intravenous infusion.

Indications—Treatment of deep vein thrombosis and pulmonary embolism; prophylaxis against postoperative deep vein thrombosis and pulmonary embolism in high-risk patients; myocardial infarction.

Contraindications—Heparin should not be given to patients with haemophilia, thrombocytopenia or peptic ulcers.

Adverse effects—Haemorrhage (treated by stopping therapy or administering a heparin antagonist such as protamine sulphate), skin necrosis, thrombocytopenia, hypersensitivity reactions, hyperkalaemia.

Therapeutic regimen—Unfractionated heparin is reserved for patients with renal failure in whom LMWHs are contraindicated or in emergencies because it has an immediate onset.

Hirudins

Mechanism of action—Derived from the medical leech, Hirudin or rather its recombinant derivatives, bivalirudin, desirudin and lepirudin, are direct thrombin inhibitors.

Route of administration—Intravenous.

Indications—Desirudin is used in patients with type II (immune) heparin-induced thrombocytopenia (HIT) and as prophylaxis of deep vein thrombosis in patients undergoing hip and knee replacement.

Lepirudin is used for thromboembolic disease in patients with type II (immune) HIT.

Bivalirudin is used in combination with antiplatelet drugs in patients undergoing coronary artery surgery.

Contraindications—Active bleeding, renal or hepatic impairment.

Adverse effects—Haemorrhage, hypersensitivity reactions.

Antiplatelet agents

Aspirin

Aspirin is acetylsalicylic acid, originally derived from the willow tree.

Mechanism of action—Aspirin blocks the synthesis of thromboxane A_2 from arachidonic acid in platelets, by acetylating and thus inhibiting the enzyme cyclooxygenase 1. Thromboxane A_2 stimulates PLC, thus increasing calcium levels and causing platelet aggregation. Aspirin also blocks the synthesis of prostacyclin from endothelial cells, which inhibits platelet aggregation. However, this effect is short lived because endothelial cells, unlike platelets, can synthesize new cyclooxygenase (Fig. 4.12).

Route of administration—Oral.

Indications—Prevention and treatment of myocardial infarction and ischaemic stroke. Aspirin is also used as an analgesic and an antiinflammatory agent (Chapter 11).

Contraindications—Children under 12 years of age (risk of Reye syndrome), during breastfeeding, haemophilia, peptic ulcers or known hypersensitivity reactions.

Adverse effects—Bronchospasm, gastrointestinal haemorrhage.

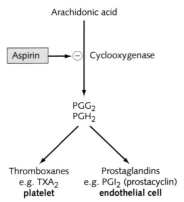

Fig. 4.12 . Inhibition of cyclooxygenase by aspirin, leading to a reduction in the formation of thromboxane and prostacyclin. *PG*, prostaglandin; *PGG2*, *PGH2*, *PGI₂*, prostacyclin; *TXA₂*, thromboxane A_2.

Dipyridamole

Mechanism of action—Dipyridamole causes inhibition of the phosphodiesterase enzyme that hydrolyses cAMP. Increased cAMP levels result in decreased calcium levels and inhibition of platelet aggregation.

Route of administration—Oral.

Indications—Prophylaxis of stroke in patients with transient ischaemic attacks (especially if given with aspirin).

Adverse effects—Hypotension, nausea, diarrhoea, headache.

Adenosine diphosphate inhibitors

These include clopidogrel, prasugrel and ticagrelor.

Mechanism of action—Ticlopidine, clopidogrel and prasugrel inhibit ADP-induced platelet aggregation by irreversible inhibition of P2Y receptors. Ticagrelor is a reversible noncompetitive inhibitor of P2Y receptors.

Route of administration—Oral.

Indications—Secondary prevention of cardiovascular and cerebrovascular events.

Adverse effects—Haemorrhage, abdominal discomfort, nausea and vomiting.

Therapeutic notes—If a patient is truly allergic to aspirin, clopidogrel can be used in its place.

Glycoprotein IIb/IIIa inhibitors

Abciximab is the main drug currently in this class.

Mechanism of action—Abciximab is an antibody fragment directed towards the glycoprotein IIb/IIIa (GPIIb/IIIa) receptor of platelets. Binding and inactivation of the GPIIb/IIIa receptor prevents platelet aggregation.

Route of administration—Intravenous.

Indications—Prevention of ischaemic cardiac complications in patients undergoing percutaneous coronary intervention; short-term prevention of myocardial infarction in patients with unstable angina.

Contraindications—Active bleeding.

Adverse effects—Haemorrhage, nausea, vomiting, hypotension.

Therapeutic notes—Tirofiban and epifibatide (peptide fragments) act by inhibiting the GPIIb/IIIa receptor. As peptides, these agents are potentially antigenic, and should only be used once.

Fibrinolytic agents

Streptokinase

Mechanism of action

Streptokinase forms a complex with, and activates, plasminogen into plasmin, a fibrinolytic enzyme.

Route of administration—Intravenous.

Indications—Life-threatening venous thrombosis, pulmonary embolism, arterial thromboembolism and acute myocardial infarction.

Contraindications—Recent haemorrhage, trauma, surgery, bleeding diathesis, aortic dissection, coma, history of cerebrovascular disease.

Adverse effects—Nausea and vomiting, bleeding.

Therapeutic regimen—Streptokinase is often used in conjunction with antiplatelet and anticoagulant drugs. The clinical preference is to use fibrinolytics with a faster onset of action, such as tissue plasminogen activators. Furthermore, streptokinase is derived from haemolytic streptococci and is thus antigenic. Repeated administration of streptokinase could result in an anaphylaxis-like reaction. If repeated fibrinolytic therapy is needed, the nonantigenic tissue-type plasminogen activators should be used.

Tissue-type plasminogen activators

Alteplase and reteplase are examples of tPAs.

Mechanism of action—tPAs are tissue-type plasminogen activators.

Route of administration—Intravenous.

Indications—Life-threatening pulmonary embolism, acute thrombotic stroke within 4 hours in selected patients and thrombosed shunts.

Contraindications—As for streptokinase.

Adverse effects—Nausea and vomiting, bleeding.

CLINICAL NOTE

Although the administration of a fibrinolytic drug could improve the life expectancy of someone suffering from an acute thrombotic stroke, it could also have disastrous effects. There are stringent criteria for administering or not administering fibrinolytic drugs. You should learn these.

Bleeding disorders

Hereditary bleeding disorders are rare. Haemophilia is a genetic disorder in which excessive bleeding occurs, owing to the absence of factor VIII (haemophilia A) or IX (haemophilia B). Abnormal bruising and mucosal bleeding characterize Von Willebrand disease.

Acquired bleeding disorders may be caused by liver disease, vitamin K deficiency or anticoagulant drugs. Caution should be taken when using the aforementioned drugs in patients with thromboembolic disease.

Treatment of bleeding disorders

Vitamin K (phytomenadione)

Mechanism of action—Vitamin K is needed for the post-transcriptional γ-carboxylation of glutamic acid residues of prothrombin (factor II) and clotting factors VII, IX and X by the liver (see Fig. 4.11). Vitamin K is also necessary for normal calcification of bone.

Route of administration—Oral, intramuscular, intravenous.

Indications—Vitamin K is used as an antidote to the effects of vitamin K antagonists, and in patients with biliary obstruction or liver disease, where vitamin K deficiency may be a problem. It is also used after prolonged treatment with antibiotics that inhibit the formation of vitamin K by intestinal bacteria and prophylaxis against haemorrhagic disease of the newborn.

Adverse effects—Haemolytic anaemia and hyperbilirubinaemia in the newborn.

Protamine

Mechanism of action—Protamine is a strongly basic protein, which forms an inactive complex with heparin, and as such is used in patients in whom heparin treatment has resulted in haemorrhage. High doses of protamine appear to have anticoagulant effects through an unknown mechanism.

Route of administration—Intravenous.

Indications—Haemorrhage secondary to heparinisation.

Adverse effects—Nausea, vomiting, flushing, hypotension.

Clotting factors

Deficiencies of clotting factors can be replaced by the administration of fresh plasma. Factors VIII and IX are available as freeze-dried concentrates.

Mechanism of action—All clotting factors are necessary for normal blood coagulation.

Route of administration—Intravenous.

Indications—Haemophilia; an antidote to the effects of oral anticoagulants.

Adverse effects—Allergic reactions, including fevers and chills.

Desmopressin

Desmopressin is a synthetic analogue of vasopressin.

Mechanism of action—Desmopressin causes the release of factor VIII. It is also used in diabetes insipidus because it has antidiuretic effects.

Route of administration—Parenteral.

Indications—Desmopressin is given for mild factor VIII deficiency and in the treatment of diabetes insipidus.

Adverse effects—Fluid retention, hyponatraemia, and headache, nausea and vomiting.

Tranexamic acid

Mechanism of action—Tranexamic acid is antifibrinolytic, inhibiting plasminogen activation and therefore preventing fibrinolysis.

Route of administration—Oral, intravenous.

Indications—Tranexamic acid agents are used in the management of haemorrhage (e.g. gastrointestinal bleed or trauma). It can also be used in patients at risk of haemorrhage (e.g. haemophilia, menorrhagia and dental extraction).

Contraindications—Thromboembolic disease.

Adverse effects—Nausea and vomiting, diarrhoea. Thromboembolic events are rare.

Aprotinin

Mechanism of action—Aprotinin inhibits the proteolytic enzymes plasmin and kallikrein, thus inhibiting fibrinolysis.

Route of administration—Intravenous.

Indications—Aprotinin is used when there is a risk of blood loss after open-heart surgery and in hyperplasminaemia.

Adverse effects—Allergy, localized thrombophlebitis.

Etamsylate

Mechanism of action—Etamsylate corrects abnormal platelet adhesion.

Route of administration—Oral, intravenous.

Indications—Etamsylate is used to reduce capillary bleeding and periventricular haemorrhage in premature infants.

Contraindications—Porphyria.

Adverse effects—Nausea, headache, rashes.

BLOOD AND FLUID REPLACEMENT

Anaemia

Anaemia is a common problem worldwide. In the young, it is commonly caused by nutritional deficiencies (vitamin B_{12}, folate and iron), in fertile women menstrual loss accounts for most cases, and in the elderly, malignancy and renal failure are the more common causes.

Iron

Ferrous sulphate, ferrous fumarate and ferrous gluconate are the commoner iron salt preparations.

Mechanism of action—Dietary supplementation of iron increases serum iron and stored iron in the liver and bone. Adequate iron is necessary for normal erythropoiesis, as well as for numerous iron-containing proteins.

Route of administration—Oral, or intravenous as second-line therapy.

Indications—Iron-deficiency anaemia.

Contraindications—Caution in pregnancy.

Adverse effects—Gastrointestinal irritation, nausea, epigastric pain, altered bowel habits.

Therapeutic notes—Iron overdose or chronic iron overload can be harmful, and either acquired or inherited in the form of haemochromatosis. The iron-chelating agent desferrioxamine can be given parenterally, which allows iron to be excreted in the urine.

Vitamin B$_{12}$

Hydroxocobalamin and cyanocobalamin are vitamin B$_{12}$ drug preparations.

Mechanism of action—Vitamin B$_{12}$ is required for deoxyribonucleic acid (DNA) synthesis and effective erythropoiesis.

Route of administration—Intramuscular, oral.

Indications—Pernicious anaemia, other macrocytic megaloblastic anaemias. Prophylactically after surgical removal of the stomach (site of intrinsic factor) or terminal ileum (site of vitamin B$_{12}$ absorption).

Contraindications—None.

Adverse effects—Itching, fever, chills, flushing, nausea.

Therapeutic notes—Initial treatment requires regular weekly injections, but once serum vitamin B$_{12}$ is normalized, injections should be given at 3-monthly intervals.

Folate

Folic acid in the form folate is administered.

Mechanism of action—Folate is required for DNA synthesis and effective erythropoiesis.

Route of administration—Oral.

Indications—Macrocytic megaloblastic anaemia, prevention of neural tube defects in pregnancy. Patients taking methotrexate (folate antagonist).

Contraindications and adverse effects—None.

Therapeutic notes—Since the introduction of folate acid supplements for pregnant women, the rate of neural tube defects in newborn babies has fallen markedly.

Erythropoietin

Epoetin is a recombinant erythropoietin. Erythropoietin is synthesized in the kidney in response to a fall in the oxygen tension of the blood passing through it.

Mechanism of action—Erythropoietin acts upon the bone marrow to stimulate stem cells to divide, to produce cells of the red cell lineage.

Route of administration—Parenteral.

Indications—Anaemia of chronic renal failure, anaemia following cancer chemotherapy, before autologous blood donation.

Contraindications—Uncontrolled hypertension.

Adverse effects—Dose-dependent increase in blood pressure and platelet count, influenza-like symptoms.

Therapeutic notes—Erythropoietin often features in the news, as an increased haemoglobin concentration most probably improves an athlete's performance, making this drug a potential drug of "misuse" in sport.

Myeloproliferative disorders

The pharmacological management of the myeloproliferative disorders is outside the scope of this text, although it relies on cytotoxic drugs. Information on these agents should be learnt from a haematology or general medical textbook.

Fluid replacement

Fluid replacement should ideally be achieved orally, although this is often not practical. Intravenous administration of fluids is commonplace in the hospital.

- Intravenous fluids are given for many reasons. In septicaemia, they are used to raise blood pressure and tissue perfusion; in those who are unable to eat or drink (e.g. unconscious or presurgery) they are used to replace water and electrolytes not being taken orally or that are lost in urine and via insensible routes. In trauma, they can help increase the blood pressure and buy time before replacing blood loss with blood products.
- There are many types of intravenous fluid. The more common fluids given intravenously are blood and the crystalloids (sodium chloride and dextrose). Supplements can be added to intravenous fluids.
- The art of fluid replacement and fluid management is best learnt from an anaesthetics or general medical textbook.

● Chapter Summary

- The heart is a pump which supplies the tissues with oxygen and nutrients via blood and removes waste.
- In heart failure, cardiac glycosides such as digoxin are used to shift the Frank-Starling ventricular function to a more favourable position. Diuretics are used to inhibit water and sodium retention.
- Anti-arrhythmic drugs can be classified as Class Ia, Ib, Ic, II, III, IV under the Vaughn-Williams classification.
- In hypertension ACE inhibitors, AIIR antagonists, calcium antagonists and diuretics can be used amongst others.
- Treatment of hyperlipidaemias can be with statins, ezetimibe, fibrates, nicotinic acids and bile acid binding resins.
- Treatment of bleeding disorders can be with vitamin K, protamine, tranexamic acid, aprotinin, etamsylate and replacement of clotting factors.

Kidney and urinary system

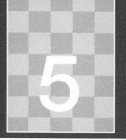

BASIC CONCEPTS

Despite making up only 1% of the total body weight, the kidneys receive approximately 25% of the cardiac output reflecting their importance to the maintenance of homeostasis.

The volume of plasma filtered by the kidneys is termed the *glomerular filtration rate* (GFR) and is equal to approximately 180 L per day for a person weighing 70 kg. This means that the entire plasma volume is filtered about 60 times a day. The kidneys have a large functional reserve and the loss of one kidney normally produces no ill-effects. The kidneys have several complex functions (see later), whereas the ureters function mainly as conduits for the transport of urine from the kidney to the bladder, where urine is stored. The bladder functions primarily as a storage sac, and urine leaves the bladder through the urethra. In women, this is a short tube that opens just in front of the vagina. In men, the tube is longer, passing through the prostate and the penis.

THE KIDNEY

Functions of the kidney

The kidney has several functions. These include the following.

- Regulation of body water content
- Regulation of body mineral content and composition
- Regulation of body pH
- Excretion of metabolic waste products, for example, urea, uric acid and creatinine
- Excretion of xenobiotics, for example, drugs
- Secretion of renin, erythropoietin and 1,25-dihydroxyvitamin D_3
- Gluconeogenesis

CLINICAL NOTE

The kidneys are the main organ by which drugs and their metabolites are eliminated from the body. When prescribing drugs in patients with impaired kidney function (e.g. the elderly) the dose must be adapted.

The nephron

Each kidney is made up of approximately one million functional units, known as *nephrons* (Fig. 5.1). Each nephron consists of a renal corpuscle, which comprizes a glomerulus and a Bowman's capsule; and a tubule, which comprizes a proximal tubule, loop of Henle, distal convoluted tubule and collecting duct system.

Blood supply

Blood reaches each kidney via the renal artery, which divides into numerous branches before forming the afferent arterioles. These afferent arterioles enter the glomerular capillaries (the glomeruli) and leave as the efferent arterioles. Leaving most nephrons is the efferent arteriole, which immediately branches into a set of capillaries known as the *peritubular capillaries*.

These branch extensively and form a network of capillaries surrounding the tubules in the cortex into which reabsorption from the tubule occurs, and from which various substances are secreted into the tubule.

Glomerular filtration

During glomerular filtration, the fluid fraction of blood in the glomerulus is forced through the capillary endothelium, a basement membrane, and the epithelium of the Bowman's capsule, to enter a fluid-filled space known as the *Bowman's space*. Approximately 20% of the plasma entering the glomerulus is filtered. The filtered fluid is known as *the glomerular filtrate* and consists of protein-free plasma.

Tubular function

The tubules are involved in reabsorption and secretion. Important components of plasma tend to be reabsorbed more or less completely, for example, sodium and glucose are 99% to 100% reabsorbed. Waste products are only partially reabsorbed, for example, approximately 45% of urea is reabsorbed.

The tubules secrete hydrogen and potassium ions, as well as organic species such as creatinine, and certain drugs such as penicillin.

Sodium and water reabsorption

Approximately 99% of filtered water and sodium is reabsorbed, but none is secreted. The Na+/K+-adenosine triphosphatase (ATPase) pump sits within the basolateral membrane of tubular cells which pumps sodium out of the cell and into the interstitium.

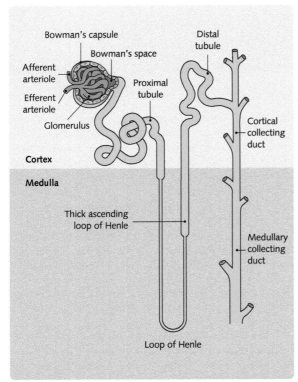

Fig. 5.1 Structure of the juxtaglomerular nephron. (Modified from Page, C., Curtis, M. Walker, M, Hoffman, B. (eds) *Integrated Pharmacology*, 3rd edn. Mosby, 2006.)

This forms a concentration gradient of sodium; high concentrations within the filtrate of the tubule lumen, and a low concentration of sodium within the cytoplasm of the tubular cells. This gradient forms the basis of most reabsorption and secretion processes that subsequently occur. Sodium reabsorption from the lumen varies according to the section of the tubule (see Figs. 5.2–5.5).

Water is reabsorbed by passive diffusion, following the movement of sodium ions, and through specific water channels (aquaporins) in the collecting tubules, which greatly increases the reabsorption of water.

Proximal tubule
The Bowman's capsule extends into the proximal tubule, which is made up of an initial convoluted section and a straight section. The proximal tubule is permeable to water and ions and is the site into which many drugs are secreted. Approximately two-thirds of the filtrate volume is reabsorbed back into the blood in the proximal tubule.

Sodium movement into the cell is coupled with that of glucose and amino acids, whereas chloride movement is by passive diffusion (see Fig. 5.2). Reabsorption of bicarbonate also takes place in the proximal tubule.

Loop of Henle
The loop of Henle consists of a descending limb, a thin ascending limb and a thick ascending limb. Some 25% of filtered sodium is reabsorbed in the thick ascending limb (see Fig. 5.3), but this portion of the tubule is impermeable to water. The increase in the solute load (sodium) in the interstitium between the ascending loop and the collecting tubules sets up an osmotic gradient which subsequently permits water reabsorption from the collecting tubules; the countercurrent multiplier system.

Juxtaglomerular apparatus
Where the afferent and efferent arterioles enter the glomerulus, a group of specialized cells, the macula densa, are situated in the juxtaglomerular apparatus.

These cells secrete renin, which is a fundamental part of the renin–angiotensin system. The renin–angiotensin system is involved directly in vascular tone and in the release of aldosterone (Chapter 4).

CLINICAL NOTE

Renal prostaglandins are vasodilators and are synthesized in response to ischaemia, angiotensin II and antidiuretic hormone (ADH). When vasoconstrictors are released, local release of renal prostaglandins (e.g. prostacyclin) compensate and preserve renal blood flow by their vasodilator action. Nonsteroidal antiinflammatory drugs (NSAIDs) inhibit prostaglandin production by inhibiting cyclooxygenase. In normal renal function, they have no effect. However, in patients in which renal blood flow is dependent on vasodilator prostaglandins (e.g. heart failure or liver cirrhosis), NSAIDs can precipitate acute renal failure. In addition, NSAIDs exacerbate salt and water retention in patients with heart failure by impairment of prostaglandin-mediated vasodilation.

Distal convoluted tubule and collecting tubule
The distal tubule is continuous with the collecting duct. The collecting duct is the site at which the tubules of many nephrons merge before draining into the renal pelvis. The renal pelvis is continuous with the ureter.

The late distal tubule and collecting duct contain two cell types (see Fig. 5.5).

- Principal cells, which incorporate sodium and potassium channels.
- Intercalated cells, which incorporate H^+-ATPases that secrete hydrogen ions.

Sodium movement into the principal cells exceeds potassium movement out of the cells so that a negative potential

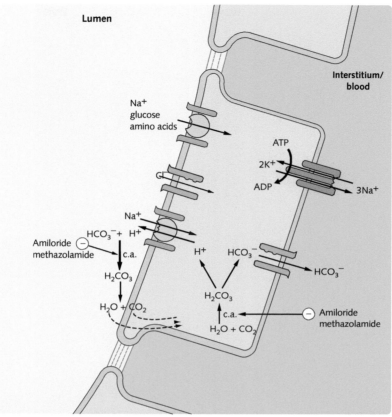

Fig. 5.2 The proximal tubule is one of the sites of bicarbonate (HCO₃-) reabsorption. Carbonic acid (H_2CO_3) is formed in the cytoplasm from the action of carbonic anhydrase (c.a.) on carbon dioxide (CO_2) and water. H_2CO_3 immediately dissociates into HCO₃-, which moves down its concentration gradient across the basolateral membrane, and H⁺, which is secreted into the lumen in exchange for Na⁺. In the lumen, H⁺ combines with filtered HCO₃- to form H_2CO_3 and subsequently CO_2 and water, which are able to diffuse back into the cell. *ADP*, Adenosine diphosphate; *ATP*, adenosine triphosphate. (Modified from Page, C., Curtis, M. Walker, M, Hoffman, B. (eds) *Integrated Pharmacology*, 3rd edn. Mosby, 2006.)

difference is established. Sodium is transported across the basolateral membrane by Na⁺/K⁺ -ATPase, and potassium is moved into the cell before being forced out by the negative potential.

This part of the tubule is the major site for potassium secretion.

The late distal tubule and collecting duct also contain mineralocorticoid receptors. When aldosterone binds to these, it produces an increase in the synthesis of Na⁺ and K⁺ channels, Na⁺/K⁺ -ATPase, and ATP, so that Na⁺ reabsorption is increased, and K⁺ and H⁺ secretion are also increased.

The collecting tubule is also the site for water reabsorption via aquaporin channels. Fine-tuning of the amount of water to be reabsorbed is controlled by the hypothalamus, which governs how much antidiuretic hormone (ADH or vasopressin) is released from the pituitary gland. The release of ADH results in more aquaporins being inserted into the luminal membrane, increasing the amount of water that is reabsorbed (Chapter 4).

Atrial natriuretic peptide, derived from the atria of the heart in response to fluid overload, is believed to act on the distal nephron causing a water and solute diuresis.

CLINICAL NOTE

ADH's release from the posterior pituitary gland results in the increased expression of aquaporin causing an increase in the passive reabsorption of water. Consequently, the urine excreted is concentrated. Note that lithium (used in the treatment of certain psychiatric conditions [Chapter 8]) can inhibit the action of ADH. Defective ADH secretion results in diabetes insipidus, an uncommon condition in which patients secrete large volumes of dilute urine.

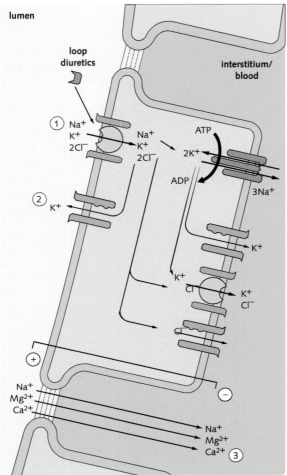

Fig. 5.3 Transport mechanism in the thick ascending loop of Henle. Loop diuretics block the $Na^+/K^+/2Cl^-$ cotransporter (1) thereby increasing the excretion of Na^+ and Cl^-. These drugs also decrease the potential difference across the tubule cell, which arises from the recycling of K^+ (2), and this leads to increased excretion of Ca^{2+} and Mg^{2+} by inhibiting paracellular diffusion (3). *ADP*, Adenosine diphosphate; *ATP*, adenosine triphosphate. (Modified from Page, C., Curtis, M. Walker, M, Hoffman, B. (eds) *Integrated Pharmacology*, 3rd edn. Mosby, 2006.)

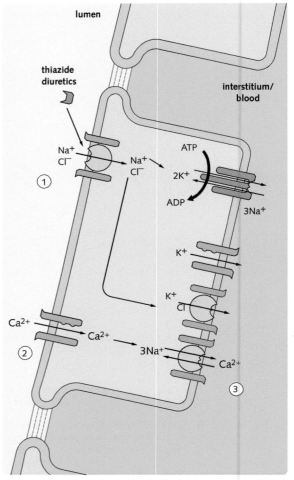

Fig. 5.4 Transport mechanisms in the early distal tubule. Thiazide diuretics increase the excretion of Na^+ and Cl^- by inhibiting the Na^+/Cl^- cotransporter (1). The reabsorption of Ca^{2+} (2) is increased by these drugs by a mechanism that may involve stimulation of Na^+/Ca^{2+} countertransport (3) caused by an increase in the concentration gradient for Na^+ across the basolateral membrane. *ADP*, Adenosine diphosphate; *ATP*, adenosine triphosphate. (Modified from Page, C., Curtis, M. Walker, M, Hoffman, B. (eds) *Integrated Pharmacology*, 3rd edn. Mosby, 2006.)

DIURETICS

Diuretics work by altering kidney function and are crucial in the management of cardiovascular disease (Chapter 4) and renal disease. Diuretics work on the kidneys to increase urine volume by reducing salt and water reabsorption from the tubules. They are prescribed for the treatment of oedema, where there is an increase in interstitial fluid volume leading to tissue swelling.

Oedema occurs when the rate of fluid formation exceeds that of fluid reabsorption from the interstitial fluid into the capillaries. The most common causes for systemic oedema are as follows.

- Congestive cardiac failure
- Hypoalbuminaemia (including liver failure and nephrotic syndrome)

Loss of fluid from the intravascular space into the interstitial compartment results in an apparent hypovolaemic state. Poor perfusion of the kidneys activates the renin–angiotensin system, which causes sodium and water retention. This exacerbates the problem of oedema.

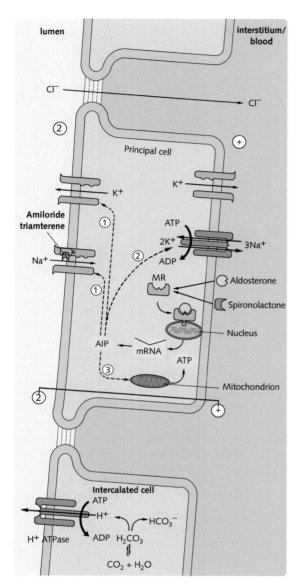

Fig. 5.5 Transport mechanisms in the late distal tubule and collecting duct. Amiloride and triamterene block the luminal Na$^+$ channels, which reduces the lumen-negative potential difference across the principal cell and decreases the driving force for K$^+$ secretion from the principal cell and H$^+$ secretion from the intercalated cell. The net effect is increased Na$^+$ excretion and decreased K$^+$ and H$^+$ excretion. Aldosterone binds to a cytoplasmic mineralocorticoid receptor (MR) stimulating the production of aldosterone-induced proteins (AIP), which (1) activate and increase the synthesis of Na$^+$ and K$^+$ channels; (2) increase the synthesis of Na$^+$/K$^+$ ATPase, and (3) increase mitochondrial production of adenosine triphosphate (ATP). The effect of aldosterone is to decrease Na$^+$ excretion and increase K$^+$ and H$^+$ excretion in urine, whereas spironolactone, an aldosterone antagonist, has the opposite effects. *ADP*, Adenosine diphosphate; *mRNA*, messenger ribonucleic acid. (Modified from Page, C., Curtis, M. Walker, M, Hoffman, B. (eds) *Integrated Pharmacology*, 3rd edn. Mosby, 2006.)

Types of diuretics

Loop diuretics

Furosemide and bumetanide are examples of loop diuretics.

Loop diuretics cause the excretion of 15% to 25% of filtered sodium as opposed to the normal 1% or less. This can result in a profound diuresis.

Site of action—Loop diuretics act at the thick ascending segment of the loop of Henle.

Mechanism of action—Loop diuretics inhibit the Na$^+$/K$^+$/2Cl$^-$ cotransporter in the luminal membrane (see Fig. 5.3). This increases the amount of sodium reaching the collecting duct and thereby increases K$^+$ and H$^+$ secretion. Calcium and magnesium reabsorption is also inhibited, owing to the decrease in potential difference across the cell normally generated from the recycling of potassium (Fig 5.6).

Loop diuretics additionally have a venodilator action, which often brings about the relief of clinical symptoms before the onset of diuresis.

Route of administration—Oral, intravenous or intramuscular. The intravenous route is used in patients with acute pulmonary oedema because the therapeutic effect is much quicker (about 30 minutes compared with 4–6 hours for an oral dose).

Indications—Used predominantly in the treatment of salt and water overload associated with acute pulmonary oedema, chronic heart failure (CHF), liver ascites and nephrotic syndrome. It can also be used in the treatment of hypertension complicated by impaired renal function.

Contraindications—Loop diuretics should not be given to those with severe renal impairment. They should be given with caution to patients receiving:

- Cardiac glycosides because the hypokalaemia caused by loop diuretics potentiates the action of cardiac glycosides and consequently increases the risk of cardiac glycoside-induced arrhythmias (Chapter 4).
- Aminoglycoside antibiotics (e.g. gentamicin) because these interact with loop diuretics and increase the risk of ototoxicity and potential hearing loss that can occur with this class of antibiotic.

Adverse effects—Hypokalaemia, hyponatraemia, hypotension and hypovolaemia. Metabolic alkalosis may occur because of increased hydrogen secretion and thus excretion. Hypocalcaemia and hypomagnesaemia are also possible. Hyperuricaemia can precipitate acute gout.

HINTS AND TIPS

Several different sodium channels exist in the renal tubule, which is why the various diuretic drugs act at different sites along its course; they have different molecular actions and different side effects. Most diuretic drugs block sodium reabsorption from the renal tubule, which leads to a high solute load in the tubule resulting in an osmotic diuresis.

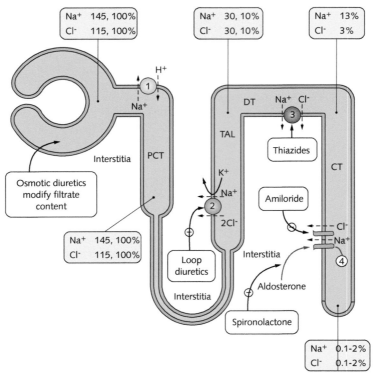

Fig. 5.6 Schematic showing the absorption of sodium and chloride in the nephron and the main sites of action of drugs. (From Ritter, J.M., Flower, R.J., Henderson, G, Rang, H.P. Rang and Dale's Pharmacology. 8th edition, 2015, p. 358, Fig. 29.4.)

Thiazide and related diuretics

Bendroflumethiazide, chlortalidone, metolazone and indapamide are examples of thiazide or related diuretics.

Thiazides produce a moderately potent diuresis, causing the excretion of 5% to 10% of filtered sodium. Although less potent than loop diuretics when prescribed alone, coadministration results in a synergistic effect and increased potency.

Site of action—Thiazide diuretics act on the early distal tubule.

Mechanism of action—Thiazide diuretics inhibit the Na^+/Cl^- cotransporter in the luminal membrane (see Fig. 5.4). Similar to loop diuretics, they increase the secretion of K^+ and H^+ into the collecting ducts, but, in contrast, they decrease Ca^{2+} excretion by a mechanism possibly involving the stimulation of a Na^+/Ca^{2+} exchange across the basolateral membrane; this is caused by reduced tubular cell sodium concentration (see Fig. 5.6).

Route of administration—Oral, having a peak effect at 4 to 6 hours.

Indications—Third-line treatment for hypertension, thiazides have been shown to reduce the risk of heart attack and strokes in patients with hypertension. Mild heart failure (loop diuretics preferred). Occasionally used for prophylaxis of calcium-containing renal stones. May be preferred in elderly patients with osteoporosis because thiazides reduce calcium excretion.

Contraindications—Hypokalaemia, hyponatraemia, hypercalcaemia. Caution when prescribing to patients taking cardiac glycosides, or to those with diabetes mellitus (thiazides may cause hyperglycaemia).

Adverse effects—Better tolerated than loop diuretics but still increase urinary frequency. Hypokalaemia, hyperuricaemia, hyponatraemia, hypermagnesaemia, hypercalcaemia and metabolic alkalosis.

CLINICAL NOTE

Mrs Hurst, 77 years old, has developed increasing dyspnoea and fatigue associated with ankle swelling preventing her from wearing her normal shoes. She has a medical history of angina, takes aspirin regularly and glyceryl trinitrate when required. Following electrocardiogram (ECG) and B-type natriuretic peptide testing, she was diagnosed as having heart failure.

Her symptoms, being caused by pulmonary and peripheral oedema, were treated with the loop diuretic furosemide with the aim of decreasing her fluid overload. Enalapril (an angiotensin-converting enzyme [ACE] inhibitor) and carvedilol (a β-blocker) were started concurrently because they have been shown to improve symptoms and decrease mortality.

Potassium-sparing diuretics

Spironolactone, amiloride and triamterene are all potassium-sparing diuretics.

Potassium-sparing diuretics produce mild diuresis and cause the excretion of 2% to 3% of filtered sodium.

Site of action—Potassium-sparing diuretics work at the late distal tubule and collecting duct (see Fig. 5.5).

Mechanism of action—There are two classes of potassium-sparing diuretics.

- Sodium-channel blockers: For example, amiloride and triamterene. These drugs block sodium reabsorption by the principal cells, thus reducing the potential difference across the cell and reducing K^+ secretion. Secretion of H^+ from the intercalated cells is also decreased.
- Aldosterone antagonists: For example, spironolactone, eplerenone. These drugs are a competitive antagonist at aldosterone receptors, and thus reduce Na^+ reabsorption and therefore K^+ and H^+ secretion. The degree of diuresis depends on aldosterone levels (see Fig. 5.6).

Route of administration—Oral.

Indications—These diuretics prolong survival in patients with heart failure (in conjunction with a loop or thiazide diuretic). They also prevent hypokalaemia, maintaining normal serum potassium levels when coadministered with other diuretics.

Aldosterone antagonists are used in the treatment of hyperaldosteronism, which can be primary (Conn syndrome) or secondary (as a result of CHF, liver disease or nephrotic syndrome).

Contraindications—Potassium-sparing diuretics interact with ACE inhibitors, increasing the risk of hyperkalaemia. They should not be given to patients with renal failure.

Adverse effects—Gastrointestinal disturbances, hyperkalaemia and hyponatraemia. Aldosterone antagonists have a wide range of adverse effects, including gynaecomastia, menstrual disorders and male sexual dysfunction because of their action on aldosterone and androgen receptors in other organs.

Therapeutic notes—Low-dose spironolactone has beneficial effects in CHF. Several preparations exist which combine a potassium-sparing diuretic with either a thiazide or a loop diuretic, for example, co-amilofruse, which contains amiloride and furosemide

Osmotic diuretics

Mannitol is an osmotic diuretic.

Site of action—Osmotic diuretics exert their effects in tubular segments that are water permeable; proximal tubule, descending loop of Henle, and the collecting ducts (see Fig. 5.6).

Mechanism of action—Osmotic diuretics are freely filtered at the glomerulus, but only partially, if at all, reabsorbed.

Passive water reabsorption is reduced by the presence of this nonreabsorbable solute within the tubule lumen. The net effect is increased water loss, with a relatively smaller loss of sodium.

Route of administration—Mannitol is administered intravenously.

Indications—Osmotic diuretics are used mainly for raised intracranial, and rarely, raised intraocular pressure (glaucoma).

Contraindications—Congestive cardiac failure and pulmonary oedema.

Adverse effects—Chills and fever.

Therapeutic notes—Osmotic diuretics are seldom used in heart failure, as an expansion of blood volume can be greater than the degree of diuresis produced.

THE URINARY SYSTEM

Urinary retention

Acute urinary retention is treated with urethral catheterisation. Chronic urinary retention is usually painless, and management depends upon the underlying cause. In men, the most common cause for chronic urinary retention is benign prostatic hyperplasia (BPH). Surgery is the definitive treatment, although many patients can be treated medically. Three classes of drugs can be used to treat bladder outflow obstruction secondary to BPH as follows.

- α-Blockers
- Parasympathomimetics
- Antiandrogens.

α-Blockers

Doxazosin and prazosin are examples of α-blockers and act by relaxing the smooth muscle at the urethra opening of the bladder, increasing the flow of urine. Because α-blockers are also used as vasodilators in cardiovascular disease (Chapter 4), postural hypotension can be a side effect, although are otherwise well tolerated.

Parasympathomimetics

Parasympathomimetics, such as bethanechol, act by increasing detrusor muscle contraction. Their effect is most marked when there is bladder outlet obstruction, and they have no role in the relief of acute urinary retention. Side effects include sweating, bradycardia and intestinal colic. They are now used infrequently, being superseded by catheterisation.

Antiandrogens—Finasteride is a specific inhibitor of the enzyme 5α-reductase, which converts testosterone to the more potent androgen dihydrotestosterone. This inhibition leads to a reduction in prostate size, and improvement of urinary flow. The antiandrogens are described in Chapter 7.

Mr Raheem, 80 years old, presents with increasing nocturia, urgency and reduced urinary flow for the past 2 years. Urinalysis was negative. Renal function and ultrasound were normal. His urine flow rate showed moderate impairment. Digital rectal examination revealed a smooth, enlarged prostate, suggestive of BPH. Prostate serum antigen was within the normal range. His symptoms were managed medically with Tamsulosin, an α-adrenergic blocker. However, in the future, he may require a transurethral resection of the prostate.

Urinary incontinence

Urinary incontinence is the involuntary leakage of urine. There are three main types of urinary incontinence.

- True incontinence (fistulous track)
- Stress incontinence (incompetent sphincter)
- Urge incontinence (detrusor instability)

Urge incontinence is the only type that is practically amenable to pharmacological intervention, mostly with muscarinic receptor antagonists.

Muscarinic receptor antagonists

Oxybutynin is the most widely used muscarinic receptor antagonist for the treatment of urge incontinence, although newer muscarinic receptor antagonists are in use (e.g. solifenacin, tolterodine).

Mechanism of action—Oxybutynin relaxes the detrusor muscle of the bladder.

Route of administration—Oral, transdermal (patches).

Indications—Urinary frequency, urgency, urge incontinence.

Contraindications—Intestinal obstruction, significant bladder outflow obstruction, glaucoma.

Adverse effects—Dry mouth, constipation, blurred vision, urinary retention, nausea and vomiting.

Therapeutic notes—The main side effects are typically caused by these drugs blocking muscarinic receptors elsewhere in the parasympathetic nervous system, and are commonly dose related.

Duloxetine

Duloxetine is a serotonin/noradrenaline reuptake inhibitor (see Chapter 8) that can be used as second-line treatment for stress incontinence, in patients who do not want, or who are unsuitable for surgery.

Desmopressin

Desmopressin is an analogue of ADH, given by mouth or by nasal spray. It can be used in the treatment of nocturnal enuresis in children or in adults with troublesome nocturia (see Chapter 4).

Mirabegron

This selective β-agonist has recently been licensed for the treatment of overactive bladder.

Erectile dysfunction

Erectile dysfunction (impotence) is a common problem worldwide and has numerous causes, including side effects arising from several prescribed medications (e.g. antipsychotics, antihypertensives and antidepressants).

The penis is innervated by autonomic (involuntary) and somatic (voluntary) nerves. Parasympathetic innervation brings about erection, and sympathetic innervation is responsible for ejaculation. Nonadrenergic, noncholinergic neurotransmission (NANC) (nitrergic) also appears to promote erection.

Nitric oxide is the neurotransmitter released by NANC nerves innervating the corpus carvenosum and is believed to be the principal mediator of inducing and sustaining an erection. Nitric oxide activates the guanylyl cyclase enzyme, which subsequently generates cyclic guanosine monophosphate (cGMP) in the vascular smooth muscle cells of the corpus carvenosum. The synthesis of cGMP, in turn, activates a protein kinase, which phosphorylates ion channels in the plasma membrane, and causes hyperpolarisation of the smooth muscle cell. Intracellular calcium ions are consequently sequestered into the endoplasmic reticulum, and further calcium influx into the cell inhibited by the closure of calcium channels. The overall effect of the fall in intracellular calcium is a relaxation of the smooth muscle and increased blood flow to the penis.

Although nitric oxide has a very short half-life and is molecularly unstable, cGMP is broken down by a specific group of enzymes, the phosphodiesterases, which subsequently results in the penis returning to its flaccid state. Inhibition of phosphodiesterase 5 found in the penis is the target of one class of drugs used in the treatment of erectile dysfunction.

Phosphodiesterase inhibitors

Sildenafil is a selective inhibitor of phosphodiesterase type 5.

Mechanism of action—Inhibition of phosphodiesterase-mediated degradation of cGMP. This enhances the vasodilator effects of nitrous oxide because of higher intracellular levels of cGMP. Thus there is the continual relaxation of penile smooth muscle and maintenance of an erection.

Route of administration—Oral.

Indications—Erectile dysfunction. There are strict guidelines in the United Kingdom as to which groups of patients can be prescribed sildenafil on the National Health Service. These include patients with erectile dysfunction resulting from diabetes, multiple sclerosis, Parkinson disease, poliomyelitis, prostate cancer, severe pelvic injury, single-gene neurological disease, spina bifida or spinal cord injury.

Contraindications—Concurrent treatment with nitrates. Conditions in which vasodilation or sexual activity are inadvisable.

Adverse effects—Many of the unwanted effects are caused by vasodilation in other vascular areas. These include hypotension, flushing and headache. In addition, dyspepsia and visual disturbances.

Therapeutic notes—Nonspecific inhibition of phosphodiesterase type 6 in the retina is responsible for occasional colour disturbances in some patient's vision. An erection will not occur unless there is sexual stimulation and a normal sexual drive.

Papaverine is a nonselective phosphodiesterase inhibitor, which is injected directly into the corpus cavernosum and causes vasodilation and thus an erection. However, most men do not like these injections.

Prostaglandin E$_1$

Alprostadil is a synthetic prostaglandin E$_1$ analogue.

Mechanism of action—It has a similar effect on penile smooth muscle as nitric oxide.

Route of administration—Direct injection into the corpus cavernosum of the penis or applied into the urethra.

Indications—Erectile dysfunction.

Contraindications—Predisposition to prolonged erection, urethral stricture and use of other agents for erectile dysfunction.

Adverse effects—Penile pain, priapism.

HINTS AND TIPS

Phosphodiesterase enzymes degrade the cyclic nucleotides cyclic adenosine monophosphate (cAMP) and cGMP. Inhibitors of the phosphodiesterases, such as sildenafil, and the less specific xanthines such as theophylline, result in accumulation of these mediators, which brings about the physiological effects of these drugs.

● Chapter Summary

- The kidneys function to regulate water, mineral content, body pH and excretion of metabolic waste products. As well as manufacturing vitamin D3.
- The kidney nephron consist of the proximal tubule, loop of Henle, juxtaglomerular apparatus, distal convoluted tubule and the collecting tubule.
- Drugs such as diuretics, loop diuretics and thiazides work on altering kidney function to increase excretion of salts.
- Urinary incontinence can be managed by muscarinic receptor antagonists like oxybutynin or mirabegron.
- Erectile dysfunction can be managed by phosphodiesterase inhibitors, and direct injection of prsotaglandin E1.

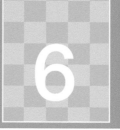

THE STOMACH

Basic concepts

The stomach stores food but also helps mechanically and chemically (through hydrochloric acid [HCL] and digestive enzymes) to break it down. Peptic ulceration and gastro-oesophageal reflux disease (GORD) are two of the common problems that can occur in the stomach.

Peptic ulceration

The gastric epithelium secretes several substances: HCl (from parietal cells), digestive enzymes (from peptic cells) and mucus (from mucus-secreting cells). The acid and enzymes convert food into a thick semi-liquid paste called *chyme*. The production of acid also kills harmful pathogens. The mucus protects the stomach from its own corrosive secretions.

Peptic ulceration results from a breach in the mucosa lining the alimentary tract. Unprotected mucosa rapidly undergoes autodigestion leading to a range of damage; inflammation or gastritis, necrosis, haemorrhage, and even perforation as the erosion deepens.

Gastric and duodenal ulcers differ in their location, epidemiology, incidence and aetiology but present with similar symptoms, and treatment is based on similar principles. Peptic ulcer disease is chronic, recurrent and common, affecting at least 10% of the population in developed countries. *Helicobacter pylori* plays a role in the pathogenesis of a significant proportion of peptic ulcer disease.

Protective factors

The mucosal defences against acid/enzyme attack consist of the following.

- The mucous barrier (approximately 500 mm thick), a mucous matrix into which bicarbonate ions are secreted, producing a buffering gradient.
- The surface epithelium and prostaglandins E_2 and I_2, synthesized by the gastric mucosa, are thought to exert a cytoprotective action by increasing mucosal blood flow.

Acid secretion

The regulation of acid secretion by parietal cells is especially important in peptic ulceration and constitutes a major target for drug action (Fig. 6.1). Acid is secreted from gastric parietal cells by a unique proton pump that catalyses the exchange of intracellular H^+ for extracellular K^+.

The secretion of HCl is controlled by the activation of three main receptors on the basolateral membrane of the parietal cell. These include the following.

- Gastrin receptors, which respond to gastrin secreted by the G cells of the stomach antrum.
- Histamine (H_2) receptors, which respond to histamine secreted from the enterochromaffin-like paracrine cells that are adjacent to the parietal cell.
- Muscarinic (M_1, M_3) receptors on the parietal cell, which respond to acetylcholine (ACh) released from neurones innervating parietal cells.

Although the parietal cells possess muscarinic and gastrin receptors, both ACh and gastrin mainly exert their acid secretory effect indirectly, by stimulating nearby enterochromaffin-like cells to release histamine. Histamine then acts locally on the parietal cells where activation of the H_2 receptor results in the stimulation of adenylyl cyclase and the subsequent secretion of acid. Excessive production of gastrin from a rare tumour, a gastrinoma, can result in excess acid production, and in peptic ulceration, a condition known as Zollinger–Ellison syndrome.

CLINICAL NOTE

Mr. Springfields is a 56-year-old city worker, who presents to A&E with epigastric pain. Normally this pain is relieved with eating or antacids, but today he vomited dark-coloured blood and had an episode of malaena. He has been taking ibuprofen for back pain over the past 2 months. He is pale and tachycardic, with a blood pressure of 110/65 mm Hg. He is stabilized with oxygen and 1 unit of blood. Upper gastrointestinal flexible endoscopy reveals a shallow ulcer overlying a blood clot. A biopsy is taken to test for *H. pylori* and returns positive. His ibuprofen is discontinued, and he is prescribed *H. pylori* eradication therapy (a proton-pump inhibitor and antibiotics) consisting of omeprazole, amoxicillin and metronidazole.

Gastrooesophageal reflux

Stomach contents are normally prevented from reentering the oesophagus by the lower oesophageal sphincter (LOS). Loss of tone of the LOS or a rise in intraabdominal pressure are the most common causes of GORD, of which heartburn

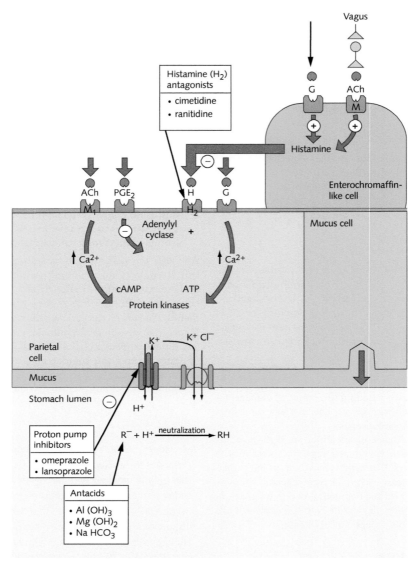

Fig. 6.1 Acid secretion from parietal cells is reduced by muscarinic antagonists, histamine (H_2) antagonists and the proton-pump inhibitors. Gastrin (G) and acetylcholine (ACh) stimulate the parietal cell directly to increase acid secretion and also stimulate enterochromaffin-like cells to secrete histamine, which then acts on the H_2 receptors of the parietal cell. Antacids raise the luminal pH by neutralising hydrogen ions. Mucosal strengtheners adhere to and protect ulcer craters and may kill *Helicobacter pylori*. *ATP*, Adenosine triphosphate; *cAMP*, cyclic adenosine monophosphate; *PGE2*, prostaglandin E2. (Modified from Page, C., Curtis, M. Walker, M, Hoffman, B. (eds) *Integrated Pharmacology*, 3rd edn. Mosby, 2006,)

is the major symptom. Conservative treatment options include raising the head of the patient's bed, avoiding excessive alcohol consumption, losing weight and smoking cessation. Patients should avoid medications, which affect oesophageal motility (e.g. nitrates or tricyclic antidepressants) or damage the mucosa (e.g. nonsteroidal antiinflammatory drugs [NSAIDs] or alendronic acid). The drugs used in the management of GORD are the same as for other acid-related disorders (Fig. 6.2).

Prevention and treatment of acid-related disease

Drugs that are effective in the treatment of peptic ulcers either reduce/neutralize gastric acid secretion or increase mucosal resistance to acid-pepsin attack. Peptic ulcers can be treated quite easily but the eradication of *H. pylori* is key to prevent recurrence.

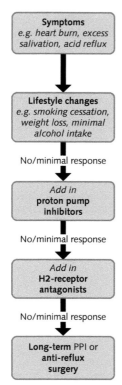

Fig. 6.2 Treatment of gastrooesophageal reflux disease: a stepwise approach. (Modified from Colledge, N.R., Walker, B., Ralston, S.H. *Davidson's Principles and Practice of Medicine*, 23rd edition, Churchill Livingstone, Edinburgh, 1999.)

Reduction of acid secretion

Proton pump inhibitors

Omeprazole, lansoprazole and pantoprazole are examples of proton-pump inhibitors (PPIs).

Mechanism of action—PPIs cause irreversible inhibition of H^+/K^+ -ATPase that is responsible for H^+ secretion from parietal cells (see Fig. 6.1). They are inactive prodrugs and are converted at acidic pH to sulphonamide, which combines covalently and thus irreversibly with -SH groups on H^+/K^+ adenosine triphosphatase (ATPase). This inhibition is highly specific and localized.

Route of administration—Oral. Some PPIs can be given intravenously.

Indications—Short-term treatment of peptic ulcers, eradication of *H. pylori,* severe GORD, confirmed oesophagitis, Zollinger–Ellison syndrome.

Contraindications—No important contraindications are reported.

Adverse effects—Gastrointestinal upset, nausea, headaches. There might be a risk of gastric atrophy with long-term treatment. Can also cause hyponatraemia.

Histamine H$_2$-receptor antagonists

Examples of H$_2$-receptor antagonists include cimetidine and ranitidine.

Mechanism of action—H$_2$-receptor antagonists competitively block the action of histamine on parietal cells (see Fig. 6.1) that inhibits gastric acid secretion.

Route of administration—Oral. Some H2-receptor antagonists can be given intravenously.

Indications—H$_2$-receptor antagonists are used in the treatment of peptic ulcer disease and GORD.

Contraindications—H$_2$-receptor antagonists may mask symptoms of gastric cancer. Before prescribing, gastric malignancy should be excluded if any "alarm features" are present.

Adverse effects—Dizziness, fatigue, gynaecomastia, rash.

Therapeutic notes—H$_2$-receptor antagonists do not reduce acid production to the same extent as PPIs but do relieve the pain of ulcer and promote healing. The drugs are administered at night when acid buffering by food is at its lowest. The usual regimen is twice daily for 4 to 8 weeks. Cimetidine inhibits the P$_{450}$ enzyme system, reducing the metabolism of drugs such as warfarin, phenytoin, theophylline and 3,4-Methylenedioxymethamphetamine (MDMA)("ecstasy"), potentiating their pharmacological effect and thus should be used with caution in patients taking these medications.

Mucosal strengtheners

Misoprostol—Mechanism of action

Misoprostol is a synthetic analogue of prostaglandin E. It imitates the action of endogenous prostaglandins (PGE$_2$ and PGI$_2$) in maintaining the integrity of the gastroduodenal mucosal barrier and promotes healing (see Fig. 6.1).

Route of administration—Oral.

Indications—Ulcer healing and ulcer prophylaxis with NSAID use.

Contraindications—Misoprostol should not be given to people with hypotension, or to women who are pregnant (causes termination) or breastfeeding.

Adverse effects—Diarrhoea, abdominal pain, spontaneous abortion in pregnancy.

Therapeutic notes—Misoprostol is most effective at correcting the deficit caused by NSAIDs that inhibit cyclooxygenase-1 and reduce prostaglandin synthesis (Chapter 11). Misoprostol can prevent NSAID-associated ulcers, and therefore is particularly useful in patients who are reliant on NSAIDs.

Chelates

Bismuth chelate and sucralfate appear to help protect the gastric mucosa by several means, including inhibiting the action of pepsin, promoting synthesis of protective prostaglandins and stimulating the secretion of bicarbonate. Chelates are sometimes used in combination regimes to treat *H. pylori*. They are administered orally and are generally well tolerated. However, they can cause blackening of the tongue and faeces. Note that sucralfate can reduce the absorption of a number of other drugs, including theophylline, tetracycline antibiotics, digoxin and amitriptyline.

Antacids

Examples of antacids include aluminium hydroxide and magnesium carbonate.

Mechanism of action—Antacids consist of alkaline aluminium (Al^{3+}) and magnesium (Mg^{2+}) salts that are used to raise the luminal pH of the stomach. They neutralize acid and, as a result, may reduce the damaging effects of pepsin, which is pH dependent (see Fig. 6.1). In addition, Al^{3+} and Mg^{2+} salts bind and inactivate pepsin.

Route of administration—Oral.

Indications—Symptomatic relief of ulcers, nonulcer dyspepsia and GORD.

Contraindications—Aluminium hydroxide and magnesium hydroxide should not be given to people with hypophosphataemia.

Adverse effects—Constipation (aluminium salts), diarrhoea (magnesium salts).

Therapeutic notes—Antacids are the simplest way to treat symptoms of excessive gastric acid secretion and can provide symptomatic relief from ulceration. Although frequent high dosing can promote ulcer healing, this is rarely practical.

Alginates

Alginate-containing antacids are administered orally and form an impenetrable raft, which floats on the surface of the gastric contents. This layer prevents gastric acid from refluxing into the oesophagus and is, therefore, most useful in GORD. This class of drug is very well tolerated but does not have any effect on acid secretion, or on preventing or healing of peptic ulcers.

Helicobacter pylori eradication regimens

H. pylori plays a significant role in the pathogenesis of peptic ulcer disease. It does not cause ulcers in everyone it infects (50%–80% of the population) but, of those who develop ulcers, 90% can be found to have an *H. pylori* infection in their antrum. It is routine practice to test for *H. pylori*, using a carbon-13 urea breath test or a stool antigen test because the eradication of this infection can promote rapid and long-term healing of the ulcer.

Treatment of peptic ulcer disease should include eradication of *H. pylori*. The rate of recurrence of duodenal ulcer after healing can be as high as 80% within 1 year when *H. pylori* eradication is not part of the treatment, but less than 5% when *H. pylori* is eradicated.

The ideal treatment for *H. pylori* eradication is not yet clear. These are the current regimens under evaluation.

- The "classic" triple therapy: 1 or 2 weeks' treatment with omeprazole, metronidazole and amoxicillin or clarithromycin. This eliminates *H. pylori* in 90% of patients but adverse effects, compliance and resistance can be problematic.
- Quadruple therapy: Omeprazole, two antibiotics and bismuth chelate.

Terlipressin

Terlipressin is a vasoactive drug that is used in the emergency treatment of oesophageal varices in patients with raised portal hypertension associated most commonly with liver cirrhosis. It causes vasoconstriction of dilated splanchnic blood vessels thus reducing blood flow and arresting the catastrophic variceal haemorrhage.

NAUSEA AND VOMITING

Basic concepts

The most common causes of nausea and vomiting are shown in Fig. 6.3. Many drugs, notably chemotherapy, opioids and general anaesthesia, cause nausea and vomiting. The act of vomiting is coordinated in the vomiting centre within the brainstem. This centre receives neuronal input from several sources, although fibres from the chemoreceptor trigger zone (CTZ) of the fourth ventricle appear fundamental in bringing about emesis (vomiting). The CTZ lies outside the blood–brain barrier and is sensitive to many stimuli, such as certain drugs, and endogenous and potentially exogenous chemical mediators. The CTZ contains numerous dopamine receptors, which partially explains why antiparkinsonian drugs (dopaminergic drugs) (Chapter 8) often induce nausea and vomiting, whereas some antidopaminergic drugs are used as antiemetics.

Emetic drugs

It is advantageous, occasionally, to induce emesis to empty the stomach of an ingested toxic substance. Ipecacuanha is given as a liquid and causes gastric irritation resulting in emesis. There is no evidence to support its use, however, and gastric lavage is the preferred method.

Antiemetic drugs

The main neurotransmitters (i.e. serotonin [5-HT], histamine and dopamine) involved in the mechanism of vomiting are target sites for many antiemetic medications.

H_1-receptor antagonists

Cyclizine, cinnarizine and promethazine are H1-receptor antagonist antiemetics.

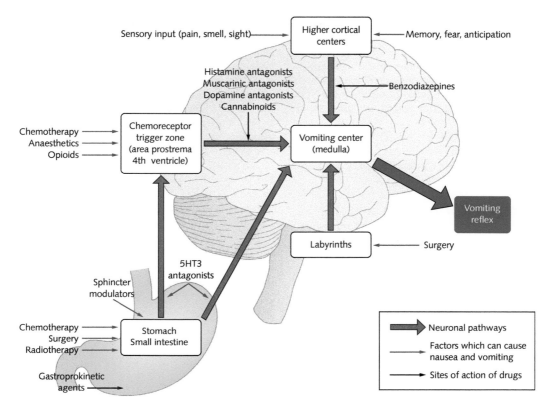

Fig. 6.3 Common causes of nausea and vomiting.

Mechanism of action—These H1-receptor antagonists have little effect on nausea and vomiting induced by substances acting directly upon the CTZ, although appear effective antiemetics in the treatment of motion sickness and vestibulocochlear disease.

Route of administration—Cyclizine: oral, intramuscular, intravenous. Cinnarizine: oral.

Indications—Motion sickness, vestibular disorders, vertigo.

Cyclizine is commonly used for morning sickness in pregnancy.

Adverse effects—Drowsiness, dry mouth, blurred vision.

Therapeutic notes—Older H1-receptor antagonists that can cross the blood–brain barrier also have significant antimuscarinic activity and should be used with caution in prostatic hypertrophy, urinary retention and glaucoma.

Phenothiazines

Prochlorperazine and chlorpromazine are the most widely used antiemetic drug in this class, although the phenothiazines are also used for their antipsychotic properties (Chapter 8).

Mechanism of action—Numerous effects. Antagonize dopamine, H1 and muscarinic receptors.

Route of administration—Oral, rectal, intramuscular.

Indications—Nausea and vomiting, vertigo, psychosis (Chapter 8).

Contraindications—May exacerbate existing parkinsonian symptoms.

Adverse effects—Sedation, postural hypotension, increased prolactin levels, extrapyramidal effects.

Dopamine antagonists

Domperidone and metoclopramide are examples of the antiemetic dopamine antagonists.

Mechanism of action—Domperidone and metoclopramide antagonize dopamine receptors and act on the CTZ. They also act peripherally on the gastrointestinal tract, increasing the motility of the oesophagus, stomach and intestine. They are not only antiemetic but also promote gastric emptying and small intestine peristalsis.

Metoclopramide also acts as a dopamine receptor antagonist elsewhere in the central nervous system, producing a number of unwanted side effects including disorders of movement, particularly in children and young adults.

Route of administration—Metoclopramide: oral, intramuscular, intravenous. Domperidone: oral, rectal.

Indications—Nausea and vomiting, functional dyspepsia/GORD.

Haloperidol and levomepromazine also act as D2 antagonists in the CTZ and can be used for acute chemotherapy-induced emesis.

Contraindications—Metoclopramide is not routinely given to patients under the age of 20 years because there is an increased risk of extrapyramidal side effects in the young.

Adverse effects—Metoclopramide can cause oculogyric crises (involuntary upward eye movement) and spasmodic torticollis (involuntary twisting of the neck). It also stimulates prolactin causing galactorrhoea and disorders of menstruation.

Domperidone can cause hyperprolactinaemia and extrapyramidal side effects, but to a lesser degree because it penetrates the blood-brain barrier much less easily than metoclopramide.

Serotonin-receptor antagonists

Ondansetron is an example of 5-HT$_3$ receptor antagonist.

Mechanism of action—Antagonism of 5-HT$_3$ receptors in the CTZ believed to be responsible for the antiemetic effects of this class of drugs.

Route of administration—Oral, rectal, intramuscular, intravenous.

Indications—Nausea and vomiting, especially postoperatively and when associated with the administration of cytotoxic drugs.

Adverse effects—Constipation, headache.

Other antiemetics

The synthetic cannabinoid nabilone has antiemetic properties where there is direct stimulation of the CTZ. Hyoscine is a muscarinic-receptor antagonist, and like the H1-receptor antagonists is most effective in the treatment of motion sickness. Betahistine dihydrochloride is used in Ménière disease, although its prime effects are assumed to be on the vestibulocochlear nerve. High dose glucocorticoids (particularly dexamethasone; see Chapter 7) can also control emesis, especially when induced by cytotoxic drugs.

THE INTESTINES

Basic concepts

Intestinal motility

Normal motility, or peristalsis, of the intestinal tract, acts to mix bowel contents thoroughly and to propel them in a caudal direction. Regulation of normal intestinal motility is under neuronal and hormonal control.

Neuronal control

Two principal intramural plexuses form the enteric nervous system.

- The myenteric plexus (Auerbach's plexus), which is located between the outer longitudinal and middle circular muscle layers.
- The submucous plexus (Meissner's plexus), which is on the luminal side of the circular muscle layer.

Together, these autonomic ganglionated plexi control the functioning of the gastrointestinal tract through complex local reflex connections between sensory neurones, smooth muscle, mucosa and blood vessels.

Extrinsic parasympathetic fibres from the vagus are excitatory and extrinsic sympathetic fibres are inhibitory. The enteric autonomic nervous system is a major target for the pharmacological therapy of gastrointestinal disorders.

Hormonal control

The activity of the gastrointestinal tract is influenced both by endocrine (e.g. gastrin) and paracrine (e.g. histamine, secretin, cholecystokinin, vasoactive intestinal peptide) secretions.

Drugs that affect intestinal motility

Four classes of drug are used clinically for their effects on gastrointestinal motility (Fig. 6.4).

- Motility stimulants
- Antispasmodics
- Laxatives (purgatives)
- Antidiarrhoeals.

Motility stimulants

Agents that increase the motility of the gastrointestinal tract without a laxative effect are used for motility disorders such as GORD and gastric stasis (slow stomach emptying). Domperidone and metoclopramide in addition to their antiemetic effects, both act to increase gastric and intestinal motility, although their mechanism of action for the latter remains unclear.

Antispasmodics

The smooth muscle relaxant properties of antispasmodic drugs may be useful as adjunctive treatment for nonulcer dyspepsia, irritable bowel syndrome and diverticular disease.

There are two classes of antispasmodic drug.

- Muscarinic receptor antagonists (antimuscarinics)
- Drugs acting directly on smooth muscle

Muscarinic receptor antagonists—Examples include atropine, propantheline and dicyclomine.

Mechanism of action—Muscarinic receptor antagonists act by inhibiting parasympathetic activity causing relaxation of the gastrointestinal smooth muscle.

Route of administration—Oral.

Indications—Nonulcer dyspepsia, irritable bowel syndrome, diverticular disease.

Contraindications—Muscarinic receptor antagonists tend to relax the lower oesophageal sphincter and should be avoided in GORD. Other contraindications include angle-closure glaucoma, myasthenia gravis, paralytic ileus and prostatic enlargement.

Adverse effects—Anticholinergic effects; dry mouth, blurred vision, dry skin, tachycardia, urinary retention.

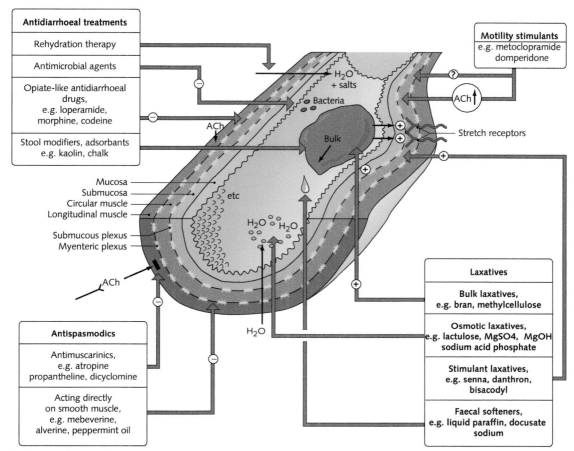

Fig. 6.4 Intestinal motility: control and site of drug action. *ACh*, Acetylcholine; *MgOH*, magnesium hydroxide; *MgSO4*, magnesium sulphate.

Drugs acting directly on smooth muscle—Mechanism of action

Mebeverine, alverine and peppermint oil are believed to be direct relaxants of smooth muscle.

Route of administration—Oral.

Indications—Irritable bowel syndrome and diverticular disease.

Contraindications—Paralytic ileus.

Adverse effects—Nausea, headache, heartburn are occasional problems.

HINTS AND TIPS

Diarrhoea can be life threatening, especially in children. Management in most cases relies on fluid replacement with oral rehydration therapy, before treating the underlying cause. Exclude other causes before treating with an antidiarrhoeal.

Laxatives

Laxatives are drugs used to hasten transit time in the gut and encourage defecation. Laxatives are used to relieve constipation (an infrequent or difficult passage of stool) and to clear the bowel before medical and surgical procedures.

It should be remembered that individuals' bowel habits vary considerably. The frequency and volume of the stool are best regulated by diet, but drugs may be necessary. The passage of food through the intestine can be hastened by:

- bulk-forming laxatives
- osmotic laxatives
- stimulant laxatives
- faecal softeners.

Bulk-forming laxatives

Bran, methylcellulose, sterculia and ispaghula husk are examples of bulk-forming laxatives.

Mechanism of action—Bulk-forming laxatives increase the volume of the nonabsorbable solid residue in the gut, distending the colon and stimulating peristaltic activity.

Route of administration—Oral.

Indications—Constipation, particularly when small hard stools are present.

Contraindications—Dysphagia, intestinal obstruction, colonic atony, faecal impaction.

Adverse effects—Flatulence, abdominal distension and gastrointestinal obstruction.

Therapeutic notes—Adequate fluid intake should be encouraged, and clinical effects may take several days to develop.

Osmotic laxatives

Examples of osmotic laxatives include lactulose, macrogols and saline purgatives.

Mechanism of action—Osmotic laxatives are poorly absorbed compounds that increase the water content of the bowel by osmosis. Lactulose is a semisynthetic disaccharide that is not absorbed from the gastrointestinal tract. Similarly, magnesium and sodium salts are poorly absorbed and are osmotically active. By producing an osmotic load, these agents trap increased volumes of fluid in the lumen of the bowel, accelerating the transfer of the gut contents through the small intestine.

Route of administration—Oral.

Indications—Constipation, hepatic encephalopathy.

Contraindications—Intestinal obstruction.

Adverse effects—Flatulence, cramps, abdominal discomfort, electrolyte disturbance.

Stimulant laxatives

Senna, danthron, Bisacodyl and sodium picosulphate are examples of stimulant laxatives.

Mechanism of action—Stimulant laxatives increase gastrointestinal peristalsis and water and electrolyte secretion by the mucosa, possibly by stimulating enteric nerves.

Route of administration—Oral.

Bisacodyl is often given by suppository. It stimulates the rectal mucosa inducing defecation in 15 to 30 mins.

Indications—Constipation and bowel evacuation before medical/surgical procedures.

Contraindications—Intestinal obstruction.

Adverse effects—In the short term, side effects of stimulant laxatives include intestinal cramp. Prolonged use can lead to damage to the nerve plexuses resulting in the deterioration of intestinal function and atonic colon. Danthron is potentially carcinogenic, hence its limited use.

Therapeutic notes—Stimulant laxatives should be given for short periods only, and danthron is indicated for use only in the terminally ill.

Faecal softeners

Liquid paraffin and docusate sodium are examples of faecal softeners.

Mechanism of action—Faecal softeners promote defaecation by softening (e.g. docusate sodium) and/or lubricating (e.g. liquid paraffin) faeces to aid their passage through the gastrointestinal tract.

Route of administration—Oral. docusate sodium can be administered rectally.

Indications—Constipation, faecal impaction, haemorrhoids, anal fissures.

Contraindications—Should not be given to children younger than 3 years.

Adverse effects—The prolonged use of liquid paraffin may impair the absorption of fat-soluble vitamins A and D and cause "paraffinomas". However, it is now seldom used clinically.

Therapeutic notes—Prolonged use of faecal softeners is not recommended.

In pregnancy, if dietary and lifestyle changes fail to control constipation, a bulk-forming laxative (ispaghula husk) should be tried first. An osmotic laxative (lactulose) or stimulant laxative (senna) may also be suitable. In children who are constipated, osmotic laxatives are first line. Lactulose is often used to soften stools and macrogols is used to clear faecal impaction.

Antidiarrhoeal drugs

Diarrhoea is the passage of frequent, liquid stools. There is an increase in the motility of the gastrointestinal tract, accompanied by an increased secretion, coupled with a decreased absorption of fluid, leading to electrolyte and water loss. Causes of diarrhoea include infections, toxins, certain drugs, chronic disease and anxiety.

There are four approaches to the treatment of severe acute diarrhoea.

- Maintenance of fluid and electrolyte balance through oral rehydration therapy (ORT)
- Use of appropriate antimicrobial drugs
- Use of opiate-like antimotility drugs
- Use of stool modifiers/adsorbents.

Maintenance of fluid and electrolyte balance through oral rehydration therapy

Oral rehydration therapy (ORT) should be the first priority in the treatment of acute diarrhoea of all causes and can be life saving.

ORT solutions are isotonic or slightly hypotonic; they vary in their composition, but a standard formula would contain sodium chloride (NaCl), potassium chloride (KCl), sodium citrate and glucose in appropriate concentrations.

Intravenous rehydration therapy is needed if dehydration is severe. In the ileum, there is cotransport of Na and glucose across the epithelial cell. The presence of glucose (in ORT) therefore enhances Na absorption and thus water uptake.

Use of antimicrobial drugs

Antibiotic treatment of diarrhoea is useful only when a bacterial pathogen has been identified or is highly suspected. Acute infectious diarrhoea is usually self-limiting. Antibiotic therapy itself carries certain risks.

- Spreading antibiotic resistance among enteropathogenic bacteria.

- Destroying normal commensal gut flora, allowing overgrowth of the bacterium *Clostridium difficile*, which can result in pseudomembranous colitis, a potentially fatal condition.

Antibiotic treatment is indicated in the following.

- Severe cholera or *Salmonella typhimurium* infection: tetracycline
- *Shigella* species infections: ampicillin
- *Campylobacter jejuni*: erythromycin or ciprofloxacin

Antibiotics are discussed in detail in Chapter 12.

Use of opiate-like antimotility drugs

Examples of opiate-like antimotility drugs include loperamide and codeine.

Mechanism of action—Opiate-like antimotility drugs act on μ-opiate receptors in the myenteric plexus, which increases the tone and rhythmic contraction of the intestine but lessens the propulsive activity. Loperamide and codeine also have an antisecretory action.

Route of administration—Oral.

Indications—Opiate-like antimotility drugs diminish propulsive activity of the intestine and thus have a constipating effect. They have a limited role to fluid and electrolyte replacement in acute diarrhoea. They are also used as adjunctive therapy in some chronic diarrhoeal conditions.

Contraindications—Opiate-like antimotility drugs should not be given to people with diarrhoeal conditions such as acute ulcerative colitis or antibiotic-associated colitis. They are not recommended for children.

Adverse effects—Nausea, vomiting, abdominal cramps, constipation, drowsiness.

Therapeutic notes—Loperamide is the most appropriate opioid for local effects on the gut and is commonly used in those with travellers' diarrhoea (often caused by *Escherichia coli)*. It has a relatively selective action on the gastrointestinal tract, reducing the frequency of abdominal cramps, decreasing the passage of faeces and shortening the duration of the illness.

Use of stool modifiers/adsorbents

Examples of stool modifiers/adsorbents include kaolin, chalk, charcoal and methylcellulose.

Mechanism of action—It has been suggested that stool modifiers/adsorbents act by absorbing toxins or by coating and protecting the intestinal mucosa, although there is no evidence to support this.

Route of administration—Oral.

Indications—There is little evidence to recommend adsorbents at all.

Contraindications—Adsorbents are not recommended for acute diarrhoea.

Adverse effects—Stool modifiers/adsorbents may reduce the absorption of other drugs.

Therapeutic notes—Adsorbents are popular "remedies" for the treatment of diarrhoea, although there is little evidence of their benefits.

Inflammatory bowel disease

The main two inflammatory bowel diseases are Crohn disease and ulcerative colitis. Crohn disease can affect the entire gut and inflammation occurs throughout the full thickness of the bowel wall, whereas ulcerative colitis affects only the large bowel and inflammation is limited to bowel mucosa. These autoimmune conditions cause relapsing and remitting symptoms.

Treatment of these conditions is not only pharmacological but also depends on psychological support, correction of nutritional deficiencies and often surgical resection.

Drug treatment is aimed at controlling inflammation and bringing about remission, and the mainstay of drug treatment for these diseases are:

- glucocorticoids
- aminosalicylates
- immunosuppressants and cytotoxics
- biologics

Glucocorticoids

Examples of glucocorticoids include prednisolone, budesonide and hydrocortisone.

Mechanism of action—Glucocorticoids have an antiinflammatory effect (Chapter 7).

Route of administration—In localized disease, glucocorticoids may be administered rectally as enemas, suppositories or foams. In extensive or severe disease, oral or intravenous therapy may be required.

Indications—Glucocorticoids are given for acute relapses of inflammatory bowel disease.

Contraindications—Bowel obstruction or perforation, or treatment for prolonged periods.

CLINICAL NOTE

An 18-year-old girl presents to her General Practitioner (GP) with a 6-week history of bloody diarrhoea associated with lower abdominal cramps and some weight loss. On direct questioning, she reports pain in her knees and that her older brother has Crohn disease. She smokes 5 cigarettes a day but only drinks alcohol socially. On examination, she is pale and has a tender abdomen. She has several investigations including blood tests, stool culture and microscopy and faecal calprotectin. An endoscopy confirms Crohn disease. A gastroenterologist starts her on oral prednisolone to induce remission. Unfortunately, she has two more inflammatory exacerbations and so azathioprine is added in. She is also advised to stop smoking.

Adverse effects—Cushingoid side effects may occur with long-term glucocorticoid use (Chapter 7).

Therapeutic notes—Budesonide is locally acting and poorly absorbed, so has fewer systemic side effects.

Glucocorticosteroids are useful for acute attacks of inflammatory bowel disease. They are also used for inducing remission in relapses of ulcerative colitis.

Aminosalicylates

Sulfasalazine, mesalazine and olsalazine are examples of aminosalicylates.

Mechanism of action—Sulfasalazine is broken down in the gut to the active component 5-aminosalicylate (5-ASA) and sulfapyridine, which transports the drug to the colon. Mesalazine is 5-ASA and olsalazine is two molecules of 5-ASA. The mechanism of action of the active molecule 5-ASA is unknown, although is postulated to act by scavenging free radicals or interfering with cytokine networks.

Route of administration—Oral, rectal.

Indications—Maintenance and long-term therapy of inflammatory bowel conditions.

Mesalazine is now the treatment of choice for induction and maintenance of remission of mild to moderate ulcerative colitis and has been shown to reduce the risk of colorectal cancer in these patients.

Contraindications—Aminosalicylates should not be given to people with salicylate hypersensitivity and renal impairment.

Adverse effects—Sulfapyridine is responsible for much of this drug's side effects. Nausea, vomiting, headache and rashes. Blood disorders and oligospermia have been reported.

Immunosuppressants and cytotoxics

In severe inflammatory bowel disease, immunosuppressant medications such as methotrexate (Chapters 11 and 13), azathioprine (Chapter 11), mercaptopurine and cyclosporine are used as adjuncts to the aforementioned therapies. Azathioprine interferes with purine synthesis and depresses antibody-mediated immune reactions. Cyclosporine can be used in severe refractory colitis and reduces the risk of surgery, although it carries a 3% mortality risk given its toxicity.

Biologics: Monoclonal antibodies

Infliximab and adalimumab block the action of the cytokine tumour necrosis factor alpha (TNF-α), which mediates inflammation in Crohn and ulcerative colitis. It is used in the treatment of severe disease or when conventional therapy cannot be used.

Obesity

Obesity is becoming increasingly common in the West and is associated with many diseases such as cardiovascular disease, diabetes mellitus, gallstones and osteoarthritis.

Dietary restriction and an exercise programme should be explored before surgical or pharmacological intervention. The most widely used antiobesity drugs act directly upon the gastrointestinal tract. There are also centrally acting appetite suppressants.

Drugs acting on the gastrointestinal tract

Orlistat and methylcellulose are examples of such antiobesity drugs.

Mechanism of action—Orlistat is a pancreatic lipase inhibitor and reduces the breakdown and subsequent absorption of fat from the gut. Methylcellulose is believed to act as a bulk-forming agent and reduces food intake by promoting early satiety (fullness).

Route of administration—Oral.

Adverse effects—Orlistat often results in oily, frequent stools, flatulence, abdominal and rectal pain. Methylcellulose may produce flatulence and abdominal distension.

Other antiobesity drugs

The centrally acting appetite suppressant sibutramine is licensed for adjunctive management of obesity but for no more than 1 year's usage; weight loss may return after cessation. Numerous other drugs are being evaluated for their antiobesity properties, including the endogenous mammalian peptide leptin, which appears to induce satiety and counteract the properties of another transmitter, neuropeptide Y, which is believed to promote feeding.

Anal disorders

Haemorrhoids, anal fissures and pruritus are commonly encountered problems. Bland ointments are the best treatment option, with careful attention to cleanliness. When necessary, topical preparations containing a local anaesthetic (Chapter 10) or corticosteroid (Chapter 7) may provide symptomatic relief. Perianal thrush can be treated with nystatin (Chapter 12). Haemorrhoids can be treated by injection with a sclerosant, commonly oily phenol.

THE PANCREAS AND GALL BLADDER

Pancreatic supplements

Pancreatic exocrine secretions contain important enzymes that break down proteins (trypsin, chymotrypsin), starch (amylase) and fats (lipase). These are essential for efficient digestion.

Pancreatin is an extract of pancreas containing protease, lipase and amylase, that is given by mouth to compensate for reduced or absent exocrine secretions in cystic fibrosis, and following pancreatectomy, total gastrectomy or chronic pancreatitis. Pancreatin is inactivated by gastric acid and so precautions must be taken to optimize delivery of the pancreatin to the duodenum.

Pancreatin preparations are best taken with food. Histamine H_2 antagonists (e.g. cimetidine) may be taken an hour before ingestion of the pancreatin to reduce gastric acid secretion, although acid-resistant (enterically coated) formulations are now available.

HINTS AND TIPS

Even though pancreatin contains peptides, which would normally be degraded in the stomach, these tablets are coated in an acid-resistant layer, and the enzymes and proenzymes within them have endogenous resistance to both acid and proteases and become active in the small intestine.

Gall bladder

Bile is secreted by the liver and is stored in the gall bladder. Bile contains cholesterol, phospholipids and bile salts. Bile salts are important for keeping cholesterol in solution. The formation of "stones" in the bile (cholelithiasis) is relatively common and can result in blockage of the draining duct, with subsequent infection and inflammation (cholecystitis). Surgical removal of the gall bladder (cholecystectomy) has largely replaced the use of drugs in the management of symptomatic gallstones, although this is suitable for patients not treatable by other means.

The dissolution of small cholesterol stones is carried out by prolonged oral administration of the bile acid ursodeoxycholic acid.

Ursodeoxycholic acid

The bile salt ursodeoxycholic acid is administered orally and handled by the body in the same fashion as endogenous bile salt. It works by decreasing secretion of cholesterol into the bile, and decreasing cholesterol absorption from the intestine.

The net effect is a reduced cholesterol concentration in the bile and a tendency for the dissolution of existing stones. It is therefore most commonly used for the dissolution of gallstones but can also be used to slow the progression of primary biliary cirrhosis.

The main side effect of ursodeoxycholic acid is diarrhoea.

Cholestyramine

This orally administered anion-exchange resin binds bile acids in the gut and prevents their reabsorption and enterohepatic recirculation. It is used in the treatment of pruritus associated with partial biliary obstruction and primary biliary cirrhosis, and in hypercholesterolaemia.

● Chapter Summary

- Peptic ulcer disease (PUD) is commonly caused by *H. pylori*. Eradication involves a proton-pump inhibitor (PPI) and antibiotics
- PPIs cause irreversible inhibition of H+/K+-ATPase: used in the treatment of peptic ulcer disease and reflux disease
- H2-receptor antagonists inhibit gastric acid secretion: used in treatment of PUD and reflux disease
- H1-receptor antagonists are used in managing motion sickness, 5-HT3 antagonists are useful postoperatively
- Misoprostol is a prostaglandin E analogue used as ulcer prophylaxis with NSAID use
- Glucocorticosteroids and aminosalicylates are the main drugs used in managing inflammatory bowel disease
- Orlistat is a pancreatic lipase inhibitor used in the management of obesity

Endocrine and reproductive systems

THE THYROID GLAND

Basic concepts

Production of thyroid hormones

The thyroid gland synthesizes and secretes three hormones: triiodothyronine (T_3), thyroxine (T_4) and calcitonin. The effects of the thyroid hormones are summarized in Box 7.1. The follicular cells of the thyroid gland synthesize and glycosylate thyroglobulin before secreting it. The iodination of thyroglobulin is catalysed by thyroid peroxidase and produces T4 and T3. The iodine required for the synthesis of T_3 and T_4 comes mainly from the diet in the form of iodide. Through the action of a thyrotrophin-dependent pump, iodide is concentrated in the follicular cells, where it is converted into iodine by thyroid peroxidase.

Control of thyroid hormone secretion

The hypothalamus contains thyroid-hormone receptors that are able to detect and respond to decreased levels of T_3 and T_4 by causing the release of thyrotropin-releasing hormone (TRH). TRH reaches the anterior pituitary via the portal circulation and stimulates TRH receptors on thyrotrophic cells, which in turn secrete thyroid-stimulating hormone (TSH).

TSH reaches the thyroid gland through the systemic circulation where it stimulates thyroid hormone secretion (Fig. 7.1). Both T_3 and T_4 bind to proteins in the plasma (mostly thyroxine-binding globulin), and less than 1% of

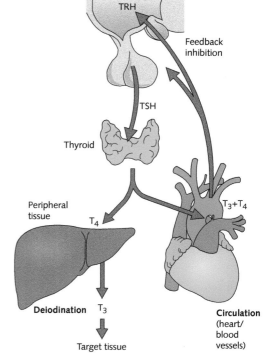

Fig. 7.1 Hypothalamic–pituitary–thyroid axis: control of thyroid hormone synthesis. T_3, Triiodothyronine; T_4, thyroxine; *TSH*, thyroid-stimulating hormone; *TRH*, thyrotropin-releasing hormone. (Modified from Page, C., Curtis, M. Walker, M, Hoffman, B. (eds) *Integrated Pharmacology*, 3rd edn. Mosby, 2006.)

total thyroid hormones are free. It is the free thyroid hormones, which exert the physiological effects. T_3 is about five times more biologically active than T_4, and T_4 is converted to T_3 in some peripheral tissues.

T_3 and T_4 both exert negative feedback on the hypothalamus and pituitary.

BOX 7.1 PHYSIOLOGICAL EFFECTS OF THYROID HORMONES

- Foetal development (physical and cognitive)
- Metabolic rate
- Body temperature
- Cardiac rate and contractility
- Peripheral vasodilatation
- Red cell mass and circulatory volume
- Respiratory drive
- Peripheral nerves (reflexes)
- Hepatic metabolic enzymes
- Bone turnover
- Skin and soft tissue effects

Modified from Page et al. 2006.

HINTS AND TIPS

Most modern laboratory thyroid function tests measure just TSH, although levels of free and total T_3 and T_4 can be measured, as well as thyroxine-binding globulin.

Thyroid dysfunction

Hypothyroidism

Hypothyroidism, thyroid insufficiency, is relatively common in adults and associated with tiredness and lethargy, weight gain, intolerance to cold, dry skin, bradycardia and mental impairment. Children with hypothyroidism manifest delayed bone growth, whereas a deficiency in utero also results in mental retardation.

Hashimoto thyroiditis is an autoimmune disease resulting in fibrosis of the thyroid gland. It is the most common cause of hypothyroidism and, similar to most autoimmune diseases is more prevalent in women. Myxoedema is also immunological in origin and represents the most severe form of hypothyroidism, sometimes causing coma.

Thyroid-hormone resistance and reduced TSH secretion will also produce the symptoms of hypothyroidism.

The causes of hypothyroidism are summarized in Table 7.1.

Management of hypothyroidism

The only effective treatment for hypothyroidism, unless it is caused by iodine deficiency (which is treated with iodide), is to administer the thyroid hormones themselves as replacement therapy.

Levothyroxine

Thyroxine is given as levothyroxine sodium for maintenance therapy. It has a half-life of 6 days and a peak onset of 9 days.

Mechanism of action—Levothyroxine is converted to T_3 in vivo to replace endogenous hormone.

Route of administration—Oral.

Indications—Hypothyroidism.

Contraindications—Levothyroxine should not be given to people with thyrotoxicosis and should be used with caution in those who have cardiovascular disease.

Adverse effects—Arrhythmias, tachycardia, anginal pain, cramps, headache, restlessness, sweating, weight loss.

Therapeutic regimen—The starting dose of levothyroxine sodium should be no greater than 100 µg daily (reduce in the elderly or those with cardiovascular disease) and increase by 25 to 50 µg every 4 weeks until a dose of 100 to 200 µg is reached.

Liothyronine sodium (L-triiodothyronine sodium)

Because liothyronine is bound only slightly by thyroid binding globulin, it has a more rapid onset of effect and a shorter duration of action than levothyroxine.

Mechanism of action—Liothyronine is rapidly metabolized in vivo to T_3. It has a half-life of 2 to 5 days and a peak onset of 1 to 2 days.

Route of administration—Oral, intravenous.

Indications—Liothyronine is given for severe hypothyroidism where a rapid effect is needed.

Contraindications—Liothyronine should not be given to people with cardiovascular disorders.

Adverse effects—Arrhythmias, tachycardia, anginal pain, cramps, headache, restlessness, sweating, weight loss.

Therapeutic regimen—The dosage of liothyronine sodium should be gradually increased as with levothyroxine sodium (20 µg liothyronine sodium is equivalent to 100 µg levothyroxine sodium). Intravenous liothyronine is the drug of choice in the emergency treatment of myxoedema (hypothyroid) coma.

Hyperthyroidism

Hyperthyroidism, thyroid excess, results either from the overproduction of endogenous hormone or exposure to excess exogenous hormone. Symptoms include increased basal metabolic rate (BMR) with consequent weight loss, increased appetite, increased body temperature, and sweating, as well as nervousness, tremor and tachycardia.

Graves disease (diffuse toxic goitre) is the most common cause of hyperthyroidism. It is an autoimmune disease caused by the activation of TSH receptors by autoantibodies. This results in an enlargement of the gland and therefore excess hormone production. Patients with Graves disease may develop classical ophthalmic changes (e.g. exophthalmos).

Toxic nodular goitre is the second most common cause of hyperthyroidism. It is caused by either a single adenoma (hyperfunctioning adenoma) or multiple adenomas (multinodular goitre).

The causes of hyperthyroidism are summarized in Box 7.2.

Table 7.1	Causes of hypothyroidism
Primary	Chronic lymphocytic thyroiditis (Hashimoto disease)
	Subacute thyroiditis
	Painless thyroiditis (postpartum thyroiditis)
	Radioactive iodine ingestion
	Postthyroidectomy
	Iodine deficiency or excess
	Inborn errors of thyroid hormone synthesis
Secondary	Pituitary disease
Target tissues	Thyroid hormone resistance

Modified from Page et al. 2006.)

Mrs Akasuki, 41 years old, presents to her General Practitioner (GP) with tremor and weight loss of 6.5 kg (1 stone) over 4 weeks, despite increased appetite. She admits to feeling hot and sweaty both day and night, which has affected her sleep. On examination, a diffuse goitre is seen. Her pulse is rapid and she has noticeable exophthalmos.

A pregnancy test is negative. A blood sample is taken and reveals an elevated serum T_3 and T_4 with suppressed TSH levels. Mrs Akasuki is diagnosed as having hyperthyroidism. She is given propranolol for her symptoms and is started on carbimazole to suppress her thyroid. She is advised to report symptoms of a sore throat and has a blood test to ensure that she has not become neutropenic, a possible dangerous side effect of carbimazole treatment. If her exophthalmos required further treatment, glucocorticosteroids are sometimes used.

BOX 7.2   CAUSES OF HYPERTHYROIDISM

- Excess exogenous thyroid hormone
- Diffuse toxic goitre (Graves disease)
- Hyperfunctioning adenoma (toxic nodule)
- Toxic multinodular goitre
- Painless thyroiditis
- Subacute thyroiditis
- Thyroid-stimulating hormone (TSH)-secreting adenoma
- Human chorionic gonadotropin (hCG)-secreting tumours

(Modified from Page et al. 2006.)

Management of hyperthyroidism

Hyperthyroidism is most commonly treated with drugs. Surgery is used only when there are mechanical problems resulting from compression of the trachea by the thyroid.

Thioureylenes

The thioureylenes are the first-line drugs for the treatment of hyperthyroidism. Carbimazole, thiamazole, and propylthiouracil (PTU) are examples of thioureylenes.

In the body, carbimazole is rapidly converted to active compound thiamazole.

Mechanism of action—The thioureylenes cause inhibition of thyroid peroxidase with a consequent reduction in thyroid hormone synthesis and storage (Fig. 7.2). The effects of PTU may take several weeks to manifest because the body has stores of T_3 and T_4. PTU also inhibits the peripheral deiodination of T_4 to T_3.

Route of administration—Oral.

Indications—Thioureylenes are used for the treatment of hyperthyroidism. Patients sensitive to carbimazole are given PTU.

Contraindications—Thioureylenes should not be given to people with a large goitre. PTU should be given at a reduced dose in patients with renal impairment.

Adverse effects—Nausea and headache; allergic reactions, including rashes; hypothyroidism and, rarely, hepatotoxicity and alopaecia. The most dangerous unwanted effects are neutropenia and agranulocytosis secondary to bone marrow suppression. This is relatively rare and is reversible on cessation of treatment.

Therapeutic regimen—Carbimazole is given at 20 to 60 mg daily until the patient is euthyroid (4–11 weeks later), then the dose is progressively reduced to a maintenance level of 5 to 15 mg daily. Treatment is usually given for 18 months. PTU is given at 300 to 600 mg daily until the patient is euthyroid, then the dose is progressively reduced to a maintenance level of 50 to 150 mg daily.

Anion inhibitors

Iodine, iodide and potassium perchlorate are examples of anion inhibitors.

Potassium perchlorate inhibits the uptake of iodine by the thyroid (see Fig. 7.2) but is no longer used owing to the risk of aplastic anaemia.

Iodide is the most rapidly acting treatment against thyrotoxicosis and is given in thyrotoxic crisis (thyroid storm). Iodide is also used for the preparation of hyperthyroid patients for surgical resection of the gland.

Mechanism of action—Iodine and iodide cause inhibition of conversion of T_4 to T_3 and inhibit hormone secretion. They also reduce the size and vascularity of the gland, which is evident after 10 to 14 days of treatment.

Route of administration—Oral.

Indications—Preoperative hyrotoxicosis and thyroid cancer.

Contraindications—Iodine and iodide should not be given to pregnant and breastfeeding women because they cause a goitre in infants.

Adverse effects—Iodine and iodide can cause hypersensitivity reactions including rashes, headache, lacrimation, conjunctivitis, laryngitis and bronchitis. With long-term treatment, depression, insomnia and impotence can occur.

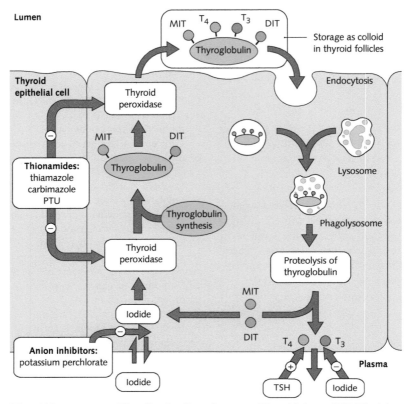

Fig. 7.2 Synthesis of thyroid hormones and the site of action of some antithyroid drugs. *DIT*, Diiodotyrosine; *MIT*, monoiodotyrosine; *PTU*, propylthiouracil; T_3, triiodothyronine; T_4, thyroxine; *TSH*, thyroid-stimulating hormone. (Modified from Page, C., Curtis, M. Walker, M, Hoffman, B. (eds) *Integrated Pharmacology*, 3rd edn. Mosby, 2006.)

Therapeutic regimen—Iodine and iodide are given 10 to 14 days before partial thyroidectomy, with either carbimazole or PTU. They should not be given long-term because iodine becomes less effective.

β-Adrenoceptor antagonists

Propranolol and atenolol are examples of β-adrenoceptor antagonists. They are used to attenuate the symptoms of increased thyroid hormone levels, and the effect of increased numbers of adrenoceptors caused by thyroid hormone. They are useful for decreasing the symptoms and signs associated with hyperthyroidism.

Mechanism of action—β-Adrenoceptor antagonists reduce tachycardia, the basal metabolic rate, nervousness and tremor.

Route of administration—Oral.

Indications—Thyrotoxic crisis; preoperatively for thyroid surgery.

Contraindications—β-Adrenoceptor antagonists should not be given to people with asthma.

Adverse effects—The side effects of β-adrenoceptor antagonists are given in Chapter 4.

Radioiodine

The use of radioactive iodine to treat hyperthyroidism is not classically considered pharmacology, although it is used in the management of thyroid disorders. The uptake of iodine isotopes is also used diagnostically as a test of thyroid function. Radioiodine emits radiation that is absorbed by the thyroid tissue enabling it to exert a powerful cytotoxic action on the thyroid follicles resulting in significant tissue destruction. Hypothyroidism will eventually occur with radioiodine but is easily managed with hormone replacement therapy.

HINTS AND TIPS

Amiodarone is rich in iodine and can cause either hyperthyroidism or hypothyroidism. Thyroid function tests should be checked before prescribing amiodarone and every 6 months during treatment. Amiodarone should be withdrawn if thyrotoxicosis or hypothyroidism are refractory to treatment.

THE ENDOCRINE PANCREAS AND DIABETES MELLITUS

Control of plasma glucose

Blood glucose levels are maintained at a concentration of about 5 mmol/L, and usually, do not exceed 8 mmol/L. A plasma glucose concentration of 2.2 mmol/L or less may result in hypoglycaemic coma and death caused by a lack of energy reaching the brain. A plasma glucose concentration of more than 10 mmol/L exceeds the renal threshold for glucose and means that glucose will be present in the urine. Osmotic diuresis then occurs.

The islets of Langerhans, located in the pancreas, contain glucose receptors and secrete the hormones glucagon and insulin. These hormones are short-term regulators of plasma glucose levels with opposite effects. In addition, their release can be influenced by gastrointestinal hormones and autonomic nerves.

Glucose receptors are also found in the ventromedial nucleus and lateral areas of the hypothalamus. These are able to regulate appetite and feeding, and also indirectly stimulate the release of a variety of hormones, including adrenaline, growth hormone and cortisol, all of which affect glucose metabolism.

The hormones involved in blood glucose regulation target the liver, skeletal muscle and adipose tissue.

Insulin

Insulin is a 51–amino acid peptide made up of an α-chain and a β-chain linked by disulphide bonds. It has a half-life of 3 to 5 minutes and is metabolized to a large extent by the liver (40%–50%), but also by the kidneys and muscles.

In response to high blood glucose levels (as occurs after a meal), as well as to glucosamine, amino acids, fatty acids, ketone bodies and sulphonylureas, the β-cells of the endocrine pancreas secrete insulin along with a C-peptide.

Insulin release is mediated by adenosine triphosphate (ATP)-dependent potassium channels located in the membrane of the β-cells. These close in response to elevated cytoplasmic ATP and decreased cytoplasmic adenosine diphosphate (ADP) levels, resulting in depolarisation of the membrane. This triggers calcium entry into the cell through voltage-dependent calcium channels, and subsequent insulin release (Fig. 7.3).

Insulin release is inhibited by low blood glucose levels, growth hormone, glucagon, cortisol and sympathetic nervous system activation.

The effects of insulin are summarized in Table 7.2.

CLINICAL NOTE

Mrs. Rait, a 52-year-old female, presents to her GP with polyuria, polydipsia and frequent infections over the past month. She is a current smoker and has high blood pressure. She has a family history of stroke. She is found to have glucose in her urine and her random venous glucose is 12 mmol/L. Her haemoglobin A1c (HbA1c) is 7%. Her renal function is normal, and she is commenced on metformin to control her glucose levels. She is advised to stop smoking, exercise more and to cut out sugary and carbohydrate high foods. She is also started on ramipril for her blood pressure. Her HbA1c is checked in 3 months and a short-acting sulfonylurea may be added if her blood sugars are still high.

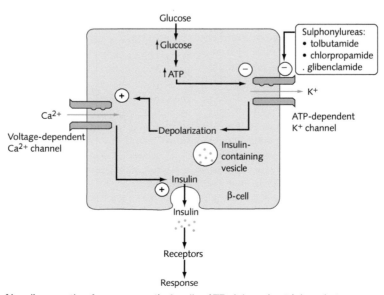

Fig. 7.3 Mechanism of insulin secretion from pancreatic β-cells. *ATP*, Adenosine triphosphate.

Table 7.2 Metabolic effects of insulin on fuel homeostasis

Carbohydrates	Increase glucose transport
	Increase glycogen synthesis
	Increase glycolysis
	Inhibit gluconeogenesis
Fats	Increase lipoprotein lipase activity
	Increase fat storage in adipocytes
	Inhibit lipolysis (hormone-sensitive lipase)
	Increase hepatic lipoprotein synthesis
	Inhibit fatty acid oxidation
Proteins	Increase protein synthesis
	Increase amino acid transport

Modified from Page, C., Curtis, M. Walker, M, Hoffman, B. (eds) Integrated Pharmacology, 3rd edn. Mosby, 2006.

Diabetes mellitus

Diabetes mellitus is characterized by an inability to regulate plasma glucose within the normal range. There is an absolute or relative insulin deficiency leading to hyperglycaemia, glycosuria (glucose in the urine), polyuria (production of large volumes of dilute urine) associated with cellular potassium depletion and polydipsia (intense thirst), in addition to weight loss.

There are two main types of diabetes mellitus.

- Type 1 diabetes (absolute insulin deficiency)
- Type 2 diabetes (insulin resistance)

In addition, pregnant women who have never had diabetes before, but who have high blood glucose levels during pregnancy are said to have gestational diabetes, affecting 4% of pregnancies. There is also maturity-onset diabetes of the young and diabetes caused by pancreatic disease or it can be medication-induced.

Patients with type 1 or type 2 diabetes have an increased risk of cardiovascular and cerebrovascular events, peripheral and autonomic neuropathy, nephropathy, and retinopathy in the long term.

Type 1 diabetes

In type 1 diabetes, pancreatic β-cells are destroyed by an autoimmune T-cell attack. This leads to a complete inability to secrete insulin. In addition to polyuria, polydipsia and weight loss, insulin deficiency causes muscle wasting through increased breakdown and reduced synthesis of proteins. In the absence of insulin, there is accelerated breakdown of fat to acetyl-CoA, which is converted to acetoacetate and β-hydroxybutyrate (which causes acidosis) and acetone (a ketone) resulting in patients with type 1 diabetes being at risk of the diabetic ketoacidosis, an acute emergency. Some untreated patients have a plasma glucose concentration of up to 100 mmol/L and the production of ketone bodies from fatty acids leads to ketonuria and

metabolic acidosis. Body fluids become hypertonic, resulting in cellular dehydration, and patients are at risk of a hyperosmolar coma.

Patients diagnosed with type 1 diabetes typically present at a young age and are not normally obese. There is often a genetic predisposition.

Type 2 diabetes

In type 2 diabetes, patients have peripheral insulin resistance and impaired insulin secretion. On average, 50% of the β-cells remain active. Patients with type 2 diabetes are often obese and physically inactive, presenting in adult life. The incidence rising progressively with age as β-cell function declines. Ketosis is less of a feature in type 2 diabetes because ketone production is suppressed by the small amounts of insulin produced by the pancreas. A hyperosmolar hyperglycaemic state is the type 2 diabetes equivalent to ketoacidosis and occurs when patients with type 2 diabetes have a concomitant illness leading to reduce fluid intake. It is characterized by hyperglycaemia, hyperosmolarity and dehydration without significant ketoacidosis. It has a high mortality rate, but if diagnosed early, responds rapidly to fluids and insulin.

Secondary diabetes mellitus

Not to be confused with type 2 diabetes, secondary diabetes mellitus accounts for less than 2% of all new cases of diabetes and is most commonly caused by pancreatic disease (pancreatitis, carcinoma, cystic fibrosis), endocrine disease (Cushing syndrome, acromegaly) or is drug-induced (following treatment with thiazide diuretics or corticosteroid therapy).

Management of diabetes mellitus

Insulin

The aim of exogenous insulin preparations is to mimic basal levels of endogenous insulin and meal-induced increases in insulin. Insulin is essential for the treatment of type 1 diabetes and often used in patients with type 2 diabetes alongside other oral antidiabetic medications.

Nowadays the most-used insulin preparation is the human (recombinant) insulin (however, insulin preparations of bovine origin are also available). Insulin is available as short-acting, intermediate-acting, and long-acting preparations (Table 7.3).

Short-acting insulins are soluble. These preparations most resemble endogenous insulin and can be given intravenously in the hospital. The rapid-acting insulins, aspart and lispro, have a faster onset and shorter duration of action than the traditional short-acting insulin. Intermediate-acting and long-acting insulins are not as soluble as the short-acting preparations. Their solubility is decreased by precipitating the insulin with zinc or protamine (a basic protein), which prolongs their release into the blood stream following subcutaneous injection of a depot preparation.

Table 7.3 Insulin preparations

Insulin preparation	Action	Peak activity (hours)	Duration (hours)
Rapid-acting insulin	Very rapid	0–2	3–4
Short-acting insulin	Rapid	1–3	3–7
Isophane insulin	Intermediate	2–12	12–22
Insulin zinc suspension	Prolonged	4–24	24–28

Mechanism of action—Insulin preparations mimic endogenous insulin.

Route of administration—Insulin must always be given parenterally (intravenously, intramuscularly or subcutaneously), because it is a peptide and thus metabolized in the gastrointestinal tract. Short-acting insulin is given intravenously in emergencies, but the administration of the insulin preparations in maintenance treatment is usually subcutaneous.

Indications—Type 1 diabetes

- Type 2 diabetes. In the long-term about one-third of patients ultimately benefit from insulin. Patients usually require insulin if maximal therapy, with a combination of oral antidiabetic medications, is not sufficiently controlling blood sugar levels.
- Gestational diabetes, if glucose is not controlled by diet alone.
- Emergency treatment of hyperkalaemia (given with glucose to lower extracellular K^+ via redistribution in cells).

Adverse effects—Local reactions, and in overdose, hypoglycaemia. Rarely, there may be immune resistance. Rebound hyperglycaemia can follow insulin-induced hypoglycaemia, because of the release of counter-regulatory hormones.

Therapeutic regimen—Different regimens are used according to the patient's needs and age.

- Short-acting insulin (e.g. lispro) three times daily (before breakfast, lunch and dinner) and intermediate-acting insulin (e.g. isophane insulin) at bedtime.
- Short-acting insulin and intermediate-acting insulin mixture twice daily before meals.
- Short-acting insulin and intermediate-acting insulin mixture before breakfast, short-acting insulin before dinner, and intermediate-acting insulin before bedtime.
- Short-acting insulin and intermediate-acting insulin mixture before breakfast are adequate for some Type 2 diabetes patients needing insulin.
- Improved glucose control can be achieved with multiple daily injections of rapid-acting insulin analogues given with meals, and a basal insulin analogue (e.g. glargine) injected once daily.

Therapeutic notes—Preparations are now available which contain mixtures of short-acting, intermediate-acting and long-acting insulins, allowing patients to inject themselves only once each time they require insulin.

Oral hypoglycaemics

Oral hypoglycaemics act to lower plasma glucose. The biguanides and the sulphonylureas are the main oral hypoglycaemics, but newer drugs are also now available and widely prescribed as summarized in Table 7.4.

Biguanides—Metformin is the only biguanide used clinically

Mechanism of action—Metformin increases the peripheral utilisation of glucose, by increasing uptake, and decreasing gluconeogenesis. It decreases hepatic glucose production by inhibiting the mitochondrial respiratory chain complex. Metformin also reduces carbohydrate absorption from the intestine and increases fatty acid oxidation. To work, metformin requires the presence of endogenous insulin; thus patients must have some functioning β-cells.

Route of administration—Oral.

Table 7.4 Summary of commonly prescribed antidiabetic medications

Family of drug	GLP-1 agonist	Biguanide	Sulfonylurea	Thiazolidinediones	DPP-4 inhibitors
Example	Exenatide	Metformin	Glibenclamide	Pioglitazone	Sitagliptin
Administration	Subcutaneous injection	Oral	Oral	Oral	Oral
Mechanism of action		Increase glucose uptake Reduced gluconeogenesis	Stimulate insulin secretion and reduce plasma glucose	Increase insulin sensitivity	Stimulate insulin secretion Potentiate endogenous incretins
Effect on weight	Weight loss	Weight loss	Weight gain	Weight gain	Weight neutral
Important adverse effects	Lactic acidosis		Hypoglycaemia	Risk of oedema, fractures and bladder cancer	Pancreatitis

GLP-1 Glucagon-like peptide-1, DPP-4, dipeptidylpeptidase-4.

Indications—Type 2 diabetes, where dieting has proved ineffective and is used off-licence in the treatment of gestational diabetes.

Metformin is associated with improved outcome in patients with diabetes and compensated heart failure.

Management of polycystic ovary syndrome, associated with insulin resistance.

Contraindications—Metformin should not be given to patients with severe hepatic or renal impairment (owing to the risk of lactic acidosis), or those in shock.

Adverse effects—Dose-related gastrointestinal disturbances (anorexia, nausea, vomiting, diarrhoea), lactic acidosis and decreased vitamin B_{12} absorption.

Therapeutic notes—metformin is given in divided doses up to a max dose of 2g. It can be used alone or in combination with other antidiabetic medications. Metformin should be taken with or after food. Metformin causes anorexia and encourages weight loss; therefore, it is a good option in patients who are overweight with type 2 diabetes.

Sulphonylureas—Gliclazide, tolbutamide, chlorpropamide and glibenclamide are examples of sulphonylureas.

Mechanism of action—Sulphonylureas block ATP-dependent potassium channels in the membrane of the pancreatic β-cells, causing depolarisation, calcium influx and insulin release. The overall effect of sulphonylureas is to stimulate insulin secretion and thus reduce plasma glucose.

Route of administration—Oral.

Indications—Sulphonylureas are used in patients with type 2 diabetes mellitus, in patients with residual β-cell activity.

Contraindications—Breastfeeding or pregnant women, or people with ketoacidosis. Long-acting sulphonylureas (chlorpropamide, glibenclamide) should be avoided in elderly people and in those with renal and hepatic insufficiency because these drugs can induce hypoglycaemia.

Adverse effects—Hypoglycaemia, which can be severe and prolonged. Weight gain; sensitivity reactions, including rashes; gastrointestinal disturbances; headache; flushing after alcohol, and although rare, bone marrow toxicity can be severe.

Therapeutic regimen—Tolbutamide is given at 500 mg, 2 or 3 times daily and lasts for 6 hours; chlorpropamide is given at 100 to 250 mg daily and lasts for 12 hours; glibenclamide is given at 2.5 to 15 mg daily and lasts for 12 hours.

DRUG INTERACTIONS

Nonsteroidal antiinflammatory drugs (NSAIDs), trimethoprim and alcohol can produce severe hypoglycaemia when coprescribed with a sulfonylurea. High doses of thiazide diuretics and glucocorticosteroids decrease the action of sulfonylureas. Therefore blood sugar levels should be monitored carefully in these instances.

α-*Glucosidase inhibitors*—Acarbose is the only available drug in this class.

Mechanism of action—Acarbose inhibits intestinal α-glucosidases, and delays the absorption of starch and sucrose, reducing postprandial increases in blood glucose.

Route of administration—Oral.

Indications—Diabetes mellitus inadequately controlled by diet alone or in combination with other oral hypoglycaemics.

Contraindications—Pregnancy, breastfeeding, bowel disease.

Adverse effects—Flatulence, diarrhoea.

Therapeutic notes—Similar to metformin, acarbose is particularly useful in the obese diabetic patient.

Thiazolidinediones—Rosiglitazone and pioglitazone belong to the thiazolidinediones. Pioglitazone is the only drug that remains in clinical use.

Mechanism of action—These agents bind to a receptor found mainly on adipose tissue (as well as in muscle and the liver) and increase lipogenesis and uptake of fatty acids and glucose. They are believed to reduce peripheral insulin resistance, leading to a reduction in plasma glucose because they act to enhance the effectiveness of endogenous insulin. Although pioglitazone takes 2 to 3 months to have maximum effect, it can reduce the need for exogenous insulin by 30%.

Route of administration—Oral.

Indications—Type 2 diabetes inadequately controlled by diet alone or in combination with either a sulphonylurea or metformin.

Contraindications—Hepatic impairment, history of heart failure, pregnancy and breastfeeding.

Adverse effects—Gastrointestinal disturbance, weight gain and fluid retention. Potentially liver failure. Increased risk of fractures, cardiovascular disease and bladder cancer with long-term use.

Therapeutic notes—Before prescribing pioglitazone, a physician experienced in treating type 2 diabetes should check liver function tests.

Gliptins—Sitagliptin, vildagliptin, saxagliptin and linagliptin are drugs that competitively inhibit dipeptidylpeptidase-4 (DPP-4).

Mechanism of action—Lower blood glucose by potentiating endogenous incretins glucagon-like-peptide-1 receptor agonist (GLP-1) and glucose depedent insulinotropic peptide (GIP) which stimulate insulin secretion.

Route of Administration—Oral.

Indications—Type 2 diabetes.

Contraindications—Ketoacidosis, acute pancreatitis.

Adverse effects—Usually well tolerated but can cause gastrointestinal upset and worsening of heart failure. Risk of pancreatitis. Weight neutral.

GLP-1 agonist—Exenatide and liraglutide are GLP-1 agonists.

Mechanism of action—Lower blood glucose by increasing insulin secretion, suppressing glucagon secretion and slowing gastric emptying.

Route of administration—Subcutaneous injection.

Indication—Obese patients with type 2 diabetes who have unsuccessfully reduced their blood glucose despite dual therapy.

Contraindication—Ketoacidosis, severe gastrointestinal disease.

Adverse effects—Gastrointestinal disturbances, pancreatitis.

Therapeutic notes—GLP-1 agonists cause modest weight loss. They are administered twice daily before meals. A modified release version can be given as a once-weekly injection and is used in combination with metformin and sulfonylurea in poorly controlled obese patients with type 2 diabetes.

Sodium glucose cotransporter 2 inhibitors—Dapagliflozin and canagliflozin are examples of a sodium glucose cotransporter (SGLT2) 2 inhibitor.

Mechanism of action—These drugs inhibit the SGLT thus allowing increased amounts of glucose to be excreted by the kidney as glucose reabsorption is inhibited.

Route of administration—Oral.

Indication—Used as dual therapy, with metformin, in adults with type 2 diabetes who cannot tolerate sulphonylureas.

Contraindications—Ketoacidosis, breastfeeding and pregnancy, severe renal impairment.

Adverse effects—Hypoglycaemia, urinary tract infections, thrush, polyuria and hypotension.

Therapeutic note—Before prescribing a SGLT2 inhibitor, renal function must be checked and should be monitored annually.

Diet and fluid replacement

Dietary control

Dietary control is important for both type 1 and type 2 diabetes.

The diet should aim to derive its energy from the following constituents, in the following amounts.

- 50% carbohydrate (slowly absorbed forms)
- 35% fat
- 15% protein.

This regimen aims to reduce total fat intake, increase protein intake, and increase the intake of high fibre foods, which slow the rate of absorption from the gut.

Simple sugars, as found in sweet drinks and cakes, should be avoided. Meals should be small and regular, thus avoiding large swings in blood glucose levels.

Rehydration therapy

Patients commonly present acutely with very high blood glucose levels and require significant fluid replacement because their fluid deficit can be as high as 7 to 8 L given the diuretic effect of hyperglycaemia. Rehydration therapy is essential to regain fluid and electrolyte balance and takes precedence over the administration of insulin.

Hyperkalaemia is a common and serious consequence of a lack of insulin associated with patients presenting with acutely high glucose levels. This is because potassium requires insulin to enter cells. As soon as insulin is administered, however, potassium follows glucose into cells, and hypokalaemia becomes the danger. Consequently, it is important to monitor plasma K^+ when treating patients in a hyperosmolar hyperglycaemic state and replace it accordingly.

Diabetic patients are also at risk of metabolic acidosis caused by excessive ketone production.

CLINICAL NOTE

A 19-year-old, with type 1 diabetes, presents to A&E feeling generally unwell with vomiting. He has recently started his second year of university and has been erratic with taking his insulin. On examination, he looks dehydrated and his breath smells sweet. His blood glucose is 20 mmol/L and he has blood ketones of 3.2 mmol/L in his urine. A venous blood gas gives a pH of 7.25, indicating acidosis. He is diagnosed with diabetic ketoacidosis and given multiple bags of intravenous fluid with sodium chloride 0.9%. In addition, he is given intravenous insulin and his glucose levels are monitored carefully. His potassium levels are also checked and once they fall into the normal range, the potassium is replaced with the fluid. Once he can eat and drink and he is no longer acidotic, he is seen by the diabetic specialist nurse who educates him on the importance of taking his insulin appropriately, and he is discharged home on his normal insulin.

Hypoglycaemia

Hypoglycaemia is relatively common in patients with diabetes who take insulin, and sulphonylureas.

The symptoms of hypoglycaemia are driven by the sympathetic nervous system and include sweating, tremor, anxiety and altered consciousness.

The history may reveal the patient has not eaten as scheduled, exercised or taken too much insulin. Check that the co-prescription of a new drug has not precipitated hypoglycaemia.

Management depends on the consciousness of the patient. If the patient is alert, glucose can be given orally as a syrup, or as simple sugar. If consciousness is altered, oral administration of glucose is dangerous, and there is a risk of the patient aspirating. In this situation, glucose should be administered intravenously, or glucagon can be given by intramuscular or intravenous injection.

Glucose (dextrose monohydrate)

Glucose is administered parenterally as dextrose monohydrate.

Mechanism of action—Dextrose mimics endogenous glucose and is used by cells.

Route of administration—Intravenous.

Indications—Hypoglycaemia, or as part of rehydration therapy.

Contraindications—Hyperglycaemia.

Adverse effects—Venous irritation, thrombophlebitis. Hypokalaemia may occur.

Therapeutic notes—Glucose is also available in numerous oral preparations, although the patient must be alert and conscious before these are administered because aspiration can occur.

Glucagon

Glucagon is a polypeptide hormone, normally secreted by the pancreatic α-cells.

Mechanism of action—Glucagon acts on the liver to convert glycogen to glucose and to synthesize glucose from noncarbohydrate precursors (gluconeogenesis). The overall effect is to raise plasma glucose levels.

Route of administration—Parenteral.

Indications—Insulin-induced hypoglycaemia.

Contraindications—Phaeochromocytoma.

Adverse effects—Nausea, vomiting, diarrhoea, hypokalaemia.

Therapeutic notes—Unlike intravenous glucose, glucagon can be administered easily by nonmedical personnel and can be carried by the patient as a prefilled syringe pen.

ADRENAL CORTICOSTEROIDS

Basic concepts

The adrenal cortex secretes several steroid hormones into the bloodstream. These are categorized by their actions into two main classes: mineralocorticoids and glucocorticoids.

Aldosterone is the main mineralocorticoid and is synthesized in the zona glomerulosa. It affects water and electrolyte balance and possesses salt-retaining activity.

Hydrocortisone (cortisol) and cortisone are the main glucocorticoids and are synthesized in the zona fasciculata and zona reticularis. These affect carbohydrate, fat and protein metabolism, and suppress inflammatory and immune responses. Cortisol and cortisone also possess some mineralocorticoid activity.

Small quantities of some sex steroids, mainly androgens, are also produced by the adrenal cortex.

Synthesis and release

Adrenal corticosteroids are not preformed but are synthesized when required from cholesterol (Fig. 7.4).

Glucocorticoids

The release of cortisol is controlled by negative feedback to the hypothalamic–pituitary–adrenal axis (see Fig. 7.4). There is a diurnal pattern of activity with an early morning peak in cortisol release.

A variety of sensorineural inputs regulate the release of corticotrophin-releasing factor (CRF) in the hypothalamus; examples include physiological and psychological "stress", injury and infection. CRF, a 41-amino-acid polypeptide, reaches the anterior pituitary in the hypothalamo-hypophysial portal system where it stimulates the release of adrenocorticotrophic hormone (ACTH). ACTH is formed from a larger molecule, proopiomelanocortin, and is released into the circulation where it stimulates the synthesis and release of cortisol from the adrenal cortex.

Natural and artificial glucocorticoids circulating in the blood exert a negative feedback effect on the production of both CRF and ACTH.

Mineralocorticoids

Aldosterone release is also partially controlled by ACTH, but other factors, especially the renin–angiotensin system (RAS), and plasma potassium levels, are more important (see Chapter 5).

Mechanism of action of corticosteroids

Endogenous and synthetic corticosteroids act in a similar way. The hormone or drug circulates to peripheral tissues where it enters cells (steroids are lipid soluble) and binds to cytosolic corticosteroid receptors. After hormone binding, these receptors are translocated to the nucleus where they interact with deoxyribonucleic acid and lead to the transcription of corticosteroid-responsive genes (CRG).

The products of these CRGs have diverse effects on the target tissues (Table 7.5). The actions of corticosteroids are divided into effects on inorganic metabolism (mineralocorticoid effects) and effects on organic metabolism (glucocorticoid effects).

Therapeutic use of corticosteroids

Corticosteroids have wide-ranging and powerful effects on human physiology. There are two main areas where these properties are taken advantage of in the therapeutic use of corticosteroids: physiological replacement therapy of corticosteroid deficiency, and antiinflammatory therapy and immunosuppression (Chapters 11 and 13).

Exogenous corticosteroids

Both naturally occurring, and a number of synthetic corticosteroids are available for clinical use. These vary in their potency, half-life and the balance between glucocorticoid versus mineralocorticoid activity (Table 7.6).

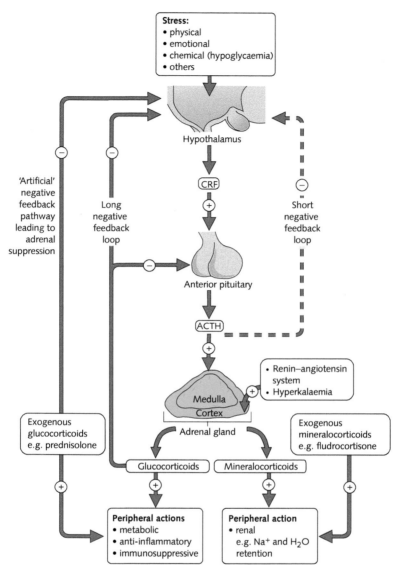

Fig. 7.4 Hypothalamic–pituitary–adrenal axis: control of adrenal corticosteroid synthesis and secretion. *ACTH*, Adrenocorticotrophic hormone; *CRF*, corticotrophin-releasing factor.

Mechanism of action—Exogenous corticosteroids imitate endogenous corticosteroids.

Indications—The therapeutic use of corticosteroids falls into the two main categories of physiological replacement therapy, and antiinflammatory therapy and immunosuppression.

Corticosteroid replacement therapy is necessary when endogenous hormones are deficient, as happens in the following.

- Primary adrenocortic destruction (Addison disease)
- Secondary adrenocortic failure caused by deficient ACTH from the pituitary or postadrenalectomy
- Suppression of the hypothalamic–pituitary–adrenal axis caused by prolonged glucocorticoid therapy.

Because all the actions of natural corticosteroids are required, a glucocorticoid with mineralocorticoid activity (cortisol) or separate glucocorticoid and mineralocorticoid are given.

The antiinflammatory and immunosuppressive effects of glucocorticoids are used to treat a wide variety of conditions (Table 7.7). In these cases, synthetic glucocorticoids with little mineralocorticoid activity are used (Chapter 11).

Contraindications—Exogenous corticosteroids should not be given to people with systemic infection unless specific antimicrobial therapy is being given.

Route of administration—Replacement therapy is given orally twice a day at physiological doses to try to mimic as

Table 7.5 Major effects of corticosteroids

Glucocorticoids	
Immunological	• Decreased production of T and B lymphocytes and macrophages, involution of lymphoid tissue • Decreased function of T and B lymphocytes, and reduced responsiveness to cytokines • Inhibition of complement system
Antiinflammatory	• Profound generalized inhibitory effects on inflammatory response • Reduced production of acute inflammatory mediators, especially the eicosanoids (prostaglandins, leukotrienes, etc.), owing to production of lipocortin, an enzyme that inhibits phospholipase A_2, thus blocking the formation of arachidonic acid and its metabolites (see Chapter 11) • Reduced numbers and activity of circulating immunocompetent cells, neutrophils, and macrophages • Decreased activity of macrophages and fibroblasts involved in the chronic stages of inflammation, leading to decreased inflammation and decreased healing
Carbohydrate metabolism	• Increased gluconeogenesis, decreased cellular uptake and use of glucose, increased storage of glycogen in the liver (hyperglycaemic actions)
Fat metabolism	• Redistribution of lipid from steroid-sensitive stores (limbs) to steroid-resistant stores (face, neck, trunk)
Protein metabolism	• Increased catabolism, decreased anabolism, leading to protein degradation
Cardiovascular	• Increased sensitivity of vascular system to catecholamines, reduced capillary permeability leading to raised blood pressure
Central nervous system	• High levels can cause mood changes (euphoria/depression) or psychotic states, perhaps caused by electrolyte changes
Anterior hypothalamus and pituitary	• Negative feedback effect of CRF and ACTH with the result that endogenous secretion of glucocorticoids is reduced, and may remain so after prolonged glucocorticoid therapy ('adrenal suppression')
Mineralocorticoids	
Kidney	• Increased permeability of the apical membrane of cells in the distal renal tubule to sodium • Stimulation of the Na^+/K^+ ATPase pump leading to reabsorption of Na^+ and loss of K^+ in the urine • Water is passively reabsorbed owing to sodium retention; thus extracellular fluid and blood volume are increased (raising blood pressure)

ACTH, Adrenocorticotrophic hormone; ATPase, adenosine triphosphatase; CRF, corticotrophin-releasing factor.

Table 7.6 Examples of therapeutically used corticosteroids

Glucocorticoids		Mineralocorticoids
'Natural hormones'	Synthetic	Synthetic
Hydrocortisone (cortisol)	Prednisolone Betamethasone Dexamethasone Beclomethasone Triamcinolone	Fludrocortisone Deoxycortone

closely as possible the level and rhythm of natural corticosteroid secretion.

When used to suppress inflammatory and immune responses, corticosteroids may be given orally or intravenously, but, depending on the condition, the topical administration of glucocorticoids is preferred, if feasible, because it can deliver high concentrations to the target site while minimising systemic absorption and adverse effects (see Table 7.7).

At high doses, even topically administered glucocorticoids can achieve systemic penetration.

Adverse effects—Overdosage or prolonged use of corticosteroids may exaggerate some of their normal physiological actions, leading to mineralocorticoid and glucocorticoid side effects. Many of these effects are similar to those seen in Cushing syndrome, a condition caused by excess secretion of endogenous corticosteroids (Fig. 7.5).

The metabolic side effects of glucocorticoids include the following.

• Central obesity and a "moon" face, as fat is redistributed
• Hyperglycaemia, which may lead to clinical diabetes mellitus, caused by disturbed carbohydrate metabolism
• Osteoporosis, caused by catabolism of protein matrix in bone

Table 7.7 Examples of conditions in which corticosteroids are used for their antiinflammatory and immunosuppressive effects

Systemic uses	Topical uses	
Acute inflammatory conditions, e.g. anaphylaxis, status asthmaticus, fibrosing alveolitis, angioneurotic oedema	Asthma	Aerosol
Chronic inflammatory conditions, e.g. rheumatoid arthritis, inflammatory bowel disease, systemic lupus erythematosus, glomerulonephritis	Allergic rhinitis	Nasal spray
Neoplastic disease myelomas, lymphomas, lymphatic leukaemias	Eczema	Ointment or cream
Miscellaneous organ transplantation	Inflammatory bowel disease	Foam enema

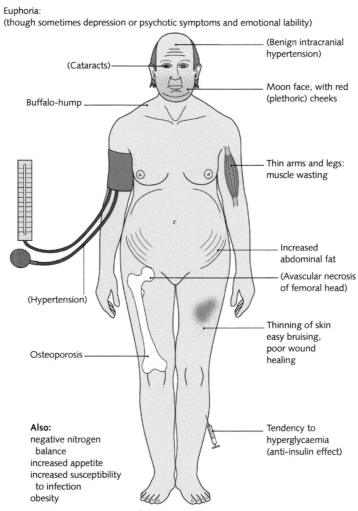

Fig. 7.5 Effects of prolonged corticosteroid use; the Cushingoid appearance.

- Loss of skin structure, with purple striae, and easy bruising, caused by altered protein metabolism
- Muscle weakness and wasting, caused by protein catabolism
- Suppression of growth in children

Corticosteroid therapy suppresses endogenous secretion of adrenal hormones via negative feedback on the hypothalamic–pituitary–adrenal axis.

Adrenal atrophy can persist for years after withdrawal from prolonged corticosteroid therapy. Replacement corticosteroid therapy is needed to compensate for the lack of sufficient adrenocortic response in times of stress (e.g. illness, surgery). Steroid therapy must be withdrawn slowly after long-term treatment because sudden withdrawal can lead to an acute adrenal insufficiency crisis.

With glucocorticoid therapy, the modification of inflammatory and immune reactions leads to an increased susceptibility to infections. This can progress unnoticed because of the suppression of normal indicators of infection, such as inflammation. Increased susceptibility occurs to usually pathogenic and opportunistic bacterial, viral and fungal organisms. Reactivation of latent infections (e.g. tuberculosis, herpes viruses) can occur.

The effects are most serious when corticosteroids are being used systemically, although topical use can exacerbate superficial skin infections, and inhaled corticosteroids can encourage oropharyngeal thrush and so on. Inhaled corticosteroids have also been recently associated with an increased risk of pneumonia, particularly in elderly patients with chronic obstructive pulmonary disease.

The other effects of glucocorticoids include mood changes (euphoria and, rarely, psychosis), peptic ulceration caused by inhibition of gastrointestinal prostaglandin synthesis, and eye problems such as cataracts and exacerbation of glaucoma.

Fluid retention, hypokalaemia and hypertension can all be side effects of any corticosteroids that possess significant mineralocorticoid activity.

HINTS AND TIPS

Corticosteroids cause several side effects, which are important to remember. These include hypertension, sodium and water retention, diabetes, osteoporosis, proximal myopathy and Cushing syndrome. In addition, they can cause skin thinning, bruising, mood disturbances and an increased risk of infections.

Therapeutic notes on specific steroid agents

Glucocorticoids

Hydrocortisone (cortisol)

- Hydrocortisone is administered orally for adrenal replacement therapy and possesses mineralocorticoid activity.
- It is administered intravenously in status asthmaticus and anaphylactic shock.
- It is applied topically for eczema, inflammatory bowel conditions and so on.

Prednisolone:

- Prednisolone is predominantly glucocorticoid in activity.
- It is the oral drug most widely used in allergic and inflammatory diseases.

Deflazacort

- Dfelazacort is derived from prednisolone, with high glucocorticoid activity.
- It is administered orally, and indicated for the treatment of inflammatory and allergic disorders.

Betamethasone and dexamethasone

- Betamethasone and dexamethasone have very high glucocorticoid activity with insignificant mineralocorticoid activity.
- They are very potent drugs used orally and by injection to suppress inflammatory and allergic disorders, and to reduce cerebral oedema; they do not possess salt-retaining or water-retaining actions.

Beclometasone

- Beclometasone is the dipropionate ester of betamethasone.
- It is a very potent drug with no mineralocorticoid activity that is useful topically because it is poorly absorbed through membranes and skin.
- It is used topically to treat asthma and allergic rhinitis, and as a cream and ointment in eczema to provide high local antiinflammatory effects with minimal systemic penetration.

Triamcinolone

- Triamcinolone is a moderately potent drug which can be used in severe asthma.
- It can also be administered by intraarticular injection for the treatment of rheumatoid arthritis.

Mineralocorticoids

Fludrocortisone

- Fludrocortisone has such high mineralocorticoid activity that glucocorticoid activity is insignificant.
- It is administered orally, in combination with a glucocorticoid, in replacement therapy.

CLINICAL NOTE

A patient presents with a gradual history of muscle weakness, weight loss and low mood. On examination, he appears slightly tanned and his blood pressure is low, with a significant postural drop. He also has a low blood sugar. His bloods show a low Na and a high K level, and a low morning cortisol, with a raised ACTH. He is diagnosed with primary adrenal insufficiency (Addison disease). He is prescribed hydrocortisone and fludrocortisone, and he is seen in endocrine follow-up regularly.

Management of Cushing syndrome

Cushing syndrome is caused by prolonged exposure to elevated levels of either endogenous or exogenous glucocorticosteroids. Patients present with symptoms as described in Fig. 7.5. Patients with Cushing syndrome as a consequence of treatment with exogenous glucocorticosteroids, must be managed by stopping the drugs slowly. Patients with excess endogenous glucocorticosteroids secondary to a pituitary adenoma require definitive management with surgical removal of their tumour.

Medical therapy includes metyrapone (a competitive inhibitor of 11B hydroxylation) and ketoconazole (inhibits 17 α-hydroxylase), which lower cortisol by directly inhibiting enzymes involved in the synthesis and secretion of cortisol in the adrenal gland.

Other medications used in the treatment of endocrine-related conditions

Somatostatin analogues

Physiologically, somatostatin is a hormone that acts on the hypothalamus to inhibit the release of growth hormone and in the pancreas to inhibit the release of glucagon and insulin.

Octreotide is a long-acting analogue of somatostatin and is used clinically to treat acromegaly (oversecretion of growth hormone causing headaches, visual field defects, enlarged hands, feet and tongue associated with cardiac features). Side effects of octreotide include gastrointestinal disturbances, gallstones and hyperglycaemia.

Dopamine receptor agonists

Bromocriptine and cabergoline are examples of dopamine receptor agonists used clinically in the treatment of prolactin-secreting tumours of the pituitary gland. Unwanted side effects include dizziness, constipation and postural hypotension.

THE REPRODUCTIVE SYSTEM

Hormonal control of the reproductive system

Physiology of the female reproductive tract

The female gonads, or ovaries, are responsible for oogenesis and the secretion of the steroid sex hormones, namely oestrogens (mainly oestradiol) and progesterone. The production of the female sex hormones is controlled by the hypothalamic–pituitary–ovarian axis (Fig. 7.6).

Gonadotrophin-releasing hormone (GnRH) is secreted by the hypothalamus and stimulates the pulsatile secretion of the gonadotrophins, follicle-stimulating hormone (FSH) and luteinising hormone (LH) by the anterior pituitary. In

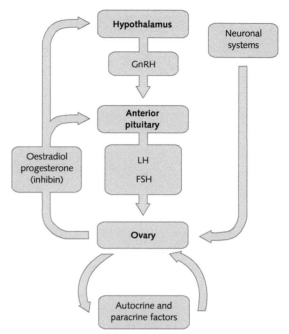

Fig. 7.6 Hypothalamic-pituitary-ovarian axis. *FSH*, Follicle-stimulating hormone; *GnRH*, gonadotrophin-releasing hormone; *LH*, luteinizing hormone.

turn, these act upon the ovaries to stimulate the release of oestradiol, progesterone and other ovarian hormones.

The ovarian hormones are able to exert a negative feedback on the hypothalamus and/or the pituitary. Some of these are selective in their inhibition; for example, inhibin selectively inhibits FSH release from the pituitary, activin selectively stimulates FSH release from the pituitary, and gonadotrophin-surge-attenuating factor selectively inhibits LH secretion from the pituitary.

Menstrual cycle

The menstrual cycle is divided into a follicular phase (days 1–14) and a luteal phase (days 14–28). The cycle proceeds as follows (numbers refer to Fig. 7.7).

1. Day 1 is the first day of menstruation, which involves the shedding of the uterine endometrium. Plasma oestrogen levels are low and thus little negative feedback occurs. As a result, the secretion of LH and FSH begins to increase.
2. Between 10 and 25 preantral follicles start to enlarge and secrete oestrogen.
3. FSH stimulates the granulosa cells to secrete oestrogen, the levels of which rise.
4. About 1 week into the cycle, one of the follicles becomes dominant, and the others undergo atresia. The dominant follicle secretes increasingly larger amounts of oestrogen.
5. Plasma oestrogen levels rise significantly as a result of increased sensitivity of the granulosa cells to FSH.

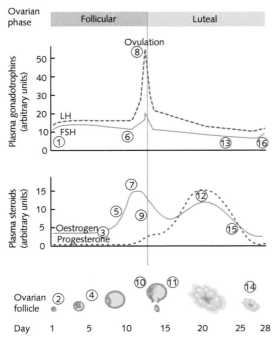

Ovarian phase

Follicular | Luteal

Ovulation ⑧

Ovarian follicle

Day 1 5 10 15 20 25 28

Fig. 7.7 The menstrual cycle. *FSH*, Follicle-stimulating hormone; *LH*, luteinizing hormone.

6. Elevated oestrogen levels provide negative feedback, and FSH secretion decreases.
7. Plasma oestrogen levels are now so high (> 200 pg/mL) that they exert a positive feedback on gonadotrophin secretion. This occurs for about 2 days, during which FSH stimulates the appearance of LH receptors on the granulosa cells.
8. An LH surge occurs. This results in a decrease in oestrogen secretion, an increase in progesterone secretion by the granulosa cells, and the resumption of meiosis in the egg.
9. Oestrogen levels decline after ovulation.
10. The first meiotic division is completed.
11. On day 14, ovulation, the release of the ovum, occurs. This is approximately 18 hours after the LH surge.
12. The granulosa cells are transformed into the corpus luteum, which secretes both oestrogen and progesterone in large quantities.
13. There is a rise in the levels of oestrogen and progesterone. As a result, FSH and LH secretion are suppressed, and their levels fall.
14. If fertilisation does not take place, the corpus luteum degenerates after about 10 days.
15. Oestrogen and progesterone levels fall; menstruation is imminent.
16. FSH and LH secretion increase once more, and the 28-day cycle begins again.

Physiology of the male reproductive tract

The male gonads, or testes, are responsible for spermatogenesis and the secretion of the steroid sex hormone testosterone. Spermatogenesis takes place in the lumen of the seminiferous tubules of the testis. The production of the male sex hormones is controlled by the hypothalamic–pituitary axis (Fig. 7.8).

The Sertoli cells are connected to one another by tight junctions and extend from the basement membrane of the seminiferous tubules into the lumen. Under the influence of FSH, these synthesize testosterone receptors and inhibin.

The Leydig cells are found in the connective tissue between the tubules. Under the influence of LH, these synthesize testosterone. Testosterone acts locally to increase sperm production, and also peripherally on the testosterone-sensitive tissues of the body.

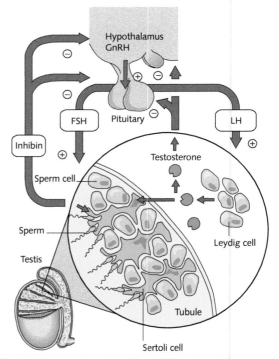

Fig. 7.8 Hormonal control of Sertoli, Leydig and sperm cell function. *FSH*, Follicle-stimulating hormone; *GnRH*, gonadotrophin-releasing hormone; *LH*, luteinizing hormone. (Modified from Page, C., Curtis, M. Walker, M, Hoffman, B. (eds) *Integrated Pharmacology*, 3rd edn. Mosby, 2006.)

Testosterone and inhibin are able to exert negative feedback control over the anterior pituitary, the former decreasing LH secretion and the latter decreasing FSH secretion. In addition, testosterone and inhibin act on the hypothalamus to decrease GnRH secretion.

Drugs that affect the reproductive system

Oral contraceptives

Combined oral contraceptive pill

The combined oral contraceptive pill (COCP) contains both an oestrogen (usually ethinylestradiol, 20–50 µg) and a progestogen (an analogue of progesterone).

COCPs provide a highly effective form of contraception. Their efficacy is reduced by some broad-spectrum antibiotics, which reduce enterohepatic recirculation of oestrogen by killing gut flora.

Mechanism of action—The levels of steroids mimic the luteal phase of the menstrual cycle, and suppress, via negative feedback effects, the secretion of gonadotrophins. Oestrogen inhibits secretion of FSH via negative feedback on the anterior pituitary and thus suppresses the development of the ovarian follicle. Progestogen inhibits secretion of LH and therefore prevents ovulation. As a result, follicular selection and maturation, the oestrogen surge, the LH surge, and thus ovulation, do not take place. In addition, the cervical mucus prevents the passage of sperm. Both progestogen and oestrogen reduce the ability of an egg implanting.

Route of administration—Oral.

Indications—Contraception and menstrual symptoms.

Contraindications—Pregnancy, breastfeeding, or those with a history of heart disease or hypertension, hyperlipidaemia or any prothrombotic coagulation abnormality, diabetes mellitus, migraine, breast or genital tract carcinoma or liver disease.

Adverse effects—Nausea, vomiting and headache, weight gain, breast tenderness, impaired liver function, impaired glucose tolerance in diabetic women, "spotting" (slight bleeding at the start of the menstrual cycle), thromboembolism and hypertension, a slightly increased risk of cervical cancer, and a possibly increased risk of breast cancer.

Therapeutic regimen—COCPs are taken for 21 days (starting on the first day of the menstrual cycle) at about the same time each day, with a 7-day break to induce a withdrawal bleed. If the delay in taking the pill is greater than 12 hours, the contraceptive effect may be lost.

Progesterone-only pill (mini pill)

The mini-pill consists of low-dose progestogen; ovulation still takes place and menstruation is normal.

Mechanism of action—The mini-pill causes thickening of cervical mucus preventing sperm penetration. It also causes suppression of gonadotrophin secretion, and occasionally ovulation, but the latter effect does not occur in the majority of women.

Route of administration—Oral.

Indications—Contraception (but less effective than the COCP). It is more suitable for heavy smokers and patients with hypertension or heart disease, diabetes mellitus and migraine, or in those who have other contraindications for oestrogen therapy.

Contraindications—Pregnancy, arterial disease, liver disease, breast or genital tract carcinoma.

Adverse effects—Menstrual irregularities, nausea, vomiting and headache, weight gain, breast tenderness.

Therapeutic regimen—The mini-pill is taken as one tablet daily, at the same time, starting on day 1 of the menstrual cycle and then continuously. If the delay in taking the pill is greater than 3 hours, the contraceptive effect may be lost.

CLINICAL NOTE

Mrs Hayat, 29 years old, recently had a pulmonary embolism on return from her holiday to Egypt. A few weeks later, she goes to her GP to enquire about oral contraception. Because she has a predisposition to venous thrombosis, the GP advises her to take oral progestogen-only contraceptives, rather than a COCP.

Other contraceptive regimens

Depot-progesterone

Examples of depot-progesterone drugs include medroxyprogesterone acetate and the etonogestrel-releasing implant. These provide long-term contraception.

Mechanism of action—Depot-progesterone causes thickening of cervical mucus. It also causes suppression of gonadotrophin secretion, and occasionally ovulation, but the latter effect does not occur in the majority of women.

Route of administration—Medroxyprogesterone acetate is administered intramuscularly. The etonogestrel-releasing implant system relies on a hormone rod placed subdermally.

Indications—Contraception.

Contraindications—Pregnancy arterial disease, liver disease, osteoporosis, breast or genital tract carcinoma.

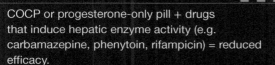

DRUG INTERACTION

COCP or progesterone-only pill + drugs that induce hepatic enzyme activity (e.g. carbamazepine, phenytoin, rifampicin) = reduced efficacy.

Both contraceptives are metabolized by hepatic cytochrome P450 enzymes, which are induced by lots of other coprescribed medications.

Adverse effects—Menstrual irregularities, nausea, vomiting and headache, weight gain, breast tenderness.

Therapeutic notes—Medroxyprogesterone acetate provides protection for about 12 weeks. The etonogestrel-implant system provides protection for 3 years.

Emergency contraception

The "morning-after" pill, levonorgestrel, provides a form of emergency contraception.

Mechanism of action—High doses of a progestogen alone or a progestogen with an oestrogen prevent implantation of the fertilized egg. Contractions of the uterine smooth muscle are induced, and these accelerate the movement of the fertilized egg into the unprepared uterine endometrium.

Route of administration—Oral.

Indications—The morning-after pill is used for emergency contraception after unprotected intercourse.

Contraindications—Preparations containing oestrogens should not be used in patients who have contraindications to oestrogens (see earlier).

Adverse effects—Nausea, vomiting and headache, dizziness, menstrual irregularities.

Therapeutic regimen—The morning-after pill regimen depends upon the type of pill being taken but commonly consists of one or two tablets within 72 hours of intercourse and one or two tablets 12 hours later.

Insertion of an intrauterine device is more effective than hormonal methods and works up to 5 days after intercourse.

Oestrogens and antioestrogens

Oestrogen agonists

The adverse symptoms of the menopause can be attributed to decreased levels of oestrogen that occur as the ovaries begin to fail. Evidence suggests that oestrogen given in low doses to menopausal women will reduce postmenopausal osteoporosis, vaginal atrophy and the incidence of stroke and myocardial infarction.

A progestogen is coadministered with oestrogen to inhibit oestrogen-stimulated endometrial growth and thus reduce the risk of uterine cancer and fibroids.

Examples of oestrogen agonists include oestradiol and oestriol.

Mechanism of action—Oestrogen agonists mimic premenopausal endogenous oestrogen levels.

Route of administration—Oral, or by transdermal patches, gels or subcutaneous implants.

Indications—Oestrogen agonists are used alone for hormone replacement therapy (HRT) in menopausal women who have undergone a hysterectomy. However, because oestrogen causes an overgrowth of cells in the uterus, it must be given in conjunction with progestogen (causes endometrial shedding) in females with a uterus to reduce the risk of endometrial cancer developing.

Also used as replacement therapy in patients with primary or secondary ovarian failure.

Contraindications—Pregnancy, oestrogen-dependent cancer, active or previous thromboembolic disease.

Adverse effects—Increased risk of endometrial cancer and possibly an increased risk of breast cancer after many years of treatment.

Therapeutic regimen—Oestrogen agonists are given for several years, starting in the perimenopausal period.

Oestrogen antagonists

Examples of oestrogen antagonists include tamoxifen, clomifene and toremifene.

Mechanism of action—Tamoxifen has an antioestrogenic effect on breast and uterine tissue.

Clomifene inhibits the negative feedback effects on the hypothalamus and anterior pituitary. This stimulates and enlarges the ovaries, increasing oestrogen secretion and inducing ovulation.

Route of administration—Tamoxifen is administered orally or by intravenous or subcutaneous injection, whereas clomifene is administered orally.

Indications—Tamoxifen is prescribed to reduce the risk of breast cancer in postmenopausal women with osteoporosis or high risk, as well as to treat breast cancer.

Clomiphene is used in the treatment of infertility.

Contraindications—Hepatic disease, ovarian cysts, endometrial carcinoma.

Adverse effects—Multiple pregnancies and hot flushes. Withdrawal causes visual disturbances and ovarian hyperstimulation.

Progestogens and antiprogestogens

Progestogen agonists

Examples of progestogen agonists include progesterone, medroxyprogesterone, dydrogesterone, hydroxyprogesterone and norethisterone.

Mechanism of action—Progestogen agonists mimic endogenous progesterone.

Route of administration—Oral, or by transdermal patches, gels or subcutaneous implants.

Indications—Progestogen agonists are given for premenstrual symptoms, severe dysmenorrhoea, menorrhagia, endometriosis, contraception and as part of HRT.

Contraindications—Pregnancy or to those with arterial disease, liver disease or breast or genital tract carcinoma.

Adverse effects—Menstrual irregularities, nausea, vomiting and headache, weight gain, breast tenderness.

Progestogen antagonists

Mifepristone is an example of a progestogen antagonist.

Mechanism of action—Progestogen antagonists bind to progesterone receptors but exert no effect. They sensitize the uterus to prostaglandins and can, therefore be used in combination with prostaglandins in the termination of early pregnancy.

Route of administration—Oral.

Indications—Progestogen antagonists are used in the termination of pregnancy.

Contraindications—Progestogen antagonists should not be given to pregnant women (64 days gestation or more), to women with adrenal failure or haemorrhagic disorders, or to those on anticoagulant or long-term corticosteroid treatment, or to smokers aged 35 years and over.

Adverse effects—Vaginal bleeding, faintness, nausea and vomiting.

Androgens and antiandrogens

Androgen agonists

Testosterone and mesterolone are examples of androgen agonists.

Mechanism of action—Androgen agonists mimic endogenous androgens.

Route of administration—Oral, intramuscularly or by implant or cutaneous patch.

Indications—Androgen agonists are given as androgen-replacement therapy in castrated men, for pituitary or testicular disease causing hypogonadism, and for breast cancer.

Contraindications—Androgen agonists should not be given to men with breast or prostate cancer, to people with hypercalcaemia, or to women who are pregnant or breastfeeding.

Adverse effects—Sodium retention causing oedema, hypercalcaemia, suppression of spermatogenesis, virilism in women and premature closure of epiphyses in prepubertal boys. The incidence of prostate abnormalities and prostate cancer is also increased.

Androgen antagonists

Cyproterone is an androgen antagonist that is a progesterone derivative. Both oestrogens and progestogens have antiandrogenic properties.

Mechanism of action—Androgen antagonists are partial agonists at androgen receptors and act on the hypothalamus to reduce the synthesis of gonadotrophins. They inhibit spermatogenesis, causing reversible infertility, but are not contraceptives.

Route of administration—Oral.

Indications—Androgen antagonists are used in the treatment of prostate cancer, acne, female hirsutism, and precocious puberty. In addition, used for male hypersexuality and sexual deviation.

Contraindications—Androgen antagonists should not be given to people with hepatic disease or severe diabetes, or to those aged 18 years and under because their bones are not fully matured.

Adverse effects—Fatigue and lethargy, and hepatotoxicity.

Therapeutic notes—Finasteride is technically an antiandrogen, although it inhibits the enzyme 5α-reductase which metabolizes testosterone to the more potent androgen dihydrotestosterone. Finasteride is indicated in benign prostatic hyperplasia and is administered orally.

Anabolic steroids

Nandrolone and stanozolol are examples of anabolic steroids.

Mechanism of action—Anabolic steroids are androgenic; stimulate protein synthesis.

Route of administration—Nandrolone is administered by deep intramuscular injection and stanozolol orally.

Indications—Anabolic steroids can be used in the management of aplastic anaemias.

Anabolic steroids, although banned, are frequently used by athletes to increase skeletal muscle bulk.

Contraindications—Hepatic impairment, men with prostate or breast cancer, pregnant women.

Adverse effects—Acne, sodium retention causing oedema, virilisation in women, amenorrhoea, inhibition of spermatogenesis, liver tumours.

Gonadotropin-releasing hormone agonists and antagonists

Agonists

Goserelin, leuprolide and buserelin are examples of GnRH agonists.

Mechanism of action—GnRH agonists are given intermittently and mimic endogenous GnRH. Continuous use desensitizes the GnRH receptors that gonadotrophs act on and inhibits gonadotrophin synthesis.

Route of administration—Buserelin is administered intranasally, whereas goserelin and leuprolide are administered by subcutaneous injection.

Indications—GnRH agonists are used for ovulation induction in those with GnRH deficiency, endometriosis, precocious puberty, and sex-hormone-dependent cancers and prostate cancer.

Adverse effects—Menopause-like symptoms, including hot flushes, palpitations, and decreased libido because of hypooestrogenism, and breakthrough bleeding.

Antagonists

Danazol and gestrinone are examples of GnRH antagonists.

Mechanism of action—GnRH antagonists inhibit the release of GnRH and the gonadotrophins. They bind to the sex steroid receptors, displaying androgenic, antioestrogenic, and antiprogestogenic effects.

Route of administration—Oral.

Indications—GnRH antagonists are given for endometriosis, menstrual disorders, including menorrhagia, cystic breast disease, gynaecomastia.

Contraindications—Pregnancy, hepatic, renal or cardiac impairment, vascular disease.

Adverse effects—Nausea and vomiting, weight gain, androgenic effects such as acne and hirsutism.

Therapeutic notes—Cetrorelix and ganirelix are luteinizing hormone-releasing hormone antagonists, inhibiting the release of the gonadotrophins. They are administered parenterally and are used for infertility in specialist centres.

Oxytocic drugs

The oxytocic drugs, oxytocin, ergometrine, prostaglandins E and F (e.g. gemeprost [PGE$_1$ analogue], dinoprostone [PGE$_2$] and carboprost [15-methyl PGF$_{2a}$]) all cause uterine contractions.

Oxytocin is a posterior pituitary hormone that acts on uterine muscle to induce powerful contractions. It does this directly and also indirectly by stimulating the muscle to synthesize prostaglandins.

In addition, prostaglandins ripen and soften the cervix, further aiding the expulsion of uterine contents.

Mechanism of action—Oxytocin acts on oxytocin receptors. The mechanism for ergometrine is not well understood but may be via partial agonist action at α-adrenoceptors or 5-hydroxytryptamine receptors. The prostaglandins act at prostaglandin receptors.

Route of administration—Gemeprost and dinoprostone are administered by vaginal pessary; dinoprostone can also be administered extraamniotically; oxytocin is administered by slow intravenous infusion, and oxytocin and ergometrine together are injected intramuscularly. Prostaglandins can be administered by intravenous infusion.

Indications—Prostaglandins are used to induce abortion. Oxytocin and dinoprostone are used for the induction of labour whereas oxytocin, ergometrine and carboprost (in those unresponsive to oxytocin and ergometrine) are used for the management of the third-stage of labour and prevention and treatment of postpartum haemorrhage.

Contraindications—Oxytocic drugs should not be given to women with vascular diseases; ergometrine should not be used to induce labour.

Adverse effects—Nausea and vomiting, vaginal bleeding, uterine pain. Oxytocin can cause hypotension and tachycardia.

BONE AND CALCIUM

Bone and calcium physiology

Bone is a tissue comprized mainly of calcium, phosphates and a protein meshwork, in addition to the components of the bone marrow.

Bone functions to provide support and enables us to carry out various physiological processes such as respiration and movement. Bone is also an active tissue and crucial in the homeostasis of calcium and phosphate.

Serum calcium is ultimately controlled by the peptide, parathyroid hormone (PTH), derived from the parathyroid glands. PTH maintains serum calcium by acting on the kidney to reabsorb calcium from the tubular filtrate, and to stimulate the activation of vitamin D. PTH also acts directly on bone, mobilising calcium. Activated vitamin D (1,25-dihydroxycholecalciferol) promotes absorption of calcium from the gut. PTH is secreted in response to low serum calcium.

Calcitonin, from the thyroid gland, inhibits calcium mobilisation from bone and decreases reabsorption from the renal tubules.

Disorders of bone and calcium

Osteoporosis is an overall loss of bone mass, and commonly occurs in women after the menopause, when oestrogens fall, and bone mobilisation slowly increases. Other causes of osteoporosis include thyrotoxicosis, and excessive glucocorticoids (exogenous or endogenous).

Osteodystrophy occurs in renal failure and is driven by secondary hyperparathyroidism. Rickets (vitamin D deficiency) is now rare in the West, although the adult variant, osteomalacia, is not uncommon. Hypercalcaemia is a medical emergency and is most often caused by malignancy.

HINTS AND TIPS

Rehydration therapy is as important in hypercalcaemia as it is in ketoacidosis (hyperglycaemia) because the fluid will be lost in the urine as a result of osmotic diuresis.

Drugs used in bone and calcium disorders

Bisphosphonates

Alendronate, disodium etidronate, pamidronate and zoledronate are examples of bisphosphonates.

Mechanism of action—Bisphosphonates inhibit and potentially destroy osteoclasts, which are responsible for mobilising calcium from bone.

Route of administration—Oral, parenteral.

Indications—Prevention of postmenopausal osteoporosis and corticosteroid-induced osteoporosis, and for the management of hypercalcaemia of malignancy.

Alendronate and risedronate for prophylaxis and treatment of osteoporosis.

Pamidronate via intravenous infusion to treat hypercalcaemia of malignancy or Paget disease

Zoledronate via intravenous infusion to treat Paget disease, selected cases of osteoporosis (often the second line) once a year.

Contraindications—Renal impairment, hypocalcaemia.

Adverse effects—Nausea, oesophagitis (with oral preparations), hypocalcaemia. Atypical femoral fractures can develop if taking long-term bisphosphonate treatment. Zoledronate can rarely cause jaw osteonecrosis; dental checks are required pretreatment.

Therapeutic note—Bisphosphonates given orally must be taken on an empty stomach with plenty of water in a sitting or standing position at least 30 minutes before breakfast because food impairs absorption and bisphosphonates can cause oesophagitis, strictures and gastric erosions.

Calcium salts

Calcium gluconate, calcium lactate and calcium carbonate are calcium salts.

Mechanism of action—Calcium supplementation replaces calcium deficiencies.

Route of administration—Oral, intravenous.

Indications—Hypocalcaemia, calcium deficiency, osteoporosis. Calcium gluconate is given intravenously as emergency treatment of hyperkalaemia to stabilize cardiac function. Calcium carbonate is used in the management of hyperphosphataemia (binds phosphate in the gut).

Contraindications—Hypercalcaemia.

Adverse effects—Mild gastrointestinal disturbance, bradycardia, arrhythmias.

Therapeutic notes—If calcium is given parenterally, serum calcium should be repeatedly monitored.

Vitamin D

Vitamin D can be administered in its inactive form as ergocalciferol, or in its active form as calcitriol.

Mechanism of action—Vitamin D acts on the gut to absorb calcium from the diet.

Route of administration—Oral, parenteral.

Indications—Vitamin D deficiency, hypocalcaemia secondary to hypoparathyroidism, renal failure and postmenopausal osteoporosis.

Contraindications—Hypercalcaemia.

Adverse effects—Symptoms of overdosage include anorexia, lassitude, nausea and vomiting, weight loss, hypercalcaemia.

Therapeutic notes—Serum calcium should be monitored closely once vitamin D therapy has started, and if symptoms of hypercalcaemia appear.

Calcitonin

Mechanism of action—Calcitonin binds specific receptors on osteoclasts inhibiting their mobilisation of bone and acts on the kidney to limit calcium reabsorption from the proximal tubules.

Route of administration—Subcutaneous or intramuscular.

Indications—Hypercalcaemia, Paget disease of bone, bone pain in neoplastic disease.

Contraindications—Caution if history of allergy, or renal impairment.

Adverse effects—Nausea, vomiting, flushing, diarrhoea, tingling of hands.

CLINICAL NOTE

Mrs Price, 73 years old, weighing 44 kg, presents with a painful, swollen and "dinner fork-like" deformity of her wrist. Radiography shows she has fractured both radial and ulnar styloid processes (Colles fracture). The doctor was concerned that she had poor bone density and sent her for a DEXA (dual energy X-ray absorptiometry) scan. The scan indicated Mrs Price had developed early osteoporosis. Her bones are manually aligned and put in a cast to be reviewed in 6 weeks. She is put on alendronate, a bisphosphonate, to increase her bone density and thus help prevent further fractures. Also, she is prescribed calcium and vitamin D supplements.

Selective oestrogen-receptor modulator

The drug is called raloxifene.

Mechanism of action—Raloxifene has both oestrogen antagonistic (uterine endometrium and breast tissue) and agonistic properties (bone and lipid metabolism). Raloxifene stimulates osteoblasts and inhibits osteoclasts.

Route of administration—Oral.

Indications—Treatment and prevention of postmenopausal osteoporosis (third line).

Contraindications—History of venous thromboembolism, undiagnosed uterine bleeding, hepatic or severe renal impairment, pregnancy, breastfeeding.

Adverse effects—Venous thromboembolism, thrombophlebitis, hot flushes, leg cramps, peripheral oedema, flu-like symptoms.

Therapeutic notes—It may reduce the incidence of oestrogen-receptor positive breast cancer and cardiovascular events, but there is no clear evidence of this.

Denosumab

Mechanism of action—Denosumab is a recombinant human monoclonal antibody that inhibits receptor activator of nuclear factor kappa B ligand (RANKL), the primary signal for bone resorption.

Route of administration—Subcutaneous injection every 6 months (or monthly for bone metastases)

Indications—Second-line treatment of osteoporosis in postmenopausal women at risk of fracture.

Men with prostate cancer at increased risk of osteoporosis because of hormone ablation.

Prevent fractures and reduce pain in patients with bone metastases from solid tumours.

Contraindications—Hypocalcaemia, pregnancy.

Adverse effects—Altered bowel habit, hypocalcaemia, recurrent infections, atypical femoral fractures.

Therapeutic notes—Dental work needs to be undertaken before treatment to reduce the risk of osteonecrosis of the jaw.

Vitamin D preparations

Ergocalciferol and alfacalcidol are examples of vitamin D preparations used in the treatment of vitamin D deficiencies, renal osteodystrophy and hypoparathyroidism. They are given orally, and the main adverse effect is hypercalcaemia.

Other drugs

Teriparatide is a recombinant parathyroid hormone. When given in small doses, teriparatide stimulates osteoblast activity and enhances bone formation. Prescribed subcutaneously by specialists to treat patients with severe osteoporosis. Well tolerated but can cause nausea, headache and arthralgias.

Strontium ranelate inhibits bone resorption and stimulates bone formation, through inhibition of osteoclasts. Treatment of severe osteoporosis by specialists only.

● Chapter Summary

- Iodide is given in thyrotoxic crises because it rapidly inhibits thyroid hormone secretion and the conversion of T_4 to T_3
- β-adrenoceptor antagonists are useful for reducing somatic symptoms associated with hyperthyroidism
- Thyroid function tests should be checked before amiodarone is prescribed and every 6 months thereafter.
- Patients with type 1 diabetes require insulin subcutaneously, whereas patients with type 2 diabetes can take oral medication
- The COCP is contraindicated in patients with migraine, diabetes or previous thromboembolism
- The progesterone-only pill is less effective but can be given to patients who smoke or have heart disease
- Bisphosphonates are commonly used in the treatment of osteoporosis

BASIC CONCEPTS

The central nervous system (CNS) consists of the brain and the spinal cord, which are continuous with one another. The brain is composed of the cerebrum (which consists of the frontal, temporal, parietal and occipital lobes), the diencephalon (which includes the thalamus and hypothalamus), the brainstem (which consists of the midbrain, pons and medulla oblongata) and the cerebellum. The brain functions to interpret sensory information obtained about the internal and external environments and send messages to effector organs in response to a situation. Different parts of the brain are associated with specific functions (Fig. 8.1).

PARKINSON DISEASE AND PARKINSONISM

Parkinsonism is characterized by a resting tremor, slow initiation of movements (bradykinesia), and muscle rigidity. A patient with parkinsonism will present with characteristic signs including the following.

- A shuffling gait
- A blank "mask-like" facial expression
- Speech impairment
- An inability to perform skilled tasks

Parkinsonism is most commonly caused by Parkinson disease, although other causes exist.

Parkinson disease is a progressive neurological disorder of the basal ganglia that occurs most commonly in elderly people.

Aetiology

The cause of Parkinson disease is unknown in most cases (idiopathic), although both endogenous and environmental neurotoxins are known to be responsible for causing parkinsonism.

Parkinson disease is progressive, with continued loss of dopaminergic neurones in the substantia nigra correlating with worsening of clinical symptoms. The possibility of a neurotoxic cause has been strengthened by the finding that 1-methyl-4-phenyl-1,2,3,6-tetrahydropyridine (MPTP), a chemical contaminant of heroin, causes irreversible damage to the nigrostriatal dopaminergic pathway. Thus this damage can lead to the development of symptoms similar to those of idiopathic Parkinson disease. Drugs that block dopamine receptors can also induce parkinsonism. Neuroleptic drugs (p. 126) used in the treatment of schizophrenia can produce parkinsonian symptoms as an adverse effect. Rare causes of parkinsonism are cerebral ischaemia (progressive atherosclerosis or stroke), viral encephalitis or other pathological damage.

HINTS AND TIPS

RATS! Symptoms of parkinsonism include rigidity, akinesia, tremor and shuffling gait.

Pathogenesis

Postmortem analysis of the brains of patients with Parkinson showed a substantially reduced concentration of dopamine (less than 10% of normal) in the basal ganglia. The basal ganglia exert an extrapyramidal neural influence that normally maintains smooth voluntary movement.

The main pathology in Parkinson disease is a progressive degeneration of the dopaminergic neurones of the substantia nigra, which project via the nigrostriatal pathway to the corpus striatum (Fig. 8.2). The inhibitory dopaminergic activity of the nigrostriatal pathway is, therefore considerably reduced (by 20%–40%) in people with Parkinson disease.

The reduction in the inhibitory dopaminergic activity of the nigrostriatal pathway results in unopposed cholinergic neurone hyperactivity from the corpus striatum, which contributes to the pathological features of parkinsonism. Frank symptoms of parkinsonism appear only when more than 80% of the dopaminergic neurones of the substantia nigra have degenerated. However, peripheral symptoms such as constipation often appear much earlier than movement disorders.

Untreated Parkinson eventually results in dementia and death.

Treatment of Parkinsonism

The treatment of parkinsonism is based on correcting the imbalance between the dopaminergic and cholinergic systems at the basal ganglia (Fig. 8.3). Two major groups of drugs are used: drugs that increase dopaminergic activity between the substantia nigra and the corpus striatum, and anticholinergic drugs that inhibit striatal cholinergic activity.

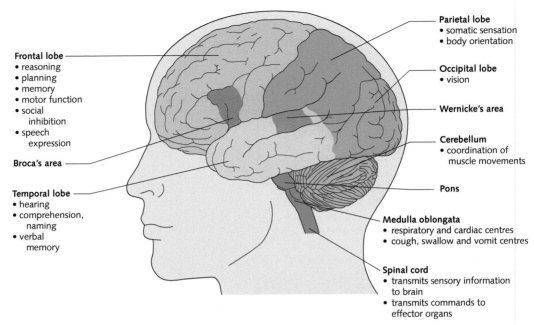

Fig. 8.1 Parts of the brain and their known functions.

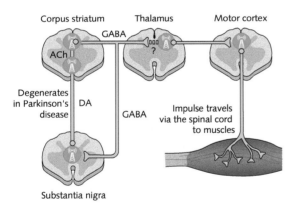

Fig. 8.2 Basal ganglia systems involved in Parkinson disease. *ACh,* Acetylcholine; *DA,* dopamine; *GABA,* γ-aminobutyric acid. (Modified from Page, C., Curtis, M. Walker, M, Hoffman, B. (eds) *Integrated Pharmacology,* 3rd edn. Mosby, 2006.)

Drugs that increase dopaminergic activity

Dopamine precursors

An example of a dopamine precursor is levodopa (L-dopa).

Mechanism of action—L-dopa is the immediate precursor of dopamine and is able to penetrate the blood–brain barrier to replenish the dopamine content of the corpus striatum. L-dopa is decarboxylated to dopamine in the brain by dopa decarboxylase, and it has beneficial effects produced through the actions of dopamine acting on D_2 re-

ceptors (see Fig. 8.3). Dopamine itself is not used, owing to its inability to cross the blood–brain barrier.

Route of administration—L-dopa is administered orally. It reaches peak plasma concentrations after 1 to 2 hours, but only 1% reaches the brain, owing to peripheral metabolism.

Indications—L-dopa is used in the treatment of parkinsonism (excluding drug-induced extrapyramidal symptoms) and is often used first line for symptom control.

Contraindications—Closed-angle glaucoma.

Adverse effects—The extensive peripheral metabolism of L-dopa means that large doses have to be given to produce therapeutic effects in the brain. Large doses are more likely to produce adverse effects including the following.

- Nausea and vomiting
- Psychiatric side effects (schizophrenia-like symptoms)
- Cardiovascular effects (hypotension)
- Dyskinesias

Nausea and vomiting are caused by stimulation of dopamine receptors in the chemoreceptor trigger zone in the area postrema, which lies outside the blood–brain barrier.

Psychiatric side effects are common limiting factors in L-dopa treatment; these include vivid dreams, confusion and psychotic symptoms more commonly seen in patients with schizophrenia. These effects are probably a result of increased dopaminergic activity in the mesolimbic area of the brain, possibly similar to that found pathologically in schizophrenia (dopaminergic overactivity is implicated in schizophrenia; see p. 125).

Hypotension is common but usually asymptomatic. Cardiac arrhythmias are caused by increased catecholamine

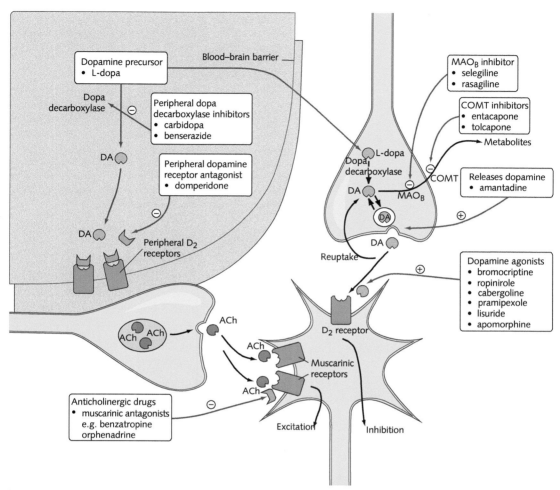

Fig. 8.3 Drugs used to treat parkinsonism and their site of action. *ACh*, Acetylcholine; *COMT*, catechol-O-methyl transferase *DA*, dopamine; *L-dopa*, levodopa; *MAO_B*, monoamine oxidase B.

stimulation following the excessive peripheral metabolism of L-dopa to noradrenaline.

Dyskinesias can often develop following treatment with L-dopa and tend to involve the face and limbs. They usually reflect overtreatment and respond to simple dose reduction.

Three strategies have been developed to optimize L-dopa treatment, to maximize the central effects of L-dopa within the brain and minimize its unwanted peripheral effects. These strategies involve coadministration of the following.

- Carbidopa (given with L-dopa as co-careldopa) or benserazide (given with L-dopa as co-beneldopa), inhibitors of dopa decarboxylase in the periphery that cannot penetrate the blood–brain barrier. Hence, extracerebral conversion of L-dopa to dopamine is inhibited.
- Domperidone, a dopamine antagonist, that does not penetrate the blood–brain barrier and can, therefore

block the stimulation of dopamine receptors in the periphery.
- Selegiline and entacapone, monoamine oxidase (MAO_B) and catechol-O-methyltransferase (COMT) inhibitors, respectively, which inhibit dopamine metabolism in the CNS.

Therapeutic notes—Initially, treatment with L-dopa is effective in 80% of patients with possible restoration of near-normal motor function. Although L-dopa restores dopamine levels in the short term, it has no effect on the underlying degenerative disease process.

As progressive neuronal degeneration continues, the capacity of the corpus striatum to convert L-dopa to dopamine diminishes. This affects the majority of patients within 5 years and manifests itself as "end of dose deterioration" (a shortening of the duration of each dose of L-dopa), and the "on-off effect" (rapid fluctuations in clinical state, varying from increased mobility and a general improvement to increased rigidity and hypokinesia). The latter effect occurs suddenly and for short periods (from a few minutes to a few hours), tending to worsen with the length of treatment.

Dopamine agonists

Examples of dopamine agonists include bromocriptine, ropinirole, cabergoline, pergolide, pramipexole, lisuride and apomorphine.

Mechanism of action—Bromocriptine, ropinirole, cabergoline (longer acting), pergolide, pramipexole, lisuride and apomorphine are dopamine agonists selective for the D_2 receptor (see Fig. 8.3). Apomorphine also has agonist action at D_1 receptors. Pramipexole has a high affinity for D_3 receptors.

Route of administration—Usually given orally but apomorphine is given via the subcutaneous route.

Indications—Dopamine agonists are used in combination with L-dopa in an attempt to reduce the late adverse effects of L-dopa therapy (end of dose deterioration and on-off effect) or when L-dopa alone does not adequately control the symptoms.

Dopamine agonists are sometimes used in the management of prolactinomas or acromegaly.

Adverse effects—The adverse effects of dopamine agonists are similar to those of L-dopa (i.e. nausea, postural hypotension, psychiatric symptoms), but they tend to be more common and more severe. Apomorphine produces profound nausea and vomiting. Ergot-derived dopamine agonists (bromocriptine, cabergoline, lisuride and pergolide) can cause fibrosis. Dopamine agonists have also been linked to the development of compulsive or disinhibited behaviours (e.g. pathological gambling or hypersexuality).

Therapeutic notes—Currently, bromocriptine is the most used of the dopamine agonists in the treatment of Parkinson disease, mainly in the treatment of younger patients with this condition. Patients and their families should be made aware of the potential disinhibited behaviours associated with dopamine agonists.

Drugs stimulating release of dopamine

Amantadine is an example of a drug that stimulates the release of dopamine (see Fig. 8.3).

Mechanism of action—Facilitation of neuronal dopamine release and inhibition of its reuptake into nerves. Amantadine has muscarinic receptor antagonist actions.

Route of administration—Oral.

Indications—Amantadine has a synergistic effect when used in conjunction with L-dopa therapy in Parkinson disease.

Adverse effects—Anorexia, nausea, hallucinations.

Therapeutic notes—Amantadine has modest antiparkinsonian effects, but it is only of short-term benefit because most of its effectiveness is lost within 6 months of initiating treatment.

Monoamine oxidase inhibitors

Selegiline is an example of a MAO_B inhibitor.

Mechanism of action—Selegiline selectively inhibits the MAO_B enzyme in the brain that is normally responsible for the metabolism of dopamine (see Fig. 8.3). By reducing the metabolism of dopamine, the actions of L-dopa are potentiated, thus allowing the dose to be reduced by up to one-third. There is also evidence to suggest that selegiline may slow the progression of the underlying neuronal degeneration in Parkinson disease.

Route of administration—Oral.

Indications—MAO_B inhibitors can be used on their own in mild cases of parkinsonism or in conjunction with L-dopa to reduce 'end-of-dose' deterioration in severe parkinsonism. Early treatment with selegiline can delay the need for levodopa therapy.

Adverse effects—The adverse effects of MAO_B inhibitors are caused by potentiation of L-dopa. Common adverse effects include a dry mouth, blurred vision and hypertension (see section under antidepressants).

> **HINTS AND TIPS**
>
> Note that with the possible exception of selegiline, none of the drugs used in the treatment of Parkinson disease affects the inevitable progressive degeneration of nigrostriatal dopaminergic neurones. The disease process is unaffected, just compensated for by drug therapy.

Catechol-*O*-methyltransferase inhibitors

Entacapone and tolcapone are examples of COMT inhibitors.

Mechanism of action—Dopamine can also be metabolized by a second pathway, in addition to that of MAO_B. The enzyme COMT can metabolize dopamine to inactive methylated metabolites. COMT inhibitors reversibly inhibit the peripheral breakdown of levodopa by the COMT enzyme.

Route of administration—Oral.

Indications—As an adjunct to L-dopa preparations when end-of-dose is problematic.

Contraindications—Phaeochromocytoma.

Adverse effects—Nausea, vomiting, abdominal pain and diarrhoea.

Therapeutic notes—Because of hepatotoxicity, tolcapone should only be prescribed under specialist supervision.

Drugs that inhibit striatal cholinergic activity

Anticholinergic agents/Muscarinic receptor antagonists

Benzatropine, procyclidine and orphenadrine are examples of anticholinergic (muscarinic receptor antagonist) agents used in the treatment of Parkinson disease.

Mechanism of action—Benzatropine, procyclidine and orphenadrine are muscarinic receptor antagonists that act at the muscarinic receptors mediating striatal cholinergic excitation (see Fig. 8.3). Their major action in the treatment of Parkinson disease is to reduce the excessive striatal cholinergic activity that characterizes the disease.

Route of administration—Oral.

Adverse effects—Typical peripheral anticholinergic effects, such as a dry mouth and blurred vision, are less common. More often, patients experience a variety of CNS adverse effects, ranging from mild memory loss to acute confusional states.

Therapeutic notes—Termination of anticholinergic treatment should be gradual because parkinsonism can worsen when these drugs are withdrawn. Anticholinergic drugs are most effective in controlling tremor rather than other symptoms of Parkinson disease.

Nonmedical options

Surgical treatment can be used for severe on-off fluctuations and drug failure. In addition, deep brain simulation has been used to reverse rigidity and tremor. Transplantation and gene therapy are potential future options.

CLINICAL NOTE

Mrs Jones, a 62-year-old barrister, presents to her General Practitioner (GP) complaining of shaking arms, the right arm more prominently so than the left. She reports that her handwriting is becoming too small to read. She is referred to a neurologist, who observes her face to be expressionless, a resting tremor and increased muscle tone. Her power, reflexes, coordination and sensation are found to be normal. Examination of her gait shows she is slow getting started and has difficulty stopping and starting. A diagnosis of Parkinson disease is made, and the implications discussed with Mrs Jones. Given that her symptoms are interfering with her daily life, she is commenced on treatment. She is given co-beneldopa and this helps to control her symptoms.

DEMENTIA AND ALZHEIMER DISEASE

Alzheimer disease is a specific process that results in dementia and is unrelated to the dementias associated with stroke, brain trauma or alcohol. Its prevalence increases markedly with age.

Alzheimer disease is progressive, and it is associated with atrophy of the brain substance, loss of neuronal tissue and deposition of amyloid plaques. The clinical features include deterioration in cognitive function, disorientation and generalized confusion.

Loss of neurones in the forebrain is most marked and a relative selective loss of cholinergic neurones most likely accounts for the features of this dementia. An obvious therapeutic approach is, therefore, restoration of cholinergic function.

Cholinesterase inhibitors

Donepezil, galantamine and rivastigmine are cholinesterase inhibitors, licensed for use for the treatment of dementia.

Mechanism of action—The cholinesterase inhibitors prevent the breakdown of acetylcholine (ACh) within the synaptic cleft, and they enhance endogenous cholinergic activity within the CNS and peripheral tissues.

Route of administration—Oral.

Indications—Mild to moderate dementia in Alzheimer disease.

Contraindications—Pregnancy, breastfeeding, hepatic and renal impairment.

Adverse effects—Nausea, vomiting, diarrhoea, anorexia and agitation.

N-Methyl-D-aspartate antagonists

Memantine is a N-Methyl-D-aspartate (NMDA) antagonist

Mechanism of action—Thought to work by selectively inhibiting excessive and pathological activation of NMDA receptor.

Route of administration—Oral.

Indication—Second-line option for patients with moderate Alzheimer disease or treatment of severe disease.

Contraindication—History of convulsions.

Adverse effects—Headache, dizziness, constipation and drowsiness.

ANXIETY AND SLEEP DISORDERS

Anxiety and anxiolytics

Anxiety is a state characterized by psychological symptoms such as a diffuse, unpleasant and vague feeling of apprehension, often accompanied by physical symptoms of autonomic arousal such as palpitations, light-headedness, perspiration, "butterflies" and, in some people, restlessness.

Although occasional anxiety is perfectly normal, it is a common and disabling symptom in a variety of mental illnesses including phobias, panic disorders and obsessive-compulsive disorders. Drugs used to treat such anxiety disorders are called anxiolytics.

SLEEP DISORDERS AND HYPNOTICS

Insomnia is a common and nonspecific disorder that may be reported by 40% to 50% of people at any given time.

Causes of insomnia include medical illness, alcohol or drugs, periodic limb movement disorder, sleep apnoea and psychiatric illness. Without an obvious underlying cause, it is known as primary or psychophysiological.

Hypnotics are drugs used to treat psychophysiological (primary) insomnia. The distinction between the treatment of anxiety and that of sleep disorders is not clear cut, particularly if anxiety is the main impediment to sleep.

γ-Aminobutyric acid receptor

The γ-aminobutyric acid (GABA) receptors of the $GABA_A$ type are involved in the actions of some classes of hypnotic/anxiolytic drugs.

- The benzodiazepines
- Newer nonbenzodiazepine hypnotics, e.g. zopiclone
- The now obsolete barbiturates

The $GABA_A$ receptor belongs to the superfamily of ligand-gated ion channels. It consists of several subunits (α, β, γ and δ), which form the GABA/Cl^- channel complex, as well as containing benzodiazepine and barbiturate modulatory receptor sites. The GABA binding site appears to be located on the α and β subunits whereas the benzodiazepine modulatory site is distinct and located on the γ subunit.

GABA released from nerve terminals binds to postsynaptic $GABA_A$ receptors, the activation of which increases the Cl^- conductance of the neurone. Occupation of the benzodiazepine sites by benzodiazepine receptor agonists enhances the actions of GABA on the Cl^- conductance of the neuronal membrane. The barbiturates similarly enhance the action of GABA, but by occupying a distinct modulatory site (Fig. 8.4).

Anxiolytic and hypnotic drugs

The pharmacotherapy of anxiety and sleep disorders involves several different classes of drug, as shown in Table 8.1, and nonpharmacological management relying on cognitive and behaviour psychotherapy.

Benzodiazepines

Benzodiazepines are drugs with anxiolytic, hypnotic, muscle relaxation and anticonvulsant actions that are used in the treatment of both anxiety states and insomnia.

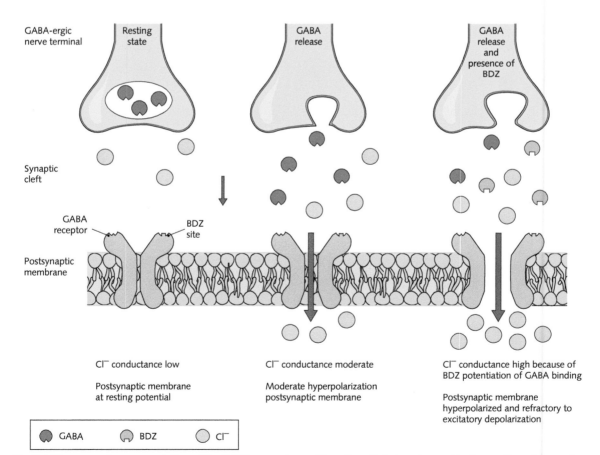

Fig. 8.4 Diagrammatic representation of the $GABA_A$ receptor and how its activity is enhanced by benzodiazepines and similarly by barbiturates. *BDZ*, Benzodiazepine; *Cl⁻*, chloride ion; *GABA*, γ-aminobutyric acid. (Modified from Page, C., Curtis, M. Walker, M, Hoffman, B. (eds) *Integrated Pharmacology*, 3rd edn. Mosby, 2006.)

Table 8.1 Drugs used to treat anxiety and sleep disorders

Anxiolytics	Hypnotics
Benzodiazepines (act on GABA$_A$ receptors) e.g. diazepam, lorazepam	Benzodiazepines (act on GABA$_A$ receptors) e.g. triazolam, temazepam, lormetazepam, nitrazepam
Acting on serotonergic receptors (act on 5-HT$_{1A}$ or 5-HT$_3$ receptors) e.g. buspirone	Nonbenzodiazepine hypnotics (act on GABA$_A$ receptors) e.g. zopiclone, zolpidem and zaleplon
Other drugs e.g. propranolol antidepressants	Other drugs e.g. chloral hydrate clomethiazole barbiturates (obsolete) sedative antidepressants sedative antihistamines

5-HT, 5-Hydroxytryptamine; GABA, γ-aminobutyric acid.

Benzodiazepines are marketed as either hypnotics or anxiolytics. It is mainly the duration of action that determines the choice of drug (see later).

Mechanism of action—Benzodiazepines potentiate the action of GABA, the primary inhibitory neurotransmitter in the CNS. They do this by binding to a site on GABA$_A$ receptors, increasing their affinity for GABA. This results in an increased opening frequency of these ligand-gated Cl$^-$ channels, thus potentiating the effect of GABA release in terms of inhibitory effects on the postsynaptic cell (see Fig. 8.4).

Indications—Benzodiazepines are used clinically in the short-term relief of severe anxiety and severe insomnia, preoperative sedation (e.g. midazolam), status epilepticus (e.g. lorazepam) and acute alcohol withdrawal (e.g. chlordiazepoxide).

Route of administration—Oral is the usual route. Intravenous, intramuscular and rectal preparations are also available.

Contraindications—Benzodiazepines should not be given to people with lung disease, and they have additive or synergistic effects with other central depressants such as alcohol, barbiturates and H1-receptor antagonists.

Adverse effects—Benzodiazepines have several adverse effects.

- Drowsiness, ataxia and reduced psychomotor performance are common; therefore care is necessary when driving or operating machinery.
- Dependence becomes apparent after 4 to 6 weeks and is both physical and psychological. The withdrawal syndrome (in 30% of patients) comprises rebound anxiety and insomnia, tremulousness and twitching.

Although in overdose, benzodiazepines alone are relatively safe when compared with other sedatives, such as barbiturates. If benzodiazepines are taken in combination with alcohol, the CNS-depressant effects are potentiated, and fatal respiratory depression can result. Treatment of a benzodiazepine-only overdose is a benzodiazepine antagonist such as flumazenil.

Therapeutic notes—Benzodiazepines are active orally, and they differ mainly with respect to their duration of action (Table 8.2). Short-acting agents (e.g. lorazepam and

Table 8.2 Approximate elimination half-lives of the benzodiazepines and their common uses

Benzodiazepine	Approximate half-life (hours)	Commonly used as
Midazolam	2–4	Anaesthesia Sedative
Temazepam	8–12	Sleeping pill Anxiolytic
Lormetazepam	10	Sleeping pill Anxiolytic
Lorazepam	12	Sleeping pill Anticonvulsant
Nitrazepam	24	Anxiolytic
Diazepam	32	Anticonvulsant Sedative

temazepam) are metabolized to inactive compounds, and these are used mainly as sleeping pills because of the relative lack of "hangover" effects in the morning. Some long-acting agents (e.g. diazepam) are converted to long-lasting active metabolites with a half-life longer than the administered parent drug. With others (e.g. nitrazepam), it is the parent drug itself that is metabolized slowly. Such drugs are more suitable for an anxiolytic effect maintained all day long, or when early morning waking is the problem. Benzodiazepines, in general, are used for acute anxiety, particularly for patients with panic disorders. Diazepam and lorazepam are often used in the acute treatment of status epilepticus.

CLINICAL NOTE

Patients with insomnia should be advised about sleep hygiene (e.g. limiting caffeine intake, avoid napping during the day, regular exercise). In addition to medical therapy, patients should be referred to psychological services for cognitive behavioural therapy.

Nonbenzodiazepine hypnotics

Zopiclone, zolpidem and zaleplon are the newer-generation hypnotics that have a short duration of action with little or no hangover effect. Although these drugs are not benzodiazepines, they act in a comparable manner to benzodiazepines on the $GABA_A$ receptor, although not at exactly the same sites. They are an effective short-term treatment for insomnia.

Anxiolytic drugs acting at serotonergic receptors

The serotonergic theory of anxiety suggests that serotonergic transmission is involved in anxiety because, in general, stimulation of this system causes anxiety whereas a reduction in serotonergic neuronal activity reduces anxiety.

The serotonergic theory prompted the development of anxiolytic drugs that act to moderate serotonergic neurotransmission while not causing sedation and incoordination.

Serotonergic agonists

Buspirone is a serotonergic ($5-HT_{1A}$) agonist.

Mechanism of action—In the raphe nucleus, the dendrites of serotonergic neurones possess inhibitory presynaptic autoreceptors of the $5-HT_{1A}$ subtype that, when stimulated, decrease the firing of 5-HT neurones. This class of anxiolytic agents called the azapirones are thought to reduce 5-HT transmission by acting as partial agonists at these $5-HT_{1A}$ receptors. Buspirone is an example.

Route of administration—Oral.

Indications—Buspirone is indicated for the short-term relief of generalized anxiety disorder. It is less effective in the management of severe anxiety states or panic attacks.

Contraindications—$5-HT_{1A}$ agonists should not be used in people with epilepsy.

Adverse effects—The adverse effects of $5-HT_{1A}$ agonists include nervousness, dizziness, headache and light headedness.

In contrast to benzodiazepines, buspirone does not cause significant sedation or cognitive impairment, and it carries only a minimal risk of dependence and withdrawal. It does not potentiate the effects of alcohol.

Therapeutic notes—The anxiolytic effect of buspirone gradually evolves over 1 to 3 weeks. Buspirone does not act in the same way as benzodiazepines; when switching, gradually reduce the benzodiazepine.

Beta-adrenoceptor blockers

Beta-adrenoceptor blockers or beta-blockers, for example, propranolol, can be very effective in alleviating the somatic manifestations of anxiety caused by marked sympathetic arousal, such as palpitations, tremor, sweating and diarrhoea.

Mechanism of action—Beta-blockers act as antagonists at beta-adrenoceptors so that excessive catecholamine release does not produce the sympathetic responses of tachycardia, sweating, and so on. Beta-blockers are also used in the treatment of cardiovascular disease (see Chapter 4).

Route of administration—Oral.

Indications—Beta-blockers are indicated in patients with predominantly somatic symptoms; this, in turn, may prevent the onset of worry and fear. Patients with predominantly psychological symptoms may obtain no benefit. Beta-blockers can be useful in patients with social phobias and to reduce performance anxiety in musicians, for whom fine motor control may be critical.

Contraindications—Beta-blockers should not be used in people with asthma.

Adverse effects—Beta-blockers can cause bradycardia, heart failure, bronchospasm and peripheral vasoconstriction.

HINTS AND TIPS

An understanding of the $GABA_A$/Cl⁻ channel complex is central to the mechanism of action of several classes of hypnotic/anxiolytic drugs. You should be aware of what these are.

Miscellaneous agents

A number of miscellaneous hypnotic agents have been used historically and are still prescribed under certain circumstances.

Chloral hydrate—Chloral hydrate is metabolized to trichloroethanol, which is an effective hypnotic. It is cheap but causes gastric irritation and there is no convincing evidence that it has any advantage over the newer benzodiazepines.

Chloral hydrate and its derivatives were previously popular hypnotics for children. Current thinking does not justify the use of hypnotics in children, and these drugs now have very limited uses.

Clomethiazole (chlormethiazole)—Clomethiazole has been used in the treatment of insomnia in elderly people because it does not cause the hangover effect. Similarly, it was used in the management of acute alcohol withdrawal, but this has been replaced by the benzodiazepine, chlordiazepoxide. In essence, this drug has been superseded and is very rarely prescribed.

Antidepressants—If the underlying cause of insomnia is associated with depression, or particularly in depressed patients exhibiting anxiety and agitation, then tricyclic antidepressants (TCAs) with sedative actions (p. 122), for example, amitriptyline, may be useful, because they act as hypnotics when given at bedtime. Alternatively, selective serotonin reuptake inhibitors (SSRIs; p. 122) may correct the mood disorder and lessen the symptoms of anxiety or insomnia.

Sedative H1-receptor antagonists (antihistamines)—The older H1-receptor antagonists, for example, diphenhydramine and promethazine, also have muscarinic receptor antagonist actions and cross the blood–brain barrier, commonly causing drowsiness and psychomotor impairment.

Proprietary brands of diphenhydramine are available over the counter to relieve temporary sleep disturbances because these drugs are relatively safe. However, promethazine has a long half-life and may result in a hangover effect.

Melatonin—Melatonin is an agonist at melatonin (MT1) receptors. Prolonged-release melatonin improves sleep onset and quality in patients aged over 55 years with persistent insomnia. It is also used in children with autism who have insomnia.

CLINICAL NOTE

Elderly people are at significant risk of falls and confusion as a result of taking hypnotics. They should, therefore be prescribed very cautiously in this population. All patients prescribed hypnotics should be advised about the risks of driving (e.g. impaired judgement).

AFFECTIVE DISORDERS

Affective disorders involve a disturbance of mood (cognitive/emotional symptoms) associated with changes in behaviour, energy, appetite and sleep (biological symptoms). Affective disorders can be thought of as pathological extremes of the normal continuum of human moods, from extreme excitement and elation (mania) to severe depressive states.

There are two types of affective disorder: unipolar affective disorders and bipolar affective disorders.

Monoamine theory of depression

The aetiology of major depressive disorders is not clear. Genetic, environmental and neurochemical influences have all been examined as possible aetiological factors.

The most widely accepted neurochemical explanation of endogenous depression involves the monoamines (noradrenaline; serotonin [5-HT]; dopamine). The original hypothesis of depression, "the monoamine theory", stated that depression resulted from a functional deficit of these transmitter amines, whereas conversely mania was caused by an excess.

The monoamine theory explains why:

- Drugs that deplete monoamines are depressant, for example, reserpine and methyldopa.
- A wide range of drugs that increase the functional availability of monoamine neurotransmitters improve mood in depressed patients, for example, TCAs and MAO inhibitors.
- The concentration of monoamines and their metabolites is reduced in the cerebrospinal fluid (CSF) of depressed patients.
- In some postmortem studies, the most consistent finding is an elevation in cortical 5-HT$_2$ binding.

However, the monoamine theory cannot explain why:

- A number of compounds that increase the functional availability of monoamines, for example, amphetamines, cocaine and L-dopa, have no effect on the mood of depressed patients.
- Some older, atypical antidepressants, for example, iprindole, worked without manipulating monoaminergic systems.
- There is a "therapeutic delay" of 2 weeks between the full neurochemical effects of antidepressants and the start of their therapeutic effect.

It is unlikely, therefore, that monoamine mechanisms alone are responsible for the symptoms of depression. Other systems that may be involved in depression include the following.

- The GABA system
- The neuropeptide systems, particularly vasopressin and the endogenous opiates
- Secondary-messenger systems also appear to have a crucial role in some treatments.

Unipolar affective disorders

A common unipolar affective disorder is depression, which is characterized by low mood, malaise, despair, guilt, apathy, indecisiveness, low energy and fatigue, changes in sleeping pattern, loss of appetite and suicidal thoughts. Attempts have been made to classify types of depression as either "reactive" or "endogenous" in origin.

Reactive depression is where there is a clear psychological cause, for example, bereavement. It involves less-severe symptoms and less likelihood of biological disturbance. It affects 3% to 10% of the population, with the incidence increasing with age, and it is more common in females.

Endogenous depression is where there is no clear cause and more severe symptoms, for example, suicidal thoughts, and a greater likelihood of biological disturbance, for example, insomnia, anorexia. Some 5% of the population experiences an episode of depression, and severe depression requiring treatment affects 1 in 4 women and 1 in 10 men. However, antidepressants are not recommended for mild depression and are generally prescribed only for moderate to severe depression.

The distinction between reactive and endogenous depression is of importance because there is some evidence that depressions with endogenous features tend to respond better to drug therapy.

Treatment of unipolar depressive disorders

The major classes of drug that are used to treat depression, and their mechanisms of action, are summarized in Table 8.3.

Tricyclic antidepressants and related drugs

Examples of TCAs and related drugs include amitriptyline, imipramine, dosulepin (dothiepin) and lofepramine.

Mechanism of action—TCAs act by blocking 5-HT and noradrenaline uptake into the presynaptic terminal from the synaptic cleft (Fig. 8.5). They also have a certain affinity for H_1 and muscarinic receptors, and for α_1- and α_2-receptors.

Contraindications—TCAs and related drugs should not be used in the following situations.

- Recent myocardial infarction or arrhythmias (especially heart block) because TCAs increase the risk of conduction abnormalities.
- Manic phase
- Severe liver disease
- Epilepsy, where TCAs lower the seizure threshold
- Patients taking other anticholinergic drugs, alcohol and adrenaline alongside TCAs potentiate the effects of these.

Lidocaine is contraindicated in combination with TCAs, owing to a potentially fatal drug interaction.

Adverse effects—Although TCAs are an effective therapy for depression, their adverse effects can reduce patient compliance and acceptability. Side effects include the following.

- Muscarinic blocking effects such as a dry mouth, blurred vision, constipation
- α-Adrenergic blocking effects causing postural hypotension
- Noradrenaline uptake block in the heart, increasing the risk of arrhythmias

- Histamine-blocking effects leading to sedation
- Weight gain

TCAs are relatively dangerous in overdose. Patients present with confusion, mania, and potentially fatal arrhythmias caused by the cardiotoxic nature of the drug.

Therapeutic notes—No individual TCA has superior antidepressant activity, and the choice of drug is usually determined by the most acceptable or desired side effects. For example, drugs with sedative actions, such as amitriptyline or trimipramine, are the TCAs of choice for patients in agitated or anxious states. The most recent TCA, lofepramine, causes fewer antimuscarinic side effects and is less dangerous if taken in overdose.

Therapeutic effects take 2 to 3 weeks to develop. TCA-related antidepressants should be withdrawn slowly.

Note that amitriptyline is sometimes used in lower doses for the treatment of neuropathic pain.

Selective serotonin reuptake inhibitors

SSRIs are the most recently introduced class of antidepressant agent. Fluoxetine (Prozac) is an SSRI. Other examples include citalopram, fluvoxamine, paroxetine and sertraline.

Mechanism of action—SSRIs act with a high specificity for potent inhibition of serotonin reuptake into nerve terminals from the synaptic cleft, while having only minimal effects on noradrenaline uptake (see Fig. 8.5). They block serotonin transporters, which belong to a class of Na^+/Cl^--coupled transporters.

Contraindications—SSRIs should not be used with MAO inhibitors because the combination can cause a potentially fatal serotonergic syndrome of hyperthermia and cardiovascular collapse.

Adverse effects—The side-effect profile of SSRIs is much better than that of TCAs and MAO inhibitors because there are no amine interactions, anticholinergic actions, adrenergic blockade or toxic effects in overdose. Adverse effects, however, caused by their effect on serotonergic nerves

Table 8.3 Major classes of antidepressant drugs and their mechanisms of action

Class of antidepressant drug	Examples	Mode of action
Tricyclic antidepressants (TCAs)	Amitriptyline imipramine lofepramine	Nonspecific blockers of monoamine uptake
Selective serotonin reuptake inhibitors (SSRIs)	Fluoxetine paroxetine sertraline	Selective blockers of 5-HT reuptake
Serotonin-noradrenaline reuptake inhibitors (SNRIs)	Venlafaxine	Selective blockers of 5-HT and noradrenaline uptake
Monoamine oxidase inhibitors (MAOIs)	Phenelzine Tranylcypromine	Noncompetitive, nonselective irreversible blockers of MAO_A and MAO_B
Reversible inhibitors of MAO_A (RIMAs)	Moclobemide	Reversibly inhibit MAO_A selectively
Atypical	Reboxetine mirtazapine	Act by various mechanisms that are poorly understood

5-HT, 5-Hydroxytryptamine; MAO, monoamine oxidase.

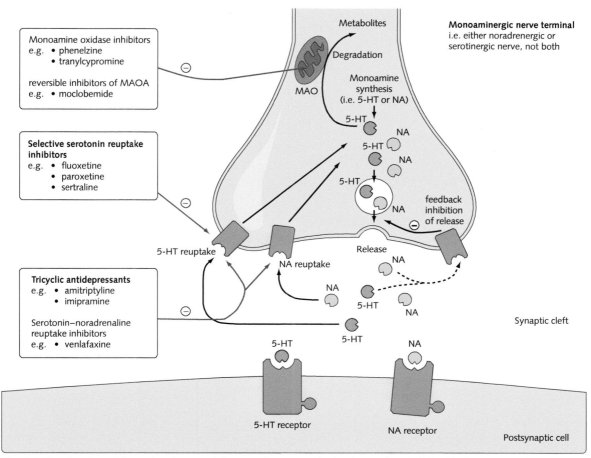

Fig. 8.5 Site of action of the major classes of drug used to treat unipolar depression. *5-HT*, 5-Hydroxytryptamine (serotonin); *MAO*, monoamine oxidase; *NA*, noradrenaline.

throughout the body, include nausea, diarrhoea, insomnia, anxiety and agitation. Sexual dysfunction is sometimes a problem.

Therapeutic notes—SSRIs have a similar efficacy to that of TCAs. It is their clinical advantages and lack of side effects that have led to their popularity. SSRIs are now the most widely prescribed antidepressants because they are first-line treatment for depression.

Serotonin-noradrenaline reuptake inhibitors

Venlafaxine is the most commonly used serotonin-noradrenaline reuptake inhibitor (SNRI)-type antidepressant.

Mechanism of action—SNRIs cause potentiation of neurotransmitter activity in the CNS, by blocking the norepinephrine and serotonin reuptake transporter (see Fig. 8.5).

Contraindications—The drug interactions of SNRIs are much like those of SSRIs; however, extra care must be taken with hypertensive patients as venlafaxine raises blood pressure.

Adverse effects—The adverse effects of SNRIs are similar to those of SSRIs, but they occur with lower frequency.

Therapeutic notes—The pharmacological effects of venlafaxine are similar to those of the TCAs, but adverse effects are reduced because it has little affinity for cholinergic and histaminergic receptors or α-adrenoceptors.

CLINICAL NOTE

Mild depression can be managed with cognitive behavioural therapies (CBT). However effective management of moderate to severe depression often requires CBT and a combination of antidepressants. In severe, life-threatening cases, electroconvulsive therapy may be used to gain fast and short-term improvement of severe symptoms when other treatment options have failed.

Monoamine oxidase inhibitors

Examples of irreversible MAO inhibitors include phenelzine, tranylcypromine and isocarboxazid, and an example of a reversible inhibitor of MAO_A (RIMAs) is moclobemide.

Mechanism of action—MAO inhibitors block the action of MAO_A and MAO_B, which are neuronal enzymes that metabolize the monoamines (noradrenaline, 5-HT and dopamine) (see Fig. 8.5). MAO has two main isoforms, MAO_A and MAO_B. Inhibition of the MAO_A form correlates best with antidepressant activity. Both nonselective irreversible blockers of MAO_A and MAO_B, and drugs that reversibly inhibit MAO_A are available.

Adverse effects—Dietary interactions may occur, such as the "cheese reaction". MAO in the gut wall and liver normally breaks down ingested tyramine. When the enzyme is inhibited, tyramine reaches the circulation, and this causes the release of noradrenaline from sympathetic nerve terminals; this can lead to a severe and potentially fatal rise in blood pressure. Patients on MAO inhibitors must, therefore avoid foods rich in tyramine, which include cheese, game and alcoholic drinks. Preparations containing sympathomimetic amines (e.g. cough mixtures and nasal decongestants) should also be avoided. MAO inhibitors are not specific, and they reduce the metabolism of barbiturates, opioids and alcohol. Side effects include CNS stimulation causing excitement and tremor, sympathetic blockade causing postural hypotension, and muscarinic blockade causing a dry mouth and blurred vision. Phenelzine can be hepatotoxic.

Therapeutic notes—Response to treatment may be delayed for 3 weeks or more. Patients with depression or phobias with atypical, hypochondriac or hysterical features are said to respond best to MAO inhibitors. MAO inhibitors are largely reserved for depression refractory to other antidepressants because of the dietary and drug interactions outlined earlier.

Atypical antidepressants

Examples of atypical antidepressants include reboxetine, mirtazapine and tryptophan.

Mechanism of action—Reboxetine is a selective inhibitor of noradrenaline reuptake, increasing the concentration of this neurotransmitter in the synaptic cleft. Mirtazapine has α_2-adrenoceptor-blocking activity, which, by acting on inhibitory α_2-autoreceptors on central noradrenergic nerve endings, may increase the amount of noradrenaline in the synaptic cleft. Tryptophan is an amino acid precursor for serotonin.

Contraindications—The contraindications for atypical antidepressants are similar to those for TCAs.

Adverse effects—Atypical antidepressants generally cause less autonomic side effects and are less dangerous in overdose, owing to their lower cardiotoxicity compared with TCAs. Mirtazapine may cause agranulocytosis. Tryptophan is associated with eosinophilic myalgia syndrome.

Therapeutic notes—Mirtazapine is a sedative, and it is, therefore used in depression when a degree of sedation is desirable.

Neither reboxetine nor mirtazapine are currently first-line drugs for the treatment of depression. Tryptophan requires specialist supervision because of the stated adverse effect.

Bipolar affective disorder

Bipolar affective disorder presents with mood and behaviour oscillating between depression and mania, and it is, previously known as manic-depressive disorder.

Bipolar affective disorder develops earlier in life than unipolar depressive disorders, and it tends to be inherited. It affects 2% of the population, and it can have associated elements of psychotic phenomena.

Treatment of bipolar affective disorders

Bipolar affective disorder is treated with a combination of mood stabilizers and antidepressants, and sometimes antipsychotics. Mood stabilizers include lithium and carbamazepine.

Lithium

Lithium is administered as lithium carbonate, and it is the most widely used mood stabilizer, with antimanic and antidepressant activity.

Mechanism of action—The mechanism of action of lithium is unclear, but it probably involves modulation of secondary-messenger pathways of cyclic adenosine monophosphate and inositol triphosphate. It is known that lithium inhibits the pathway for recapturing inositol for the resynthesis of polyphosphoinositides. It may exert its effect by reducing the concentrations of lipids important in signal transduction in neurones in the brain.

Indications—Lithium salts are mainly used in the prophylaxis and treatment of bipolar affective disorder (usually second line), but also in the prophylaxis and treatment of acute mania, and in the prophylaxis of resistant recurrent depression.

Contraindications—Some drugs may interact causing a rise in plasma lithium concentration and so should be avoided. Such drugs include antipsychotics, nonsteroidal antiinflammatory drugs (NSAIDs), diuretics and cardioactive drugs. Lithium is excreted via the kidney, and caution should be used in patients with renal impairment.

Adverse effects—Lithium has a long plasma half-life and a narrow therapeutic window; therefore side effects are common and plasma concentration monitoring is essential. Early side effects include thirst, nausea, diarrhoea, tremor and polyuria; late side effects include weight gain, oedema, acne, nephrogenic diabetes insipidus and hypothyroidism. Toxicity/overdose (serum level > 2–3 mmol/L) effects include vomiting, diarrhoea, tremor, ataxia, confusion and coma.

Therapeutic notes—Careful monitoring after initiation of treatment is essential.

Carbamazepine

Carbamazepine is as effective as lithium in the prophylaxis of bipolar affective disorder and acute mania, particularly in rapidly alternating bipolar affective disorder. However, it is most commonly prescribed as an anticonvulsant (see later).

Mechanism of action—Carbamazepine is a GABA agonist, and this may be the basis of its antimanic properties. The relevance of its effect in stabilising neuronal sodium and calcium channels is unclear.

Adverse effects—Drowsiness, diplopia, nausea, ataxia, rashes and headache; blood disorders such as agranulocytosis and leukopenia; and drug interactions with lithium, antipsychotics, TCAs and MAO inhibitors. Many other drugs can be affected by the effect of carbamazepine on inducing hepatic enzymes. Diplopia, ataxia, clonus, tremor and sedation are associated with acute carbamazepine toxicity.

Therapeutic notes—At the start of treatment with carbamazepine, plasma concentrations should be monitored to establish a maintenance dose.

PSYCHOTIC DISORDERS

Psychotic disorders are characterized by a mental state that is out of touch with reality, involving a variety of abnormalities of perception, thought and ideas.

Psychotic illnesses include the following.

- Schizophrenia
- Schizoaffective disorder
- Delusional disorders
- Some depressive and manic illnesses.

Neuroleptics, or antipsychotics, are drugs used in the treatment of psychotic disorders.

Schizophrenia

Epidemiology

Schizophrenia characteristically develops in people aged 15 to 45 years; it has a relatively stable cross-cultural incidence affecting 1% of the population, with a greater proportion being male.

Symptoms and signs

Schizophrenia is a psychotic illness characterized by multiple symptoms affecting thought, perceptions, emotion and volition.

Symptoms fall into two groups (positive and negative) that may have different underlying causes.

Positive symptoms include:

- Delusions: false personal beliefs held with absolute conviction
- Hallucinations: false perceptions in the absence of a real external stimulus; most commonly, these are auditory (hearing voices) and occur in 60% to 70% of patients with schizophrenia, but they can be visual, tactile or olfactory.
- Thought alienation and disordered thought: belief that one's thoughts are under the control of an outside agency (e.g. aliens, MI5). This type of belief is common, and thought processes are often incomprehensible.

Negative symptoms include:

- Poverty of speech: restriction in the amount of spontaneous speech
- Flattening of affect: loss of normal experience and expression of emotion
- Social withdrawal
- Anhedonia: inability to experience pleasure
- Apathy: reduced drive, energy, and interest
- Attention deficit: inattentiveness at work or at home

The distinction between the positive and negative symptoms found in schizophrenia is of importance because neuroleptic drugs tend to have the most effect on positive symptoms, whereas negative symptoms are fairly refractory to treatment and carry a worse prognosis.

Theories of schizophrenia

The cause of schizophrenia remains mysterious. Any theory of the cause of schizophrenia must take into account the strong, although not invariable, hereditary tendency (50% concurrence in monozygotic twins), as well as the environmental factors known to predispose towards its development.

Many hypotheses have been suggested to explain the manifestations of schizophrenia at the level of neurotransmitters in the brain. The potential role of excessive dopaminergic activity, in particular, has attracted considerable attention. Evidence for this theory includes the following.

- Most antipsychotic drugs block dopamine receptors, the clinical dose being proportional to the ability to block D_2 receptors.
- Single photon emission computed tomography (SPECT) ligand scans show that there are increased D_2 receptors in the nucleus accumbens of patients with schizophrenia.
- Psychotic symptoms can be induced by drugs that increase dopaminergic activity, (e.g. antiparkinsonian agents).

However, there is much evidence that the dopaminergic theory fails to explain. Current research indicates a likely role for other neurotransmitters in schizophrenia, including 5-HT, GABA and glutamate. Although the dopamine theory cannot explain many of the features and findings in schizophrenia, most current pharmacological treatment (typical neuroleptics) is aimed at dopaminergic transmission (Table 8.4).

Table 8.4 Classes of dopamine receptor

Type	2nd messenger + cellular effects	Location in CNS and postulated function
D_1	cAMP increase	Mainly postsynaptic inhibition Functions unclear
D_2	cAMP decrease K^+ conductance up Ca^{2+} conductance down	Mainly presynaptic inhibition of dopamine synthesis/release in nigrostriatal, mesolimbic and tuberoinfundibular systems Affinity of neuroleptics for D_2 receptors correlates with antipsychotic potency
D_3	Unknown	Localized mainly in limbic and cortical structures concerned with cognitive functions and emotional behaviour Not clear whether antipsychotic effects of neuroleptics are mediated by the D_3 type
D_4	Unknown	Similar to D_3 type; clozapine has particular affinity for D_4 receptors

cAMP, Cyclic adenosine monophosphate; CNS, central nervous system.

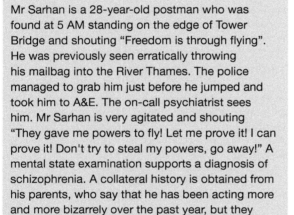

CLINICAL NOTE

Mr Sarhan is a 28-year-old postman who was found at 5 AM standing on the edge of Tower Bridge and shouting "Freedom is through flying". He was previously seen erratically throwing his mailbag into the River Thames. The police managed to grab him just before he jumped and took him to A&E. The on-call psychiatrist sees him. Mr Sarhan is very agitated and shouting "They gave me powers to fly! Let me prove it! I can prove it! Don't try to steal my powers, go away!" A mental state examination supports a diagnosis of schizophrenia. A collateral history is obtained from his parents, who say that he has been acting more and more bizarrely over the past year, but they just thought it was caused by stress. Shortly after admission, he began shouting abuse and pushing past staff with the intention of leaving despite their discouragement. He was rapidly tranquillized using haloperidol and sectioned under section 2 of the Mental Health Act.

Treatment of schizophrenia

The treatment of schizophrenia and all other psychotic illnesses involves the use of antipsychotic medication, the neuroleptic drugs. Neuroleptic drugs produce a general improvement in all the acute positive symptoms of schizophrenia, but it is less clear how effective they are in the treatment of chronic schizophrenia and negative symptoms.

Mechanism of action—Antipsychotic drugs have a variety of structures and fall into various classes (Tables 8.4 and 8.5). There is a strong correlation between clinical potency and affinity for D_2 receptors among the typical neuroleptics.

Neuroleptics take days or weeks to work, suggesting that secondary effects (e.g. increases in the number of D_2 receptors in limbic structures) may be more important than a direct effect of D_2 receptor block.

Most neuroleptics also block other monoamine receptors, and this is often the cause of some of the side effects of these drugs.

The distinction between typical and atypical groups is not clearly defined, but it rests partly on the incidence of extrapyramidal motor side effects, and partly on receptor specificity. Atypical neuroleptics are less prone to producing motor disorders than other drugs, and they tend to have different pharmacological profiles with respect to dopamine and other receptor specificity.

Route of administration—All the neuroleptic drugs can be given orally, although some of the typical drugs can be given by the intramuscular route, which prolongs their release and aids drug compliance.

Typical neuroleptics

Phenothiazines

This class of compounds is subdivided into three groups by the type of side chain attached to the pharmacophore (the phenothiazine ring) (see Table 8.5). Side-effect patterns vary with the different side chains.

- Propylamine side chains: for example, in chlorpromazine, produce strong sedation, a moderate muscarinic block, and moderate motor disturbance. Indicated for violent patients, owing to their sedative effect.
- Piperidine side chains: for example, in thioridazine, produce moderate sedation, strong muscarinic block and low motor disturbance. Favoured for use in elderly patients.
- Piperazine side chains: for example, in fluphenazine, produce low sedation, low muscarinic block and strong motor disturbance. Contraindicated for use in elderly patients, owing to the motor effects.

Table 8.5 Classes of neuroleptic drugs

Class	Chemical classification	Examples

Typical antipsychotics	Phenothiazines:
	    propylamine side chains
	    piperidine side chains
	    piperazine side chains
	Butyrophenones
	Thioxanthines
		Chlorpromazine
		Thioridazine
		Fluphenazine
		Haloperidol
		Flupentixol

Atypical antipsychotics	Dibenzodiazepines
	Dopamine/5-HT blockers:
	    diphenylbutylpiperidines
	    substituted benzamides
	    benzixasoles
		Clozapine,
		olanzapine
		Pimozide
		Sulpiride
		Risperidone

5-HT, 5-Hydroxytryptamine

Butyrophenones and thioxanthenes

The butyrophenone and thioxanthene groups of compounds have the same profile of low sedation, low muscarinic block and high incidence of motor disturbance.

An example of a butyrophenone compound is haloperidol; flupentixol is an example of the thioxanthenes.

Atypical neuroleptics

Dibenzodiazepines

Dibenzodiazepines such as clozapine and olanzapine have a low affinity for the D_2 receptor and a higher affinity for D_1 and D_4 receptors.

Indications—Olanzapine is recommended as first-line treatment of patients with schizophrenia. Clozapine is prescribed in refractory cases given the 1% risk of potentially fatal neutropenia.

Adverse effects—Clozapine has a low incidence of adverse motor effects because of its low affinity for the D_2 receptor. Side effects of dibenzodiazepines include hypersalivation, sedation, weight gain, tachycardia and hypotension.

Therapeutic notes—Olanzapine is similar to clozapine, although it carries less risk of agranulocytosis.

HINTS AND TIPS

Antipsychotic medications are used in the treatment of acute mania and schizophrenia. Olanzapine, quetiapine, risperidone and haloperidol are commonly prescribed. If a combination of two antipsychotics is ineffective or not tolerated, then lithium is added. In cases where lithium is inappropriate, sodium valproate is sometimes used.

Dopamine/5-HT blockers

Examples of dopamine/5-HT blockers include the diphenylbutylpiperidines (e.g. pimozide and sulpiride) and the benzoxazoles (e.g. risperidone).

Sulpiride, and the newer agent pimozide show high selectivity for D_2 receptors compared with D_1 or other neurotransmitter receptors. Both drugs are effective in treating schizophrenia but sulpiride is claimed to have less tendency to cause adverse motor effects. Pimozide appears to be similar to conventional neuroleptic agents, but it has a longer duration of action, allowing once-daily medication.

Benzoxazoles such as risperidone show a high affinity for 5-HT receptors and a lower affinity for D_2 receptors. With this class of drugs, extrapyramidal motor side effects occur with less frequency than with "classic" neuroleptics.

Quetiapine fumarate is a dibenzothiazepine derivative that acts as an antagonist at the D_1, D_2, 5-HT_{1A} and 5-HT_2 receptors.

Aripiprazole appears to mediate its antipsychotic effects primarily by partial agonism at the D_2 receptor. It is also a partial agonist at 5-HT_{1A} receptors, and similar to the other atypical antipsychotics, aripiprazole displays an antagonist profile at the 5-HT_{2A} receptor, as well as a moderate affinity for histamine and α-adrenergic receptors.

Zotepine has good efficacy against negative symptoms of schizophrenia. This is thought to be caused by its noradrenaline reuptake inhibition. It also has a high affinity for the dopamine D_1 and D_2 receptors. It also affects the 5-HT_{2A}, 5-HT_{2C}, 5-HT_6 and 5-HT_7 receptors.

Adverse effects of neuroleptics

Neuroleptic drugs cause a variety of adverse effects (Box 8.1). The majority of the unwanted effects of neuroleptics can be inferred from their pharmacological actions, such as the disruption of dopaminergic pathways (the major action of most neuroleptics) and the blockade of monoamine and other receptors, including muscarinic receptors, α-adrenoceptors and histamine receptors.

BOX 8.1   ADVERSE EFFECTS OF THE NEUROLEPTICS

- Acute neurological effects: acute dystonia, akathisia, parkinsonism
- Chronic neurological effects: tardive dyskinesia, tardive dystonia
- Neuroendocrine effects: amenorrhoea, galactorrhoea, infertility
- Idiosyncratic: neuroleptic malignant syndrome
- Anticholinergic: dry mouth, blurred vision, constipation, urinary retention, ejaculatory failure
- Antihistaminergic: sedation
- Antiadrenergic: hypotension, arrhythmia
- Miscellaneous: photosensitivity, heat sensitivity, cholestatic jaundice, retinal pigmentation

(Modified from Page et al. 2006.)

In addition, individual drugs may cause immunological reactions or have their own characteristic side-effect profile.

Adverse effects on the dopaminergic pathways

There are three main dopaminergic pathways in the brain (Fig. 8.6).

- Mesolimbic and/or mesocortical dopamine pathways running from groups of cells in the midbrain to the nucleus accumbens and amygdala. This pathway affects thoughts and motivation.
- Nigrostriatal dopamine pathways running from the midbrain to the caudate nuclei. This pathway is important in smooth motor control.
- Tuberoinfundibular neurones running from the hypothalamus to the pituitary gland, the secretions of which they regulate.

Antagonism of dopamine receptors leads to interference with the normal functioning of these pathways, bringing about unwanted side effects, as well as the desired antipsychotic effect. This antagonism is the cause of the most serious side effects associated with neuroleptic use.

- Psychological effects because of D_2 receptor blockade of the mesolimbic/mesocortical pathway.
- Movement disorders because of D_2 receptor blockade of the nigrostriatal pathways.
- Neuroendocrine disorders because of D_2 receptor blockade of the tuberoinfundibular pathway.

Neuroleptics are thought to exert their antipsychotic effects by antagonism of dopaminergic nerves in the mesolimbic mesocortical pathway. However, as a side effect of mesolimbic and mesocortical dopaminergic inhibition, sedation and impaired performance are common.

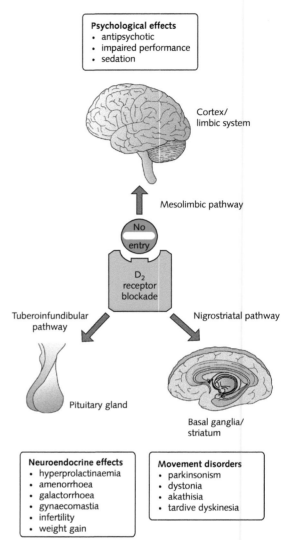

Psychological effects
- antipsychotic
- impaired performance
- sedation

Cortex/limbic system

Mesolimbic pathway

No entry

D_2 receptor blockade

Tuberoinfundibular pathway

Nigrostriatal pathway

Pituitary gland

Basal ganglia/striatum

Neuroendocrine effects
- hyperprolactinaemia
- amenorrhoea
- galactorrhoea
- gynaecomastia
- infertility
- weight gain

Movement disorders
- parkinsonism
- dystonia
- akathisia
- tardive dyskinesia

Fig. 8.6 Effect of D_2 dopamine receptor blockade on the dopaminergic pathways in the brain.

Blocking of dopamine receptors in the basal ganglia (corpus striatum) frequently results in distressing and disabling movement disorders. Two main types of movement disorder occur. Acute reversible parkinsonian-like symptoms (tremor, rigidity and akinesia) are treated by dose reduction, anticholinergic drugs or switching to an atypical neuroleptic. Slowly developing tardive dyskinesia, often irreversible, and manifesting as involuntary movements of the face, trunk and limbs, appear months or years after the start of neuroleptic treatment. It may be a result of proliferation or sensitization of dopamine receptors. Incidence is unpredictable, and it affects approximately 20% of long-term users of neuroleptics. Treatment is generally unsuccessful. The newer atypical neuroleptics may be less likely to induce tardive dyskinesia.

By reducing the negative feedback on the anterior pituitary, oversecretion of prolactin can result (hyperprolactinaemia). This can lead to gynaecomastia, galactorrhoea, menstrual irregularities, impotence and weight gain in some patients (see Fig. 8.6).

Adverse effects from nonselective receptor blockade

The adverse effects of neuroleptics from nonselective receptor blockade include the following.

- Anticholinergic effects caused by muscarinic-receptor antagonism, such as dry mouth, urinary retention, constipation, blurred vision, and so on.
- Adverse effects caused by α-adrenoceptor antagonism. Many neuroleptics have the capacity to block α-adrenoceptors and cause postural hypotension.
- Adverse effects caused by antagonism of central histamine H_1 receptors may contribute to sedation.

Adverse effects caused by individual drugs or immune reactions

The neuroleptic drug clozapine can cause neutropenia as a result of toxic bone marrow suppression, whereas pimozide can cause sudden death secondary to cardiac arrhythmia.

Immune reactions to neuroleptic drugs can include dermatitis, rashes, photosensitivity and urticaria. Such reactions are more common with the phenothiazines, which can also cause deposits in the cornea and lens.

Neuroleptic malignant syndrome

This is the most lethal adverse effect of neuroleptic use. It is an idiosyncratic reaction of unknown pathophysiology. Symptoms include fever, extrapyramidal motor disturbance, muscle rigidity and coma. Urgent treatment is indicated.

HINTS AND TIPS

Neuroleptics have many side effects, some related to their principal mechanism of action (dopamine receptor antagonism) and some unrelated to this. Learn these well because they are a popular examination topic.

Drugs used for attention deficit hyperactivity disorder

Amphetamines

Dexamphetamine is an example.

Mechanism of action—Amphetamines act by releasing monoamines (dopamine and noradrenaline) in the brain. The main central effects of amphetamine-like drugs are increased stamina, anorexia and insomnia.

Route of administration—Oral.

Indications—Used to treat attention deficit hyperactivity disorder (ADHD) in children. Occasionally used in the treatment of narcolepsy.

Contraindications—Moderate to severe hypertension, structural cardiac disease, hyperthyroidism.

Adverse effects—Gastrointestinal upset, palpitations and weight loss. Hallucinations, paranoia and aggressive behaviour can also occur if taken for a long time.

Methylphenidate

Methylphenidate is also given orally in the treatment of ADHD. It produces a profound and sustained elevation of extracellular noradrenaline and dopamine.

EPILEPSY

Epilepsy is a chronic disease, in which seizures result from the abnormal high-frequency discharge of a group of neurones, starting focally and spreading to a varying extent to affect other parts of the brain. According to the focus and spread of discharges, seizures may be classified in two ways.

- Partial (focal), which originate at a specific focus and do not spread to involve other cortical areas.
- Generalized, which usually have a focus (often in the temporal lobe) and then spread to other areas.

Different epileptic syndromes can be classified on the basis of seizure type and pattern, with other clinical features (such as age of onset), anatomic location of focus, and aetiology taken into account.

Common types of epileptic syndrome

Epileptic syndromes result from either generalized seizures or focal seizures (Table 8.6).

Generalized seizures involve loss of consciousness, and it may be convulsive or nonconvulsive.

- Tonic-clonic (grand-mal seizures): convulsive generalized seizures characterized by periods of tonic muscle rigidity followed later by jerking of the body (clonus).

Table 8.6 Classification of common epileptic syndromes

Partial (local, focal) seizures	Generalized seizures
Psychomotor (temporal lobe) epilepsy	Tonic-clonic seizure or grand-mal epilepsy
Partial motor epilepsy	Absence seizure or petit-mal epilepsy

- Absence (petit-mal seizures): generalized seizures characterized by changes in consciousness lasting less than 10 seconds. They occur most commonly in children, where they can be confused with day-dreaming.

The effect on the body of focal seizures depends on the location of the abnormal signal focus: for example, involvement of the motor cortex will produce convulsions whereas involvement of the brainstem can produce unconsciousness. Psychomotor or temporal lobe epilepsy results from a partial seizure with cortical activity localized to the temporal lobe. Such seizures are characterized by features including impaired consciousness or confusion, amnesia, emotional instability, atypical behaviour and outbursts.

Partial motor seizures have their focus in cortical motor regions and they present with convulsive or tonic activity corresponding to the neurones involved, for example, the left arm.

Another type of epileptic syndrome is status epilepticus. This is a state in which seizures follow each other without consciousness being regained or if a seizure is prolonged. Status epilepticus constitutes a medical emergency because of the risk of respiratory arrest and hypoxia.

Causes of epilepsy

The aetiology of epilepsy is unknown in 60% to 70% of cases, but a family history is an important factor. Damage to the brain, for example, by tumours, head injury, infections or cerebrovascular accident, may subsequently cause epilepsy.

The neurochemical basis of the abnormal discharges in epilepsy is not known, but it may involve altered GABA metabolism.

HINTS AND TIPS

Remember that epilepsy is simply aberrant electrical activity spreading throughout an area of, or the whole of, the brain. Antiepileptic medications limit the propagation of this spread and inhibit the development of symptoms.

Treatment of epilepsy

Drugs used to treat epilepsy are termed antiepileptics; the term anticonvulsant is also used.

The aim of pharmacological treatment of epilepsy is to minimize the seizure activity/frequency, without producing adverse drug effects.

Mechanisms of action of antiepileptics

Antiepileptic drugs act generically to inhibit the rapid, repetitive neuronal firing that characterizes seizures. There are three established mechanisms of action by which the antiepileptic drugs achieve this (Fig. 8.7).

Inhibition of ion channels involved in neuronal excitability

Drugs such as phenytoin, carbamazepine and valproate inhibit the "fast" sodium current. These drugs bind preferentially to inactivated (closed) sodium channels, preventing them from opening. The high-frequency repetitive depolarisation of neurones during a seizure increases the proportion of sodium channels in the inactivated state susceptible to the blockade. Eventually, sufficient sodium channels become blocked so that the fast neuronal sodium current is insufficient to cause a depolarization. Note that neuronal transmission at normal frequencies is relatively unaffected because a much smaller proportion of the sodium channels are in the inactivated state.

Absence seizures involve oscillatory neuronal activity between the thalamus and the cerebral cortex. This oscillation involves "T-type" calcium channels, which produce low-threshold spikes and consequently cause groups of cells to fire in bursts. Ethosuximide inhibits T-type low-threshold and reduces the fast-inactivating calcium current, dampening the thalamocortical oscillations that are critical in the generation of absence seizures.

Inhibition of excitatory transmission

Drugs that block excitatory amino acid receptors (NMDA antagonists) have been shown to be antiepileptic in animal models. Such drugs may prove useful in the clinical treatment of epilepsy in the future. Lamotrigine, one of the newer antiepileptic agents, inhibits the release of glutamate as one of its actions, and this may contribute to its antiepileptic activity.

Enhancement of GABA-mediated inhibition

This can take any of the following forms.

- Enhancement by direct GABA agonist properties, for example, by gabapentin, another of the newer antiepileptics, agent which has been designed to mimic GABA in the CNS.
- Potentiation of chloride currents through the $GABA_A$/ Cl^- channel complex, for example, by benzodiazepines and barbiturates. The increased postsynaptic inhibitory chloride current at $GABA_A$ receptors hyperpolarizes neurones and makes them refractory to excitation (see Table 8.1).
- Inhibition of GABA degradation in the CNS, for example, by vigabatrin, which is an irreversible inhibitor of GABA transaminase (GABAT), the enzyme normally responsible for the metabolism of GABA in the neurone. Inhibition of $GABA_T$, therefore leads to an increase in synaptic levels of GABA and so enhances GABA-mediated inhibition.

Antiepileptic drugs (anticonvulsants)

Antiepileptic drugs can be classified according to their mechanism of action (see Fig. 8.7), but in clinical practice, it is useful to think of the drugs according to their use (Table 8.7).

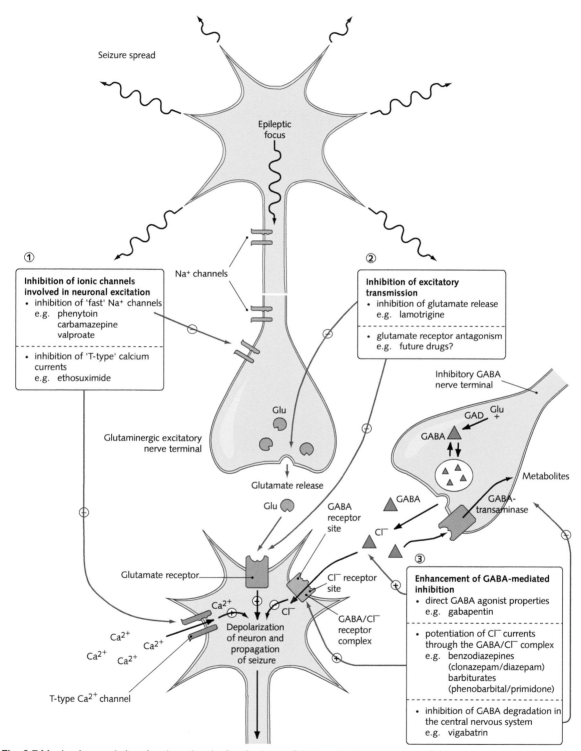

Fig. 8.7 Mechanism and site of action of antiepileptic drugs. *GABA*, γ-Aminobutyric acid; *GAD*, glutamic acid decarboxylase; *Glu*, glutamate.

Table 8.7 Drugs used for epilepsy classified by clinical use

Seizure type	Primary drugs	Secondary drugs
Partial and/or generalized tonic-clonic seizures	Sodium valproate Carbamazepine	Phenytoin Vigabatrin Gabapentin Lamotrigine Phenobarbital
Absence seizures	Ethosuximide Sodium valproate Lamotrigine	Phenobarbital
Status epilepticus	Lorazepam	Diazepam Clonazepam

Phenytoin

Mechanism of action—Phenytoin blocks use-dependent, voltage-gated sodium channels. Phenytoin reduces the spread of a seizure. However, it does not prevent the initiation of an epileptic discharge, but it does stop it spreading and causing overt clinical symptoms.

Route of administration—Oral, intravenous.

Indications—Phenytoin is indicated in all forms of epilepsy.

Contraindications—Phenytoin has many contraindications, mainly because it induces the hepatic cytochrome P_{450} oxidase system, increasing the metabolism of oral contraceptives, anticoagulants, dexamethasone and pethidine.

Adverse effects—Dose-related effects of phenytoin include ataxia, blurred vision and hyperactivity secondary to the cerebellovestibular system being affected. Acute toxicity causes sedation and confusion. The nondosage-related effects include effects on collagen such as gum hypertrophy and coarsening of facial features; allergic reactions, for example, rash, hepatitis and lymphadenopathy; haematological effects, for example, megaloblastic anaemia; endocrine effects, for example, hirsutism (hair growth); and teratogenic effects (it may cause congenital malformations).

Therapeutic notes—The use of phenytoin is further complicated by its zero-order pharmacokinetics, characteristic toxicities, and the necessity for long-term administration. Phenytoin has a narrow therapeutic index, and the relationship between dose and plasma concentration is nonlinear. This is because phenytoin is metabolized by a hepatic enzyme system saturated at therapeutic levels. Small dosage increases may therefore produce large rises in plasma concentrations with acute side effects. Monitoring of plasma concentration of phenytoin greatly assists dosage adjustment. Because of its adverse effects and narrow therapeutic window, phenytoin is no longer a first-line treatment for any of the seizure syndromes.

Sodium valproate

Mechanism of action—Sodium valproate has two mechanisms of action: similar to phenytoin, it causes a use-dependent block of voltage-gated sodium channels; it also increases the GABA content of the brain when given over a prolonged period.

Route of administration—Oral, intravenous.

Indications—Sodium valproate is useful in all forms of epilepsy.

Contraindications—Sodium valproate should not be given to people with acute liver disease or a history of hepatic dysfunction.

Adverse effects—Sodium valproate has fewer side effects than other antiepileptics; the main problems are gastrointestinal upset and, importantly, liver failure. Hepatic toxicity appears to be more common when sodium valproate is used in combination with other antiepileptics.

Therapeutic notes—Sodium valproate is well absorbed orally and has a half-life of 10 to 15 hours. Sodium valproate is now the first-line drug for most types of seizure syndromes.

Antiepileptic medication should be avoided in pregnancy unless there is no safer alternative and only after the risks have been discussed with the patient. Prescribers should ensure that women of childbearing age are using effective contraception throughout treatment because of the risk of major congenital malformations.

Carbamazepine

Mechanism of action—Similar to phenytoin, carbamazepine causes a use-dependent block of voltage-gated sodium channels. Oxcarbazepine, another antiepileptic, is structurally a derivative of carbamazepine. It has an extra oxygen atom on the dibenzazepine ring, which helps reduce the impact on the liver of metabolising the drug, and also prevents the serious forms of anaemia occasionally associated with carbamazepine. It is thought to have the same mechanism of action as carbamazepine.

Route of administration—Oral, rectal.

Indications—Carbamazepine can be used in the treatment of all forms of epilepsy except absence seizures. It can also be used to treat neuralgic pain (p. 150, Chapter 10.).

Contraindications—Like phenytoin, carbamazepine is a strong enzyme inducer in the liver and so causes similar drug/drug interactions.

Adverse effects—Ataxia, nystagmus, dysarthria, vertigo, sedation.

Therapeutic notes—Carbamazepine is well absorbed orally with a long half-life (25–60 hours) when first given. Enzyme induction subsequently reduces this half-life.

Ethosuximide

Mechanism of action—Ethosuximide exerts its effects by inhibition of low-threshold calcium currents (T-currents).

Route of administration—Oral.

Indications—Ethosuximide is the drug of choice in simple absence seizures and is particularly well tolerated in children.

Contraindications—Ethosuximide may make tonic-clonic attacks worse.

Adverse effects—The adverse effects of ethosuximide include gastrointestinal upset, drowsiness, mood swings and skin rashes. Rarely, it causes serious bone marrow depression.

Vigabatrin

Mechanism of action—Vigabatrin exerts its effects by irreversible inhibition of GABA transaminase.

Route of administration—Oral.

Indications—Vigabatrin is indicated in epilepsy not satisfactorily controlled by other drugs.

Contraindications—Vigabatrin should not be used in people with a history of psychosis because of the side effect of hallucinations.

Adverse effects—Drowsiness, dizziness, depression, visual hallucinations and visual field defects.

Therapeutic notes—Vigabatrin is a new drug, used as an adjunct to other therapies. It should be prescribed by a specialist and not given in patients with absence seizures because it can worsen this type of epilepsy.

Lamotrigine

Mechanism of action—Lamotrigine appears to act via an effect on sodium channels and inhibits the release of excitatory amino acids.

Route of administration—Oral.

Indications—Monotherapy and adjunctive treatment of partial seizures, and generalized tonic-clonic seizures.

Contraindications—Hepatic impairment.

Adverse effects—Rashes, fever, malaise and drowsiness. Rarely, hepatic dysfunction and bone marrow failure.

Gabapentin

Mechanism of action—Gabapentin is a lipophilic drug that was designed to mimic GABA in the CNS (agonist), although it does not appear to have GABA-mimetic actions. Its mechanism of action remains elusive, but its antiepileptic action almost certainly involves voltage-gated calcium-channel blockade.

Route of administration—Oral.

Indications—Monotherapy and adjunctive therapy in partial epilepsy with or without secondary generalisation, and in the treatment of neuropathic pain.

Contraindications—Avoid sudden withdrawal, in elderly patients and in those with renal impairment.

Adverse effects—Somnolence, dizziness, ataxia, fatigue and, rarely, cerebellar signs.

Barbiturates

Examples of barbiturates include phenobarbital and primidone (which itself, is largely converted to phenobarbital).

Mechanism of action—Barbiturates cause potentiation of chloride currents through the $GABA_A/Cl^-$ channel complex.

Route of administration—Oral, intravenous.

Indications—Barbiturates are used in all forms of epilepsy (except absence seizures), including status epilepticus.

Contraindications—Barbiturates should not be used in children, elderly people, and people with respiratory depression.

Adverse effects—The main side effect of barbiturates is sedation, which limits their use clinically, along with the danger of potentially fatal CNS depression in overdose. Phenobarbital is an inducer of cytochrome P_{450}, and so interacts with many medications.

Therapeutic notes—Only the long-acting barbiturates are antiepileptic. Phenobarbital has a plasma half-life of 10 hours. The strong sedating nature of these drugs now limits their use in the management of epilepsy.

Benzodiazepines

Examples of benzodiazepines include lorazepam, diazepam, midazolam, clonazepam and clobazam.

Mechanism of action—Benzodiazepines cause potentiation of chloride currents through the $GABA_A/Cl^-$ channel complex (see Table 8.1). Clonazepam is unique in that it acts at the $GABA_A$ receptor and inhibits T-type calcium channels.

Route of administration—Oral, intravenously.

Indications—Clonazepam is occasionally used for tonic-clonic and partial seizures. Lorazepam and diazepam are effective in the management of status epilepticus because they act very rapidly when compared with other antiepileptics.

Contraindications—Benzodiazepines should not be used in people with respiratory depression.

Adverse effects—The most common adverse effect of the benzodiazepines is sedation and respiratory depression.

Therapeutic notes—The repeated seizures of status epilepticus can damage the brain and be potentially life-threatening, so they should be controlled by administration of a benzodiazepine (e.g. rectal diazepam, buccal midazolam or intravenous lorazepam). Note that lorazepam has a longer half-life than diazepam.

Other anticonvulsants

Other agents used as antiepileptics include tiagabine, topiramate, acetazolamide and piracetam. Their indications and side-effect profiles can be obtained from the *British National Formulary (BNF)*.

Emmett Hezz, a 19-year-old student car mechanic is brought to A&E following a collapse while waiting for a taxi. His fiancée was with him at the time and tells staff that he fell to the ground suddenly and that his breathing appeared to stop for about 30 seconds. He then developed jerking movements of his arms and legs and by this time, his face had turned blue. He was incontinent of urine and on regaining consciousness was drowsy, confused and complaining of aching muscles. In hospital, he was able to explain that 8 months ago, he experienced a similar episode when in a park, but was too embarrassed to tell anybody.

On examination, his pulse is 76 beats per minute and regular. No abnormalities are found, other than a bleeding tongue. The history is very indicative of a tonic-clonic (grand mal) seizure. He is admitted for 24 hours and sent for blood investigations, electrocardiogram (ECG), head computed tomography (CT) and electroencephalogram (EEG). EEG reveals generalized spike-and-wave activity, but no other abnormality. He is warned not to drive or operate heavy machinery until he has been seizure-free for a year. Emmett agrees to start taking the anticonvulsant sodium valproate and return for a follow-up appointment.

Status epilepticus

Intravenous benzodiazepines (lorazepam or diazepam) are first-line drugs in the treatment of status epilepticus. If these fail to bring an end to seizure activity, intravenous phenytoin should be administered. Alternatively, intravenous fosphenytoin, a prodrug of phenytoin, can be given more rapidly but requires ECG monitoring. Thiopental (and other muscle relaxants) can be used as a final option.

THE EYE

The eyeball is a 25-mm sphere made up of two fluid-filled compartments (the aqueous humour and the vitreous humour) separated by a translucent lens, all encased within four layers of supporting tissue (Fig. 8.8). There are four layers.

- The cornea and sclera
- The uveal tract, comprising the iris, ciliary body and choroid
- The pigment epithelium
- The retina (neural tissue containing photoreceptors).

Light entering the eye is focused by the lens onto the retina, and the signal reaches the brain via the optic nerve.

Glaucoma

Glaucoma describes a group of disorders characterized by a loss in the visual field associated with cupping of the optic disc and optic nerve damage. Glaucoma is the second most common cause of blindness in the world and the most common cause of irreversible blindness. Glaucoma is generally associated with raised intraocular pressure (IOP) but can occur when the IOP is within normal limits.

There are two types of glaucoma: open-angle and closed-angle.

Open-angle glaucoma is the most common type of glaucoma and it may be congenital. It is caused by pathology of the trabecular meshwork that reduces the drainage of the aqueous humour into the canal of Schlemm. Treatment involves either reducing the amount of aqueous humour produced (Fig. 8.9) or increasing its drainage.

In closed-angle glaucoma, the angle between the iris and the cornea is very small, and this results in the forward ballooning of the iris against the back of the cornea.

Chronic open-angle glaucoma is of insidious onset and often picked up at a routine check-up, whereas acute closed-angle glaucoma symptoms include painful, red eyes and blurred vision. Acute closed-angle glaucoma is a medical emergency and requires admission to save sight. It is difficult for the patient to notice a gradual loss of visual fields associated with chronic open-angle glaucoma and so regular check-ups are vital for at-risk groups, such as elderly people.

Treatment of open-angle glaucoma

The most effective way of preventing damage to the eye is by lowering the IOP. Most drugs used to treat eye disease can be given topically in the form of drops and ointments. To enable these drugs to penetrate the cornea, they must be lipophilic or uncharged.

Drugs used to inhibit aqueous production

Beta-adrenoceptor antagonists and prostaglandin analogues are the current choice for first-line treatment.

Beta-adrenoceptor antagonists

Timolol and betaxolol are examples of beta-adrenoceptor antagonists used in glaucoma.

Mechanism of action—Beta-adrenoceptor antagonists block β_2-receptors on the ciliary body and on ciliary blood vessels, resulting in vasoconstriction and reduced aqueous production (see Fig. 8.9).

Route of administration—Topical.

Indications—Open-angle glaucoma. beta-adrenoceptor antagonists are also used in the treatment of cardiovascular disease (Chapter 4).

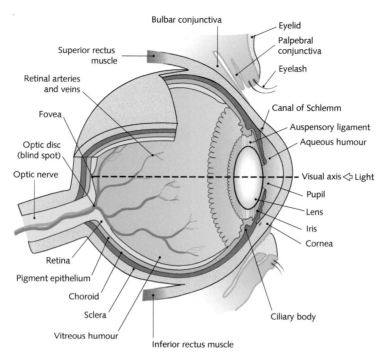

Fig. 8.8 Anatomy of the eye. (Modified from Page, C., Curtis, M. Walker, M, Hoffman, B. (eds) *Integrated Pharmacology*, 3rd edn. Mosby, 2006.)

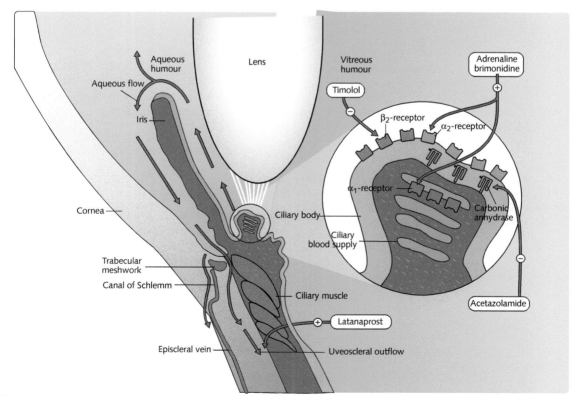

Fig. 8.9 Production and drainage of the aqueous humour. (Modified from Page, C., Curtis, M. Walker, M, Hoffman, B. (eds) *Integrated Pharmacology*, 3rd edn. Mosby, 2006.)

Contraindications—Beta-adrenoceptor antagonists should not be given to patients with asthma, bradycardia, heart block or heart failure.

Adverse effects—Systemic side effects include bronchospasm in asthmatic patients, and potentially bradycardia owing to their nonselective action on beta-receptors. Other side effects include transitory dry eyes and allergic blepharoconjunctivitis.

Prostaglandin analogues
Examples include latanoprost and travoprost.

Mechanism of action—Promote outflow of aqueous from the anterior chamber via an alternative drainage route, called the uveoscleral pathway.

Indications—Open angle glaucoma, ocular hypertension.

Contraindication—Pregnancy.

Adverse effects—Brown pigmentation of the iris may occur.

Sympathomimetics (adrenoceptor agonists)
Adrenaline, dipivefrine and brimonidine are commonly used sympathomimetics.

Mechanism of action—Agonism at α-adrenoceptors is thought to be the principal means by which these agents reduce aqueous production from the ciliary body. Adrenaline may also increase drainage of aqueous humour (see Fig. 8.9).

Route of administration—Topical.

Indications—Open-angle glaucoma. Sympathomimetics are also used in the management of cardiac (Chapter 4) and anaphylactic emergencies and in the treatment of reversible airways disease (Chapter 3).

Contraindications—Closed-angle glaucoma, hypertension, heart disease.

Adverse effects—Pain and redness in the eye.

Therapeutic notes—Adrenaline is not very lipophilic, and therefore it does not penetrate the cornea effectively. This can be overcome by administering dipivefrine hydrochloride, a prodrug that crosses the cornea and that is metabolized to adrenaline once inside the eye.

Carbonic anhydrase inhibitors
Acetazolamide and dorzolamide are carbonic anhydrase inhibitors (CAIs).

Mechanism of action—CAIs inhibit the enzyme carbonic anhydrase, which catalyses the conversion of carbon dioxide and water to carbonic acid, which dissociates into bicarbonate and H^+. Bicarbonate is required by the cells of the ciliary body, and underproduction of bicarbonate limits aqueous secretion (see Fig. 8.9). CAIs given systemically also have a weak diuretic effect (Chapter 5).

Route of administration—Oral, topical, intravenous.

Indications—Open-angle glaucoma.

Contraindications—Hypokalaemia, hyponatraemia, renal impairment. These effects can be reduced if the drug is given in a slow-release form.

Adverse effects—Irritation of the eye, nausea, vomiting, diarrhoea, diuresis.

Drugs used to increase the drainage of aqueous humour

Miotics–muscarinic agonists
Pilocarpine is a muscarinic agonist.

Mechanism of action—Pilocarpine causes contraction of the constrictor pupillae muscles of the iris, constricting the pupil, and allowing aqueous to drain from the anterior chamber into the trabecular meshwork (see Fig. 8.9).

Route of administration—Topical.

Indications—Open-angle glaucoma.

Contraindications—Acute iritis, anterior uveitis.

Adverse effects—Eye irritation, headache and brow ache, blurred vision, hypersalivation. May exacerbate asthma.

Treatment of closed-angle glaucoma

Drugs to treat closed-angle glaucoma are used in emergencies as a temporary measure to lower IOP.

Pilocarpine and a CAI are often first-line treatments, with mannitol and glycerol being administered systemically to reduce IOP for resistant or more serious cases.

YAG (yttrium-aluminium-garnet) laser surgery provides a permanent cure for closed-angle glaucoma. A hole is made in the iris (iridectomy) to allow increased flow of aqueous humour.

HINTS AND TIPS

Stimuli that cause the pupils to dilate, such as sitting awake in a dark room, increase the tightness of the angle between the iris and the cornea and can thus precipitate an attack of acute closed-angle glaucoma.

Examining the eye

Mydriatic drugs dilate the pupil, that is, cause mydriasis, whereas cycloplegic drugs cause paralysis of the ciliary muscle, that is, cycloplegia. Mydriatic and cycloplegic drugs are used in ophthalmoscopy to allow a better view of the interior of the eye.

Mydriasis and cycloplegia reduce the drainage of the aqueous humour, and they should therefore be avoided in patients with closed-angle glaucoma.

Muscarinic antagonists
The most effective mydriatics are the muscarinic receptor antagonists. These block the parasympathetic control of the iris sphincter muscle.

Table 8.8 Mydriatic and cycloplegic effects of the commonly used muscarinic antagonists

Drug	Duration (h)	Mydriatic effect	Cycloplegic effect
Tropicamide	1–3	++	+
Cyclopentolate	12–24	+++	+++
Atropine	168–240	+++	+++

The type of muscarinic receptor antagonist chosen will depend on the length of the procedure and on whether or not cycloplegia is required.

The most commonly used muscarinic receptor antagonists, their duration of action, and their mydriatic and cycloplegic effects are summarized in Table 8.8.

α-Adrenoceptor agonists

α-Adrenoceptor agonists can cause mydriasis by stimulating the sympathetic control of the iris dilator muscle. The sympathetic system does not control the ciliary muscle, however, and, therefore these drugs do not produce cycloplegia. The α-agonist most commonly used to produce mydriasis is phenylephrine.

Muscarinic agonists and α-antagonists

A muscarinic agonist such as pilocarpine, or an α-receptor antagonist such as moxisylyte may be used to reverse mydriasis at the end of an ophthalmic examination, although this is not usually necessary.

● Chapter Summary

- Medications used in Parkinson disease correct the imbalance between the dopaminergic and cholinergic systems within the basal ganglia
- Benzodiazepines and hypnotic drugs should only be prescribed as a short course in the treatment of insomnia or anxiety
- Beta-blockers are useful in the treatment of somatic symptoms associated with anxiety
- SSRIs are the most commonly prescribed antidepressant, but patients must be informed that their effect can take up to 4 weeks
- Tricyclic antidepressants are harmful in overdose and can cause muscarinic blocking side effects including a dry mouth, blurred vision and constipation
- Lithium is an effective mood stabilizer but has a narrow therapeutic window and patients require substantial monitoring whilst taking it
- Beta-adrenoceptor antagonists and prostaglandin analogues are used to reduce the intraocular pressure associated with glaucoma

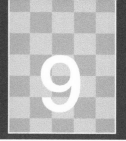

Drug misuse 9

DEFINITIONS

Drug misuse

Drug misuse is defined as the use of drugs that cause actual physical or mental harm to an individual or to society, or that is illegal. Therefore drug misuse includes alcohol, nicotine, and prescription medications taken in excess, as well as the more obvious illicit drugs such as ecstasy, heroin, cocaine or amphetamines.

Drug dependence

Drug dependence is defined as the compulsion to take a drug repeatedly, with distress being caused if this is prevented. Dependence on drugs is often caused by the rewarding effects but is also related to psychological and physical effects. These are not exclusive and there is a mixture of both in most people who are dependent on drugs. Psychological dependence is when the rewarding effects (positive reinforcement) predominate to cause a compulsion to continue taking the drug. Physical dependence is when the distress on stopping the drug (negative reinforcement) is the main reason for continuing to take it, that is, avoidance of symptoms associated with the withdrawal.

Drug tolerance

Drug tolerance is the necessity to increase the dose of an administered drug progressively to maintain the effect produced by the (smaller) original doses. Drug tolerance is a phenomenon that develops with chronic administration of certain drugs.

Many different mechanisms can give rise to drug tolerance, although they are rather poorly understood. They include the following.

- Downregulation of receptors
- Changes in receptor coupling
- Exhaustion of biological mediators or transmitters
- Increased metabolic degradation (enzyme induction)
- Physiological adaptation.

Withdrawal

Withdrawal is the term used to describe the syndrome of effects caused by stopping administration of a drug. It results from the change of (neuro) physiological equilibrium induced by the presence of the drug.

DRUGS OF MISUSE

Drugs with a high potential for misuse fall into many distinct pharmacological categories. They may or may not be used therapeutically, and they may be illegal or legal (Table 9.1). Controlled drugs are categorized into three classes (Table 9.2).

> **HINTS AND TIPS**
>
> Always use the correct chemical name when describing drugs of misuse, for example, amphetamines rather than lay street terms such as *whizz* or *speed*.

Central stimulants

Amphetamines

Other names—"Speed", "whizz", "billy", "base".

Mechanism of action—Amphetamines cause the release of monoamines and the inhibition of monoamine reuptake, especially of dopamine and noradrenaline in neurones.

Route of administration—Amphetamines are administered orally, or "snorted" as a powder nasally; sometimes used intravenously.

Effects—Increased motor activity; euphoria and excitement; anorexia and insomnia; peripheral sympathomimetic effects, such as hypertension and inhibition of gut motility; stereotyped behaviour and psychosis, which develop with prolonged usage. Stimulant effects last for a few hours and are followed by depression and anxiety.

Clinical uses—The clinical uses of amphetamines are for narcolepsy and for attention deficit hyperactivity disorder in children.

Tolerance, dependence and withdrawal—Tolerance to the peripheral sympathomimetic stimulant effects of amphetamines develops rapidly, but it develops much more slowly to other effects such as locomotor stimulation. Amphetamines cause strong psychological dependence but no real physical dependence. After stopping chronic use, the individual will usually enter a deep, long sleep ("REM rebound") and awake feeling tired, depressed and hungry. This state may reflect the depletion of the normal monoamine stores.

Adverse effects—Acute amphetamine toxicity causes cardiac arrhythmias, hypertension and stroke. Chronic toxicity

Table 9.1 Drugs with high potential for misuse

Drug class	Examples
Central stimulants	Cocaine
	Amphetamines
	MDMA (ecstasy)
	Nicotine
Central depressants	Alcohol
	Benzodiazepines
	Barbiturates
Opioid analgesics	Morphine
	Heroin (diamorphine)
	Methadone
Cannabinoids	Cannabis
	Tetrahydrocannabinoids (THCs)
Hallucinogens	LSD
	Mescaline
	Psilocybin
Dissociative anaesthetics	Ketamine
	Phencyclidine

LSD, Lysergic acid diethylamide; MDMA, methylenedioxymethamphetamine

Table 9.2 Classes of controlled drugs

Class A drugs	Class B drugs	Class C drugs
Cocaine MDMA (ecstasy) Diamorphine (heroin) and other strong opioids LSD class B substance when prepared for injection Others	Amphetamines Barbiturates Some weak opioids Others	Benzodiazepines Cannabis Androgenic and anabolic steroids Human chorionic gonadotrophin Others

LSD, Lysergic acid diethylamide; MDMA, methylenedioxymethamphetamine

causes paranoid psychosis, vasoconstriction, tissue anoxia, damage at sites of injection or snorting and damage to the foetal brain in utero.

Cocaine

Other names—"Coke", "Charlie", "snow", "crack".

Mechanism of action—Cocaine strongly inhibits the re-uptake of catecholamines into noradrenergic neurones, and thus strongly enhances sympathetic activity.

Route of administration—Cocaine hydrochloride is usually snorted nasally. Crack is the free base, which is more volatile, and which does not decompose on heating. It can, therefore be smoked, producing a brief intense "rush".

Effects—The behavioural effects produced by cocaine are similar to those produced by amphetamines, such as euphoria. The euphoric effects may be greater, and there is less of a tendency for stereotypic behaviour and paranoid delusions.

The effects of cocaine hydrochloride (lasting about an hour) are not as long lasting as those of amphetamine, whereas those obtained from crack are brief (minutes).

Clinical uses—Cocaine is no longer used clinically

Tolerance, dependence and withdrawal—Cocaine causes strong psychological dependence but no real physical dependence. Withdrawal causes a marked deterioration in motor performance, which is restorable on the provision of the drug.

Adverse effects—Acute cocaine toxicity causes toxic psychosis, cardiac arrhythmias, hypertension and stroke. Chronic toxicity causes paranoid psychosis, vasoconstriction, tissue anoxia and damage at sites of injection or snorting. Cocaine used by pregnant mothers impairs foetal development and damages the foetal brain.

CLINICAL NOTE

Cocaine can cause cardiac toxicity because it has a direct effect on the heart. Cocaine will increase myocardial contractility as a result of sympathomimetic effects mediated by B1 receptors, but the heart is unable to meet the demand because of a decrease in coronary artery blood flow (caused by sympathomimetic effects on α1 receptors). First-line treatment of cocaine-induced arrhythmias is usually benzodiazepines, which moderate the effects of cocaine on the central nervous system (CNS) and cardiovascular system. The use of β-blockers are contraindicated because the resultant unopposed alpha effect can precipitate a dangerous hypertensive crisis in patients who have cocaine induced chest pain.

Methylenedioxymethamphetamine

Other names—"Ecstasy", "E", "disco biscuits", "pills".

Mechanism of action—Methylenedioxymethamphetamine (MDMA) is an amphetamine derivative that has a mechanism of action similar to that of amphetamines (release of monoamines, inhibition of monoamine reuptake). MDMA also acts on serotonergic neurones, potentiating the effects of serotonin (5-HT).

Route of administration—MDMA is usually taken as a pill containing other psychoactive drugs, such as amphetamine or ketamine.

Effects—MDMA has mixed stimulant and hallucinogenic properties, especially in its pure form. Euphoria, arousal and perceptual disturbances are common. Uniquely, MDMA has the effect of creating a feeling of euphoric empathy, so that social barriers are reduced.

Clinical uses—MDMA has no clinical use.

Tolerance, dependence and withdrawal—It is not currently known to what extent tolerance and dependence occur with MDMA. The withdrawal syndrome is similar to that with amphetamines.

Adverse effects—The most serious acute consequences of acute MDMA toxicity appear to be hyperthermia and exhaustion caused indirectly by the hyperexcitability that is induced. Acute hyperthermia results in damage to skeletal muscle and renal failure. MDMA causes users to consume large amounts of water and in addition, MDMA causes inappropriate secretion of antidiuretic hormone leading to overhydration and hyponatraemia ("water intoxication").

Ketamine

Other names—"Special K", "Cat valium"

Mechanism of action—N-methyl-D aspartic acid (NMDA) receptor antagonist.

Route of administration—Ketamine is typically injected or snorted when misused.

Effects—Ketamine causes an overwhelming feeling of relaxation, "a full body buzz" and out of body experience, as well as hallucinations. It is known as a *dissociative anaesthetic*.

Clinical uses—Ketamine is sometimes used as a general anaesthetic.

Tolerance, dependence and withdrawal—Ketamine can cause users to develop cravings and dependence on the drug.

Adverse effects—Ketamine eliminates pain therefore several misusers cause themselves significant injuries. In addition, depression, amnesia and hallucinations can occur. Importantly, ketamine causes thickening of the bladder and urinary tract. Long-term addicts can develop problems with passing urine and severe bladder dysfunction.

Nicotine

Nicotine is found in cigarettes, cigars, pipes and chewing tobacco.

Mechanism of action—Nicotine exerts its effects by acting as an agonist at nicotinic receptors, thus mimicking some of the actions of acetylcholine, both in the CNS and in the periphery.

Route of administration—Nicotine is usually inhaled, although it can be chewed or applied topically via "patches" as part of treating nicotine withdrawal.

Effects—Nicotine has both stimulant and relaxant properties. Physiologically, nicotine increases alertness, decreases irritability and relaxes skeletal muscle tone. Peripheral effects caused by ganglionic stimulation include tachycardia, increased blood pressure and decreased gastro-intestinal motility.

Clinical uses—Nicotine has no clinical use.

Tolerance, dependence and withdrawal—Tolerance to nicotine occurs rapidly, first to peripheral effects but later to central effects.

Nicotine is highly addictive, causing both physical and psychological dependence. Withdrawal from tobacco often leads to a syndrome of craving, irritability, anxiety and increased appetite for approximately 2 to 3 weeks.

Adverse effects—Acute nicotine toxicity causes nausea and vomiting. Chronic toxicity caused by smoking leads to more morbidity in the United Kingdom than all other drugs combined, predisposing to all the following diseases, often greatly so.

- Cardiovascular diseases, including atherosclerosis, hypertension and coronary heart disease
- Cancer of the lung, bladder and mouth
- Respiratory diseases such as bronchitis, emphysema (chronic obstructive pulmonary disease) and asthma
- Foetal growth retardation

The most successful treatments for nicotine addiction combine psychological and pharmacological treatments. Pharmacological options largely rely on nicotine replacement, once the patient has stopped smoking, with a gradual reduction in nicotine. The latest drug to be used to help cigarette smokers is bupropion (Zyban), which is derived from an antidepressant.

CLINICAL NOTE

Note that nicotine consumption during pregnancy is associated with miscarriage, ectopic and foetal growth restriction, placental abruption, stillbirth and premature delivery. Patients should be advised to stop smoking if they are trying to conceive or if they are already pregnant. This would also include the cessation of using the newer e-cigarettes because the vaporized nicotine causes similar problems, in addition to nicotine toxicity.

Nicotine replacement products

Mechanism of action—Measured doses of nicotine are used to replace nicotine derived from cigarettes once the patient has stopped smoking, meeting the physical nicotine needs. The dose of nicotine is gradually reduced over 10 to 12 weeks.

Route of administration—Oral (chewing gum, sublingual tablets), transdermal (patches), nasal (spray), inhalation.

Indications—Adjunct to smoking cessation.

Contraindications—Severe cardiovascular disease, recent cerebrovascular accident, pregnancy, breastfeeding.

Adverse effects—Nausea, dizziness, headache and cold, influenza-like symptoms, palpitations.

Therapeutic notes—Nicotine replacement products are available over the counter or General Practitioners (GPs) can prescribe them for patients intending to stop smoking.

Bupropion (Zyban)

Mechanism of action—Bupropion is a selective inhibitor of the neuronal uptake of noradrenaline and dopamine. This is believed to reduce nicotine craving and withdrawal symptoms.

Route of administration—Oral.

Indications—Adjunct to smoking cessation.

Contraindications—History of epilepsy (bupropion lowers seizure threshold) and eating disorders, pregnancy, breastfeeding.

Adverse effects—Dry mouth, gastrointestinal disturbances, insomnia, tremor and impaired concentration.

Therapeutic notes—Bupropion is available on the National Health Service.

Varenicline (Champix)

Mechanism of action—A partial agonist at nicotinic acetylcholine receptors. The stimulatory effect produces a weak nicotine-like effect, which reduces the craving for nicotine itself, while the blocking effect inhibits the pleasurable effect derived from smoking. Hence varenicline is thought to mediate the rewarding effects of smoking.

Route of administration—Oral

Indication—Cessation of smoking, prevent relapse.

Contraindication—Pregnancy, history of psychiatric illness as increased risk of suicidal thoughts.

Adverse effects—Nausea, abnormal dreams, headaches, flatulence.

Irritability, depression, insomnia can occur on abrupt cessation of varenicline.

Therapeutic notes—Should be started 1 to 3 weeks before the target stop date and should be prescribed alongside psychological support. Available only on prescription.

Central depressants

Ethanol

Mechanism of action—Ethanol, or alcohol, acts in a similar way to volatile anaesthetic agents, as a general CNS depressant. The cellular mechanisms involved may include inhibition of calcium entry, hence the reduction in transmitter release, as well as potentiation of inhibitory gamma-aminobutyric acid (GABA) transmission.

Route of administration—Ethanol is administered orally.

Effects—The familiar effects of ethanol intoxication range from increased self-confidence and motor incoordination through to unconsciousness and coma. Peripheral effects include a self-limiting diuresis and vasodilatation.

Clinical uses—Ethanol is used as an antidote to methanol poisoning.

Tolerance, dependence and withdrawal—Tolerance and physical and psychological dependence all occur with ethanol, such that there were 100,000 hospital admissions relating to alcohol consumption where an alcohol related disease, injury or condition was the primary reason.

There are two stages of alcohol withdrawal.

- Early stage ("hangover"), which is common and starts 6 to 8 hours after cessation of drinking. It involves tremulousness, nausea, retching and sweating.
- Late stage (delirium tremens), which is much less common and starts 48 to 72 hours after cessation of drinking. It involves delirium, tremor, hallucinations and confusion.

Management of these late withdrawal symptoms involves benzodiazepines (such as chlordiazepoxide).

Adverse effects—Acute ethanol toxicity causes ataxia, nystagmus, coma, respiratory depression and death. Chronic ethanol toxicity causes neurodegeneration (potentiated by vitamin deficiency), dementia, liver damage, pancreatitis, and so on, and accompanying psychiatric illness-depression/psychosis is common.

CLINICAL NOTE

Wernicke encephalopathy is a classic triad of confusion, ataxia and ophthalmoplegia caused by thiamine deficiency related to alcohol abuse. On admission to hospital, patients who consume excess alcohol are prescribed vitamins, including thiamine to reduce the risk of this occurring.

Supportive treatment for ethanol dependency

Disulfiram is an aldehyde dehydrogenase inhibitor taken as tablets.

Mechanism of action—Alcohol is usually broken down into acetaldehyde and then removed from the body. Disulfiram blocks aldehyde dehydrogenase enzyme which breaks down the acetaldehyde which leads to high levels of acetaldehyde in the blood, causing a number of unpleasant effects. These include a throbbing headache, flushed face, vomiting and palpitations.

Indication—It should be prescribed alongside psychological support and must only be given to patients who have stopped drinking and who require a deterrent to drinking further alcohol.

Benzodiazepines

Mechanism of action—Benzodiazepines exert their effects by potentiation of inhibitory GABA transmission.

Route of administration—Benzodiazepines are administered orally.

Effects—Benzodiazepines are widely abused drugs as they induce a feeling of calm and reduced anxiety, creating a "dream-like" effect.

Clinical uses—Benzodiazepines are prescribed as anxiolytics and hypnotics.

Tolerance, dependence and withdrawal—Benzodiazepines have a potential for misuse; tolerance and dependence are common.

A physical withdrawal syndrome can occur in patients given benzodiazepines, even for short periods. Symptoms include rebound anxiety and insomnia with depression, nausea and perceptual changes that may last from weeks to months.

Adverse effects—The adverse effects of acute benzodiazepine toxicity include hypotension and confusion. Cognitive impairment occurs in chronic benzodiazepine toxicity.

CLINICAL NOTE

Mr Alrum, a 45-year-old male is brought to A&E following a fall in the road. He is confused and smells strongly of alcohol. Some minor cuts and bruises are noted on his right arm and leg. Blood tests reveal a macrocytic anaemia, elevated γ-glutamyl transferase and alanine aminotransferase (liver transaminases) indicating alcohol misuse. Given that he is disorientated, sweating and trembling, he is given chlordiazepoxide and vitamins. He is seen by the alcohol specialist nurse who discovers that Mr Alrum has recently lost his job because of poor performance and that he is feeling low in mood and hopeless. A set of screening questions confirms a diagnosis of alcohol dependence and Mr Alrum is offered psychological support.

Opioid analgesics

Diamorphine (heroin) and other opioids

Other names—"Smack", "H", "gear", "junk", "jack", "brown".

Mechanism of action—Opioids show agonist action at opioid receptors. Strong opioids produce a sense of euphoria and wellbeing by reducing anxiety and stress. These effects contribute to their analgesic effect in the clinical management of pain but also account for the illicit use of these drugs by addicts.

Route of administration—Opioids are generally taken intravenously by misusers because this produces the most intense sense of euphoria (rush).

Effects—Opioids produce feelings of euphoria and wellbeing. Other effects are mentioned in Chapter 10.

Clinical uses—Opioids are used as analgesia for moderate to severe pain.

Tolerance, dependence and withdrawal—Tolerance to opioid analgesics develops quickly in addicts and results in larger and larger doses of the drug being needed to achieve the same effect.

Dependence involves both psychological factors and physical factors. Psychological dependence is based on the positive reinforcement provided by euphoria.

There is a definite physical withdrawal syndrome in addicts following cessation of drug treatment with opioids. This syndrome comprizes a complex mixture of irritable and sometimes aggressive behaviour, combined with autonomic symptoms such as fever, sweating, yawning, pupillary dilatation, and piloerection that gives the state its colloquial name of *cold turkey*. Patients are extremely distressed and restless and strongly crave the drug. Symptoms are maximal at 2 days and largely disappear in 7 to 10 days.

Treatment of withdrawal—Methadone is a long-acting opiate, active orally, used to wean addicts from their addiction. The withdrawal symptoms from this longer-acting compound are more prolonged but less intense than, for example, those of heroin. Treatment usually involves substitution of methadone followed by a slow reduction in dose over time.

Clonidine, an α_2-adrenoceptor agonist, inhibits firing of locus coeruleus neurones, and it is effective in suppressing some components of the opioid withdrawal syndrome, especially nausea, vomiting and diarrhoea.

Adverse effects—Acute opioid toxicity causes the following.

- Confusion, drowsiness and sedation. Initial excitement is followed by sedation and finally coma on overdose.
- Shallow and slow respiration caused by a reduction of sensitivity of the respiratory centre to carbon dioxide.
- Vomiting caused by stimulation of the chemoreceptor trigger zone.
- Autonomic effects such as tremor and pupillary constriction.
- Bronchospasm, flushing and arteriolar dilatation caused by histamine release.

Acute toxicity may be countered by use of an opioid antagonist such as naloxone. The adverse effects of direct chronic toxicity are minor (see Chapter 10).

HINTS AND TIPS

Heroin addicts are able to tolerate 300- to 600-mg doses several times per day. This is 30 to 60 times the normal dose needed to produce an analgesic effect. A nonaddict given this would die of respiratory depression.

Cannabinoids

Cannabis

There are two forms of cannabis: marijuana is the dried leaves and flowers of the cannabis plant, and hashish is the extracted resin of the cannabis plant.

Other names—"Hash," "weed", "skunk", "pot", "dope", "gear", "grass", "ganja", "blow".

Mechanism of action—How cannabis exerts its effects is not clearly defined, but it includes both depressant, stimulant and psychomimetic effects. The active constituent of cannabis is D^9-tetrahydrocannabinol (THC), although metabolites that also have activity may be important.

Route of administration—Cannabis is usually smoked, although it may be eaten.

Effects—Cannabis has several effects.

- Subjectively, users feel relaxed and mildly euphoric.
- Perception is altered, with the apparent sharpening of sensory experience.
- Appetite is enhanced.
- Peripheral actions include vasodilatation and bronchodilation, and a reduction in intraocular pressure.

Clinical uses—Cannabis is not currently licensed for use in the United Kingdom. However, cannabis extract is used to treat spasticity in patients with multiple sclerosis. In some patients with chronic disease or malignancy, cannabis is used as an antiemetic.

Tolerance, dependence and withdrawal—Tolerance to cannabis occurs to a minor degree. It is not dangerously addictive, with only moderate physical and psychological withdrawal effects noted, such as mild anxiety/dysphoria and sleep disturbances.

Adverse effects—Acute cannabis toxicity causes confusion and hallucinations. Chronic toxicity may cause flashbacks, memory loss and "demotivational syndrome". There is a clear correlation between cannabis use and schizophrenia.

Psychotomimetic drugs or hallucinogens

Examples of psychotomimetic drugs include lysergic acid diethylamide (LSD), mescaline and psilocybin.

Street names—"Acid", "trips", "magic mushrooms".

Mechanism of action—How LSD, mescaline and psilocybin produce changes in perception is not well understood, but it seems to involve serotonin. LSD appears to affect serotonergic systems by acting on 5-HT_2 inhibitory autoreceptors on serotonergic neurones to reduce their firing. Whether LSD is an agonist, an antagonist or both is not clear.

Route of administration—Psychotomimetic drugs are administered orally as a liquid, pills or paper stamps.

Effects—Psychotomimetic drugs cause a dramatically altered state of perception-vivid and unusual sensory experiences combined with euphoric sensations. Hallucinations, delusions and panic can occur; this is known as a "bad trip" and it can be terrifying.

Clinical uses—Psychotomimetic drugs have no clinical uses.

Tolerance, dependence and withdrawal—Tolerance to, dependence on, and withdrawal from psychotomimetic drugs are not significant.

Adverse effects—Acute toxicity from psychotomimetic drugs causes frightening delusions or hallucinations that can lead to accidents or violence. In chronic toxicity, "flashbacks" (a recurrence of hallucination) may occur long after the "trip". Other psychotic symptoms may also occur.

● Chapter Summary

- Dependence is defined as the compulsion to take a drug repeatedly
- Physical dependence is the result of avoiding symptoms associated with drug withdrawal
- Drug tolerance is the necessity to increase the dose of an administered drug progressively to maintain the desired effect
- Amphetamines, taken orally or snorted nasally, cause the release of monoamines, resulting in stereotypical behaviours and paranoid delusions
- Cocaine strongly inhibits the reuptake of catecholamines into neurones causing euphoria
- MDMA acts on serotonergic neurones, potentiating the effects of 5-HT and creates a feeling of euphoric empathy
- MDMA causes water intoxication and exhaustion
- Opioid withdrawal results in cold turkey symptoms including fever, piloerection and irritability
- Nicotine replacement products are available to help patients stop smoking
- Ethanol abuse can result in Wernicke encephalopathy

BASIC CONCEPTS

Pain, which may be acute or chronic, is defined as an unpleasant sensory and emotional experience associated with actual or potential tissue damage. Pain is a subjective experience, as a patient's experience of pain is individual.

An analgesic drug is one that effectively removes (or at least lessens) the sensation of pain. The principles of pain relief are as follows.

1. Careful assessment
2. Diagnosis of the cause of the pain
3. Use of analgesics in accordance with the analgesic ladder (Fig. 10.1)
4. Regular review of the effectiveness of the prescribed drug

Pain perception

Pain perception is best viewed as a three-stage process; activation of nociceptors (pain-specific receptors), followed by the transmission and onward passage of pain information.

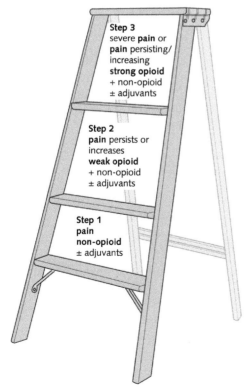

Fig. 10.1 The World Health Organization (WHO) analgesic ladder for chronic pain.

Activation of nociceptors in the peripheral tissues

Noxious thermal, chemical or mechanical stimuli can trigger the firing of primary afferent fibres (type C/Aδ), through the activation of nociceptors in the peripheral tissues (Fig. 10.2).

Transmission of pain information

Transmission of pain information from the periphery to the dorsal horn of the spinal cord is inhibited or amplified by a combination of local (spinal) neuronal circuits and descending tracts from higher brain centres. This constitutes the "gate-control mechanism".

- The primary afferent fibres synapse in lamina I and II of the dorsal horn of the spinal cord.
- Transmitter peptides (substance P, calcitonin gene-related peptide, bradykinin, glutamate) and nitric oxide are involved in the ascending pain pathways.
- The activity of the dorsal horn relay neurons is modulated by several inhibitory inputs. These include: local inhibitory interneurons, which release opioid peptides; descending inhibitory noradrenergic fibres from the locus ceruleus area of the brainstem, which are activated by opioid peptides; and descending inhibitory serotonergic fibres from the nucleus raphe magnus and periaqueductal grey areas of the brainstem, which are also activated by opioid peptides (see Fig. 10.2).

Onward passage of pain information

The onward passage of pain information is via the spinothalamic tract, to the higher centres of the brain. The higher centres of the brain coordinate the cognitive and emotional aspects of pain and control appropriate reactions. Opioid peptide release in both the spinal cord and the brainstem can reduce the activity of the dorsal horn relay neurons and cause analgesia (see Fig. 10.2).

Opioid receptors

All opioids, whether endogenous peptides, naturally occurring drugs, or chemically synthesized drugs, interact with specific opioid receptors to produce their pharmacological effects.

Drugs interact with opioid receptors as either full agonists, partial agonists, mixed agonists (full agonists on one opioid receptor but partial agonists on another) or as antagonists. Opioid analgesics are agonists.

There are three major opioid receptor subtypes: μ, δ and κ.

- μ receptors are thought to be responsible for most of the analgesic effects of opioids and for some major adverse effects for example, respiratory depression. Most of the analgesic opioids in use are μ receptor agonists.

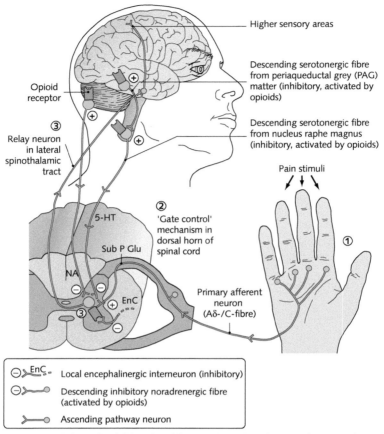

Fig. 10.2 Nociceptive pathways and sites of opioid action. (1) Activation of nociceptors in the peripheral tissues; (2) transmission of pain information; (3) onward passage of pain information to higher centres. *5-HT*, 5-Hydroxytryptamine (serotonin); *Glu*, glutamate; *NA*, noradrenaline; *Sub P*, substance P.

- δ receptors are probably more important in the periphery, but they may also contribute to analgesia.
- κ receptors contribute to analgesia at the spinal level, and may elicit sedation and dysphoria, but they produce relatively few adverse effects, and do not contribute to physical dependence.

- σ receptors are not selective opioid receptors, but they are the sites of action of psychomimetic drugs, such as phencyclidine (PCP). They may account for the dysphoria produced by some opioids.

Opioid receptor activation has an inhibitory effect on synapses in the central nervous system (CNS) and in the gut (Table 10.1).

Table 10.1 Actions mediated by opioid receptor subtypes			
Action	μ/δ	κ	σ
Analgesia	Supraspinal and spinal	Spinal	—
Respiratory depression	Marked	Slight	—
Pupil	Constricts	—	Dilates
GIT mobility	Reduced (constipating)	—	—
Mood/effect	Euphoria inducing but also sedating	Dysphoria inducing mildly sedating	Marked dysphoric and psychomimetic actions
Physical dependence	+++	+	—

GIT, Gastrointestinal tract.

Secondary-messenger systems associated with opioid receptor activity include the following.

- μ/δ receptors, the activation of which causes hyperpolarisation of a neuron by opening potassium channels and inhibiting calcium channels
- κ receptors, the activation of which inhibits calcium channels

Activation of all opioid receptors by endogenous or exogenous opioids results in the following.

- Inhibition of the enzyme adenylate cyclase and thus a reduction in cyclic adenosine monophosphate (cAMP) production
- Inhibition of voltage-gated calcium-channel opening
- Potassium-channel activation, which causes hyperpolarisation of the cell membrane

Endogenous opioids

Physiologically, the CNS has its own "endogenous opioids" that are the natural ligands for opioid receptors. There are three main families of endogenous opioid peptides occurring naturally in the CNS.

- Endorphins
- Dynorphins
- Enkephalins

They are derived from three separate gene products (precursor molecules), but all possess homology at their amino end. The expression and anatomic distribution of the products of these three precursor molecules within the CNS are varied, and each has a distinct range of affinities for the different types of opioid receptor (Table 10.2). Although it is known that the endogenous opioids possess analgesic activity, they are not used therapeutically.

Table 10.2 Endogenous opioid peptides

Precursor molecules	Products	Relative opioid receptor affinity
Pro-opiomelanocortin (POMC)	Endorphins e.g. β-endorphin and other nonopioid peptides e.g. ACTH	μ
Proenkephalin	Enkephalins e.g. Leu^5 enkephalin, Met^5 enkephalin, extended Met^5 enkephalins	δ μ μ
Prodynorphin	Dynorphins, e.g. dynorphin A	κ

ACTH, adrenocorticotrophic hormone.

OPIOID ANALGESIC DRUGS

Opioid analgesics are drugs, either naturally occurring (e.g. morphine) or chemically synthesized, that interact with specific opioid receptors to produce analgesia.

Mechanism of action—Opioid analgesic drugs work by agonist action at opioid receptors (see earlier).

The sense of euphoria produced by strong opioids contributes to their analgesic activity by helping to reduce the anxiety and stress associated with pain. This effect also accounts for the illicit use of these drugs.

Route of administration—Oral, rectal, intravenous, intramuscular, transdermal and transmucosal (as lozenges).

Oral absorption is irregular and incomplete, necessitating larger doses; 70% is removed by first-pass hepatic metabolism. Fentanyl is available in a transdermal drug delivery system as a self-adhesive patch, which is changed every 72 hours. Transdermal fentanyl is particularly useful in patients prone to nausea, sedation or severe constipation with morphine. Fentanyl is also useful for breakthrough pain when given as lozenges and helpful in patients with renal impairment because it is mainly metabolized by the liver. Morphine is the drug of choice for severe nociceptive pain.

Indications—Strong opioids (Table 10.3) are used in moderate to severe pain. They are commonly used preoperatively and postoperatively in patients with cancer, myocardial infarction or acute pulmonary oedema.

Weak opioids (see Table 10.3) are used in the relief of mild to moderate pain, as antitussives (Chapter 3) and as antidiarrhoeal agents (Chapter 6), taking advantage of the side effects of opioid analgesics.

Contraindications—Opioid analgesics should not be given to people in acute respiratory depression, with acute alcohol intoxication, or with head injuries before neurological assessment (because they can affect a patient's conscious level).

CLINICAL NOTE

Mrs Moore is a 60-year-old patient with bone pain secondary to advanced metastatic breast cancer, while receiving chemotherapy. She has been on several analgesics for the pain, including nonsteroidal antiinflammatory drugs (NSAIDs). NSAIDs were effective initially, but over the following months, the pain increased. In addition to regular NSAIDs, she was given co-codamol, a compound analgesic containing codeine and paracetamol. Compound analgesics contain both an opioid and a nonopioid and can be effective in controlling pain. Nevertheless, a palliative care specialist is asked to review Mrs Moore's pain and advise that she may require morphine in the future.

Table 10.3 Opioid analgesics

Weak opioid analgesics	Strong opioid analgesics
Pentazocine	Morphine
Codeine	Diamorphine
Dihydrocodeine	Phenazocine
Dextropropoxyphene	Pethidine
	Buprenorphine
	Nalbuphine

Adverse effects—Opioid analgesics share many adverse effects. These can be subdivided into central and peripheral adverse actions.

Central adverse actions include the following.

- Drowsiness and sedation, in which initial excitement is followed by sedation and finally a coma
- Reduction in sensitivity of the respiratory centre to carbon dioxide, leading to shallow and slow respiration
- Tolerance and dependence (Chapter 9)
- Suppression of a cough, an effect exploited clinically in antitussives (Chapter 3)
- Vomiting caused by stimulation of the chemoreceptor trigger zone (CTZ)
- Pupillary constriction caused by stimulation of the parasympathetic third cranial nerve nucleus
- Hypotension and reduced cardiac output, which are partly caused by reduced hypothalamic sympathetic outflow

Peripheral adverse actions include the following.

- Constipation, is partly caused by stimulation of cholinergic activity in the gut wall ganglia which results in smooth wall spasm
- Contraction of smooth muscle in the sphincter of Oddi and in the ureters, which results in an increase in blood amylase and lipase caused by pancreatic stasis
- Histamine release, which produces bronchospasm, flushing and arteriolar dilatation
- Lowered sympathetic discharge and direct arteriolar dilatation, which results in lowered cardiac output and hypotension

Adverse effects of opioids tend to limit the dose that can be given, and the level of analgesia that can be maintained. The most serious of all these effects is respiratory depression, which is the most common cause of death from opioid overdose.

Constipation and nausea are also common problems and clinically it is common to coadminister laxatives and an antiemetic (Chapter 6).

Tolerance and dependence—Tolerance to opioid analgesics can be detected within 24 to 48 hours from the onset of administration, and it results in increased doses of the drug being needed to achieve the same clinical effect.

Dependence involves μ receptors and is both physical and psychological in nature and is discussed in Chapter 9. If physical dependence develops, it is characterized by a definite withdrawal syndrome following cessation of the drug. This syndrome comprises a complex mixture of irritable, and sometimes aggressive behaviour combined with extremely unpleasant autonomic symptoms such as fever, sweating, yawning and pupillary constriction. The withdrawal syndrome is relieved by the administration of μ receptor agonists (e.g. naloxone) and worsened by the administration of μ receptor antagonists.

Psychological dependence of opioid analgesics is based on the positive reinforcement provided by euphoria.

In the clinical context, especially in terminal care, where tolerance and dependence can be monitored, they are not inevitably problematic. However, the fear of tolerance and dependence often leads to overcaution in the use of opioid analgesics, and inadequate pain control in some patients.

Therapeutic notes—Strong opioid analgesics include morphine, diamorphine (heroin), pethidine and buprenorphine.

- Morphine remains the most valuable drug for severe pain relief, although it frequently causes nausea and vomiting. It is the drug of choice for severe pain in terminal care. Morphine is the standard against which other opioid analgesics are compared.
- Diamorphine (heroin) is twice as potent as morphine, owing to its greater penetration of the blood–brain barrier. It is metabolized to 6-acetylmorphine and thence morphine in the body. Diamorphine causes less nausea and hypotension than morphine, but more euphoria. It has a rapid onset of action and thus is useful for breakthrough pain.
- Pethidine is more lipid soluble than morphine, and it has a rapid onset and short duration of action, making it useful in labour. Pethidine is equianalgesic compared with morphine, but it produces less constipation. Interaction with monoamine inhibitors is serious, causing fever, delirium and convulsions or respiratory depression.
- Buprenorphine has both agonist and antagonist actions at opioid receptors, and it may precipitate withdrawal symptoms in patients dependent on other opioids. It has a longer duration of action than morphine and its lipid solubility allows sublingual administration. Buprenorphine is commonly given as a patch for patients with long-term opioid analgesic requirements. Unlike most opioid analgesics, the effects of buprenorphine are only partially antagonized by naloxone owing to its high-affinity attraction to opioid receptors.

Weak opioid analgesics include pentazocine, codeine, dihydrocodeine and dextropropoxyphene.

- Pentazocine has both κ/σ receptor agonist and μ antagonist actions, and it may precipitate withdrawal symptoms in patients dependent on other opioids. Pentazocine is weak orally, but, by injection, it has a potency between that of morphine and codeine. It is not recommended because of the side effects of thought disturbances and hallucinations, which probably are caused by its action on σ receptors.

- Codeine has about one-twelfth of the analgesic potency of morphine but is commonly prescribed as a weak opioid analgesic. The incidence of nausea and constipation limit the dose and duration that can be used. Codeine is also used for its antitussive and antidiarrhoeal effects.
- Dihydrocodeine has an analgesic efficacy similar to that of codeine. It may cause dizziness and constipation.
- Dextropropoxyphene has an analgesic efficacy about one-half that of codeine (i.e. very mild), and so it is often combined with aspirin or paracetamol. Such mixtures can be dangerous in overdose, with dextropropoxyphene causing respiratory depression and acute heart failure and the paracetamol being hepatotoxic.

CLINICAL NOTE

Opioids are renally excreted so should be used cautiously in patients with renal impairment. If opioid analgesia is required, oxycodone or fentanyl is safer to prescribe.

Opioid antagonists

Examples of opioid antagonists include naloxone and naltrexone.

Mechanism of action—These drugs act by specific antagonism at opioid receptors: μ, δ and κ receptors are blocked more or less equally. They block the actions of endogenous opioids as well as of morphine-like drugs.

Naloxone is short acting (half-life: 2–4 hours) whereas naltrexone is long acting (half-life: 10 hours).

Route of administration—Intravenous.

Indications—Opioid antagonists are given to reverse opioid-induced analgesia and respiratory depression rapidly, mainly after overdose, or to improve the breathing of newborn babies who have been affected by opioids given to the mother.

Adverse effects—Precipitation of withdrawal in those with physical dependence on opioids. Reversal of analgesic effects of opiate agonist.

HEADACHE AND NEURALGIC PAIN

Headache

A headache is a very common presenting symptom, yet one which can be difficult to manage. The most common causes of a headache include the following.

- Tension-type headache
- Migraine
- Headache associated with eye or sinus disease

More sinister causes of a headache (including meningitis and tumours) are less common, and these can often be excluded by the history and examination.

The pathophysiology underlying a headache is unclear, although symptomatic relief is often obtained from NSAIDs and paracetamol. Some headaches are related to stress and anxiety, and these patients may benefit from antidepressant drugs (Chapter 8).

The management of a migraine includes the treatment and prophylaxis of acute attacks. Drugs used for acute migrainous attacks.

- NSAIDs and paracetamol (see p. 159)
- Antiemetics (Chapter 6)
- Serotonin (5-HT$_1$) agonists

Drugs used in migraine prophylaxis include the following.

- Histamine (H1)/5-HT antagonists
- β-receptor antagonists (Chapter 4)
- Tricyclic antidepressants (Chapter 8)

Serotonin agonists

Sumatriptan and rizatriptan are 5-HT$_1$ agonists.

Mechanism of action—Serotonin agonists are believed to reverse the dilatation of cerebral blood vessels in the acute attack, which may be responsible for some of the symptoms of a migraine.

Route of administration—Oral, intranasal, subcutaneous.

Indications—Acute migraine attacks.

Contraindications—Caution in coronary artery disease (may cause vasoconstriction of coronary vessels), hepatic impairment, pregnancy and breastfeeding.

Adverse effects—Sensations of tingling, heat, chest tightness.

H1 receptor/serotonin antagonists

Pizotifen is the main drug in this class.

Mechanism of action—Unlike the serotonin agonists, pizotifen appears to limit the initial proinflammatory and vascular changes which precede migrainous episodes.

Route of administration—Oral.

Indications—Prevention of migraine and cluster headache.

Contraindications—To be used cautiously in patients with urinary retention, angle-closure glaucoma, renal impairment, pregnancy, breastfeeding.

Adverse effects—Antimuscarinic effects (urinary retention, dry mouth), drowsiness, increased appetite.

Neuralgic pain

Neuralgic pain is a pain in the distribution of a particular nerve or nerve root. The most common pathologies are sciatica, herpetic neuralgia and trigeminal neuralgia.

Neuralgia commonly occurs because of compression or entrapment of the nerve or nerve root, and definitive management relies on the surgical release of the nerve.

Pharmacological options can be used when surgery is ill advised, or ineffective, or as an adjunct. NSAIDs are not effective for neuralgic pain. Antidepressants, in particular, amitriptyline, often have an "analgesic" effect in neuralgic pain, and often at a dose lower than their antidepressant effect (Chapter 8).

The other main class of drug used orally in neuralgic pain are the anticonvulsants, notably carbamazepine, phenytoin and more recently lamotrigine (Chapter 8). These potentially stabilize the neurones involved and limit their activation.

Local anaesthesia of the nerve in question can provide relief for some patients, although nerve ablation with drugs (e.g. bupivacaine) or by surgical means can be performed to alleviate symptoms.

LOCAL ANAESTHESIA

Basic concepts

Local anaesthetics are drugs used to inhibit pain sensation. These drugs work by reversibly blocking nerve conduction.

Chemistry
All local anaesthetics have the same basic structure.

- An aromatic group (lipophilic end) linked to a basic side chain (hydrophilic end) by an ester or amide bond (Fig. 10.3)
- The basic side chain (usually a secondary or tertiary amine) is important because only the uncharged molecule can enter the nerve axoplasm.

Potency and duration of action are correlated with high lipid solubility.

Pharmacokinetics
Elimination of local anaesthetics depends on the nature of the chemical bond.

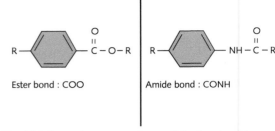

Fig. 10.3 General structure of ester-linked and amide-linked local anaesthetics.

- Local anaesthetics with ester bonds are inactivated by plasma cholinesterases.
- Local anaesthetics with amide bonds are degraded by N-dealkylation in the liver.

Metabolites can often be pharmacologically active.

Mechanism of block

Importance of pH and ionization
Local anaesthetics are weak bases ($pK_a = 8$–9). Only the uncharged form can penetrate lipid membranes; thus, quaternary ammonium compounds, which are fully protonated, must be injected directly into the nerve axon if they are to work.

The proportion of uncharged local anaesthetic is governed by the pH, the pK_a and the Henderson–Hasselbalch equation (Chapter 1).

$$B + H^+ = BH^+$$
$$pK_a = pH + \log\left[BH^+\right]/\left[B^-\right]$$

A local anaesthetic with a pK_a of 8 will be 10% uncharged at pH 7, 50% uncharged at pH 8, and 5% uncharged at pH 6.

Routes of block

Most local anaesthetics block by two routes (Fig. 10.4).

- The hydrophobic route, the uncharged form enters the membrane and blocks the channel from a site in the protein membrane interface.
- The hydrophilic route, the uncharged form crosses the membrane to the inside where the charged form blocks

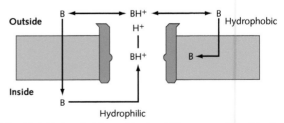

Fig. 10.4 Hydrophobic and hydrophilic routes of the block for local anaesthesia.

the channel. This pathway depends on the channel being open and, therefore this type of block is use dependent. Use dependency is especially important in the antiarrhythmic action of local anaesthetics.

- Nerve block occurs when the number of noninactivated channels (those unaffected by the drug) is insufficient to bring about depolarisation to the threshold.

CLINICAL NOTE

Mr Hadeed is a 34-year-old metal grinder who presents to an Eye Hospital A&E with an acute onset of left eye pain, which occurred while at work. He has never had any pain like this before. Slit-lamp examination revealed a fairly superficial foreign body in his left eye. To remove the foreign body, the eye is prepared with the application of lidocaine (local anaesthetic) eye drops and then the foreign body is removed with a needle.

Routes of administration

Surface anaesthesia
In surface anaesthesia, the local anaesthetic is applied directly to the skin and mucous membranes, for example, cornea, bronchial tree, oesophagus and genitourinary tract. The local anaesthetic, for example, lidocaine, must be able to penetrate the tissues easily. Problems occur when large areas, for example, the bronchial tree, are anaesthetized.

Infiltration anaesthesia
Infiltration anaesthesia involves direct injection of a local anaesthetic into tissue. Often, a vasoconstrictor such as adrenaline is used with the local anaesthetic to prevent the spread of the local anaesthetic into the systemic circulation. Vasoconstrictors must never be used at extremities as ischaemia could result.

Nerve block anaesthesia
In nerve block anaesthesia, a local anaesthetic is injected close to the appropriate nerve trunk, for example, the brachial plexus. The injection must be accurate in location. Nerve block anaesthesia can be useful in the reduction of limb dislocations or fractures.

Spinal and epidural anaesthesia
Spinal anaesthesia involves the injection of a local anaesthetic into the cerebrospinal fluid (CSF) in the subarachnoid space.

In epidural anaesthesia, the local anaesthetic is injected into the space between the dura mater and the spinal cord.

In both spinal and epidural anaesthesia, the local anaesthetic acts by blocking spinal roots, as opposed to the spinal cord itself. Problems arise from the block of preganglionic sympathetic fibres supplying the vasculature (causing vasodilatation) and the heart (causing bradycardia), both leading to hypotension. Rostral spread can lead to the blocking of intercostal and phrenic nerves and result in respiratory depression. Tilting the patient can control the amount the anaesthetic spreads.

HINTS AND TIPS

In inflamed tissues, the pH is acidic, resulting in a greater proportion of the charged form of the anaesthetic, thus delaying or preventing its onset of action.

Unwanted effects

Unwanted effects of local anaesthetics are mainly associated with the spread of the drug into the systemic circulation.

- Effects on the CNS, such as restlessness, tremor, confusion, agitation. At high doses, CNS depression can occur. Procaine is worse than lidocaine or bupivacaine for causing CNS depression and is seldom used.
- Respiratory depression
- Possible effects on the cardiovascular system, including myocardial depression and vasodilatation
- Visual disturbances and twitching
- Severe toxicity causes convulsions and coma

HINTS AND TIPS

Fentanyl should not be used in patients who have been on monoamine inhibitors in the previous 14 days. The interaction between these drugs can produce an accumulation of serotonin and the patient may become delirious and violent, or may develop severe hypertension, dysrhythmias or fatal respiratory depression.

Properties and uses

Table 10.4 shows the properties and uses of the main local anaesthetics, and Table 10.5 lists other compounds that block sodium channels.

GENERAL ANAESTHESIA

Basic concepts

General anaesthesia is the absence of sensation associated with a reversible loss of consciousness.

Table 10.4 Properties and uses of the main local anaesthetics

	Rate of onset	Duration	Tissue penetration	Chemistry	Common use
Cocaine	Rapid	Moderate	Rapid	Ester bond	ENT
Procaine	Moderate	Short	Slow	Ester bond	Little used, CNS effects
Tetracaine (amethocaine)	Slow	Long	Moderate	Ester bond	Topical, prevenepuncture
Oxybuprocaine (benoxinate)	Rapid	Short	Rapid	Ester bond	Surface, ophthalmology
Benzocaine	Very slow	Very long	Rapid	Ester bond, no basic side chain	Surface ENT
Lidocaine (lignocaine)	Rapid	Moderate	Rapid	Amide bond	Widely used in all applications, EMLA
Prilocaine	Moderate	Moderate	Moderate	Amide bond	Many uses, IVRA, EMLA. Low toxicity
Bupivacaine	Slow	Long	Moderate	Amide bond	Epidural and spinal anaesthesia

CNS, Central nervous system; EMLA, eutectic mixture of local anaesthetics; ENT, ear, nose and throat; IVRA, intravenous regional anaesthetic.

Table 10.5 Naturally occurring and synthetic sodium channel blockers

Compound	Source	Type of block
Tetrodotoxin	Puffer fish	Outside only
Saxitoxin	Plankton	Outside only
μ-Conotoxins	Piscivorous marine snail	Affects inactivation
μ-Agatoxins	Funnel web spider	Affects inactivation
α-, β- and γ-toxins	Scorpions	Complex
QX314 and QX222	Synthetic, permanently charged local anaesthetics	Inside only (hydrophobic pathway)
Benzocaine	Synthetic, uncharged local anaesthetic	From within the membrane (hydrophilic pathway)
Local anaesthetics	Plant (cocaine), others synthetic	Inside and from within the membrane

General anaesthetics are used as an adjunct to surgical procedures to render the patient unaware of, and unresponsive to, painful stimuli. Modern anaesthesia is characterized by the so-called balanced technique, in which drugs and anaesthetic agents are used specifically to produce analgesia, sleep/sedation and muscle relaxation and the abolition of reflexes.

No one drug or anaesthetic agent can produce all these effects, and so a combination of agents is used in the three clinical stages of surgical general anaesthesia. The three stages are premedication, induction and maintenance.

Some may argue that a fourth stage exists, in which drugs are used to reverse the action of agents given in the previous three stages.

Premedication

Premedication is often given on the ward before the patient is taken to the operating theatre (Table 10.6), and it has four component aims.

- Relief from anxiety
- Reduction of parasympathetic bradycardia and secretions
- Analgesia
- Prevention of postoperative emesis.

Table 10.6 General anaesthetic agents

Premedication	Induction/ intravenous agents	Maintenance/ inhalation agents
Relief from anxiety, e.g. diazepam, lorazepam	Barbiturates, e.g. thiopental	Nitrous oxide Halothane
Reduction of parasympathetic bradycardia and secretions, e.g. atropine, hyoscine	Nonbarbiturates, e.g. propofol, ketamine	Enflurane Isoflurane Sevoflurane
Analgesia, e.g. NSAIDs, fentanyl		
Postoperative antiemesis, e.g. metoclopramide, prochlorperazine		

NSAIDs, Nonsteroidal antiinflammatory drugs.

Relief from anxiety

Oral benzodiazepines, for example, diazepam and midazolam (Chapter 8), are most effective and they perform three useful functions.

- Relieve apprehension and anxiety before anaesthesia
- Lessen the amount of general anaesthetic required to achieve and to maintain unconsciousness
- Possibly, sedate postoperatively.

Reduction of parasympathetic bradycardia and secretions

Muscarinic antagonists, for example, atropine and hyoscine (Chapter 2), are used to prevent salivation and bronchial secretions, and importantly to protect the heart from arrhythmias, particularly bradycardia caused by some inhalation agents and neuromuscular blockers.

Analgesia

Opioid analgesics, for example, fentanyl, are often given before an operation: although the patient is unconscious during surgery, adequate analgesia is important to stop physiological stress reactions to pain. NSAIDs are useful alternatives and adjuncts to opiates, although are likely to be inadequate for severe postoperative pain used alone.

Postoperative antiemesis

Drugs that provide postoperative antiemesis include metoclopramide and prochlorperazine. Nausea and vomiting are common after general anaesthesia, often because of the administration of opioid drugs perioperatively and postoperatively. Antiemetic drugs can be given with the premedication to inhibit this.

Induction

Intravenous agents (see Table 10.6) are used to produce a rapid induction of unconsciousness. Patients, in general, prefer intravenous agents because some patients find having a mask placed over the face unpleasant.

Prevention of acid aspiration in emergency and obstetric operations is crucial, and it relies on the administration of either an H_2-receptor antagonist or a proton-pump inhibitor before induction (Chapter 6).

Maintenance

Inhalation anaesthetic agents (see Table 10.6) are used to maintain a state of general anaesthesia after induction in most patients, although intravenous agents can be used via a continuous pump.

Anaesthetic agents

Anaesthetic agents depress all excitable tissues including central neurones, cardiac muscle and smooth and striated muscle. Different parts of the CNS have different sensitivities to anaesthetics, and the reticular activating system, which is responsible for consciousness, is among the most sensitive. Hence, it is possible to use anaesthetics at a concentration that produces unconsciousness without unduly depressing the cardiovascular or respiratory centres of the brain or the myocardium. However, for the majority of anaesthetics, the margin of safety is small.

Intravenous anaesthetics

Intravenous anaesthetics, for example, thiopental, propofol and ketamine, are all CNS depressants. They produce anaesthesia by relatively selective depression of the reticular activating system of the brain. They may be used alone for short surgical procedures, but they are used mainly for the induction of anaesthesia, and, therefore, it is rapidity of onset that is the desirable feature.

Intravenous anaesthetics are all highly lipid-soluble agents and cross the blood–brain barrier rapidly; their rapid onset (< 30 seconds) results from this rapid transfer into the brain and high cerebral blood flow. Duration of action is short (minutes) and terminated by redistribution of the drug from the CNS into less-well-perfused tissues (Fig. 10.5); drug metabolism is irrelevant to recovery.

Thiopental

Mechanism of action—Thiopental is a highly lipophilic member of the barbiturate group of CNS depressants that act to potentiate the inhibitory effect of GABA on the $GABA_A/Cl^-$ receptor channel complex.

Route of administration—Intravenous.

Indications—Rapid induction of general anaesthesia.

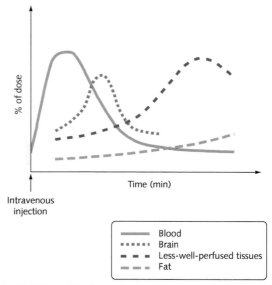

Fig. 10.5 Redistribution of intravenous anaesthetic agents to less-well-perfused tissues causes a short central duration of action. (Modified from Rang HP, et al. *Pharmacology,* 7th edition. Churchill Livingstone 2012.)

Contraindications—Thiopental should not be given to a patient with a previous allergy to it or who has porphyria.

Adverse effects—Respiratory depression, myocardial depression (bradycardia), vasodilatation and anaphylaxis. There is a risk of severe vasospasm if thiopental is accidentally injected into an artery.

Therapeutic notes—Thiopental is a widely used induction agent, but it has no analgesic properties. It provides smooth and rapid (< 30 seconds) induction but, owing to its narrow therapeutic margin, overdosage with consequent cardiorespiratory depression occur. Thiopental is given as the sodium salt, which is unstable in solution and so it must be made up immediately before use.

Propofol

Mechanism of action—Propofol is similar to thiopental in its mechanism of action.

Route of administration—Intravenous.

Indications—Induction or maintenance of general anaesthesia or sedation in intensive care units.

Contraindications—Propofol should not be given to patients with a previous allergy to it.

Adverse effects—Convulsions, anaphylaxis, and delayed recovery from anaesthesia have occasionally been reported as side effects.

Therapeutic notes—Propofol is associated with rapid recovery without nausea or hangover, and it is very widely used. Propofol is the drug of choice if an intravenous agent is to be used to maintain anaesthesia by a continuous infusion.

CLINICAL NOTE

Dina is a 17-year-old student who presents to A&E, looking very unwell and with severe pain in her right iliac fossa. She reports that the pain had originally started around her belly button a couple of hours ago and that she has vomited twice since. Examination reveals a tender abdomen with guarding. A computed tomography scan shows an inflamed appendix. She is rushed to theatre. Midazolam is given as sedation because she is rather anxious about the sudden forthcoming operation. Hyoscine is given before the operation because it dries bronchial and salivary secretions. Domperidone is also given beforehand for antiemesis. General anaesthesia is induced with propofol and maintained with isoflurane. The muscle relaxant rocuronium and the analgesic fentanyl (intravenous) are also given for the operation. Rocuronium is stopped before completion of the operation, but a small dose of neostigmine is required to fully reverse the effect of rocuronium.

Etomidate

Mechanism of action—The mechanism of action of etomidate is similar to that of thiopental.

Route of administration—Intravenous.

Indications—Rapid induction of general anaesthesia.

Contraindications—Etomidate should not be given to patients with a previous allergy to it.

Adverse effects—Extraneous muscle movement and pain on injection, possible adrenocortical suppression.

Therapeutic notes—Etomidate is an induction agent that gained favour over thiopental because of its larger therapeutic margin and faster metabolism leading to fewer hangover effects. Etomidate is more prone to causing extraneous muscle movement and pain on injection compared with other agents.

Ketamine

Mechanism of action—Ketamine produces full surgical anaesthesia, but the form of the anaesthesia is known as *dissociative anaesthesia* because the patient may remain conscious although amnesic and insensitive to pain. This effect is probably related to an action on N-methyl-D-aspartate (NMDA)-type glutamate receptors. Ketamine is a derivative of the street drug PCP (angel dust) (Chapter 9).

Route of administration—Intravenous, intramuscular.

Indications—Ketamine is used in the induction and maintenance of anaesthesia, especially in children.

Contraindications—Ketamine should not be given to people with hypertension or psychosis.

Adverse effects—These include cardiovascular stimulation, tachycardia and raised arterial blood pressure, as well as transient psychotic sequelae such as vivid dreams and hallucinations.

Therapeutic notes—Ketamine is not often used as an induction agent, owing to the high incidence of dysphoria and hallucinations during recovery in adults. These effects are much less marked in children, and ketamine, in conjunction with a benzodiazepine, is often used for minor procedures in paediatrics.

Inhalation anaesthetics

Examples of inhalation anaesthetics include halothane, enflurane, isoflurane, sevoflurane and desflurane. Nitrous oxide also has anaesthetic properties.

Inhalation anaesthetics may be gases or volatile liquids. They are commonly used for the maintenance of anaesthesia after induction with an intravenous agent.

Mechanism of action

It is not known exactly how inhalation anaesthetic agents produce their effects. Unlike most drugs, inhalation anaesthetics do not all belong to one recognizable chemical class. It seems that the pharmacological action of inhalation anaesthetics is dependent on the physiochemical properties of the molecule. Anaesthetic potency is closely linked to lipid solubility–anaesthetics dissolve in the membrane lipid and cause volume expansion. There is evidence to suggest that anaesthetics may also act by binding to discrete hydrophobic domains of membrane proteins. Anaesthetics are thought to enhance the activity of inhibitory $GABA_A$ receptors and other ion gated channels, particularly potassium channels.

HINTS AND TIPS

Similar to the benzodiazepines and barbiturates, thiopental and propofol act via the $GABA_A/Cl^-$ receptor in causing CNS depression.

Pharmacokinetic aspects

The depth of anaesthesia produced by inhalation anaesthetics is directly related to the partial pressure (tension) of the agent in the arterial blood because this determines the concentration of an agent in the CNS. The concentration of anaesthetic in the blood is in turn determined by the following.

- The concentration of anaesthetic in the inspired gas (alveolar concentration)
- The solubility of the anaesthetic in the blood (blood/gas partition coefficient)
- Cardiac output
- Alveolar ventilation.

Rapid induction and recovery are important properties of an anaesthetic agent, allowing flexible control over the arterial tension (and hence brain tension) and, therefore the depth of anaesthesia. The speed at which induction of anaesthesia occurs is determined by two properties of the anaesthetic: its solubility in blood (blood/gas partition coefficient) and its solubility in fat (lipid solubility).

- Agents of low blood solubility (e.g. nitrous oxide, enflurane) produce rapid induction and recovery because relatively small amounts are required to saturate the blood, and so the arterial tension (and hence brain tension) rises and falls quickly (Fig. 10.6).
- Agents of high blood solubility (e.g. halothane) have much slower induction and recovery times because much more anaesthetic solution is required before the arterial anaesthetic tension approaches that of the inspired gas (see Fig. 10.6).
- Agents with high lipid solubility (e.g. ether) accumulate gradually in the body fat during prolonged anaesthesia and so may produce a prolonged hangover if used for a long surgical procedure (see Fig. 10.6).

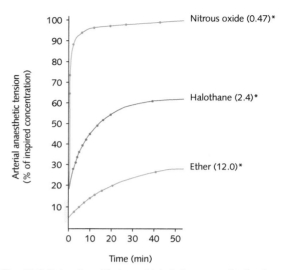

Fig. 10.6 Rate of equilibrium of inhalation anaesthetics in humans. (Modified from Papper EM, Kitz R. *Uptake and Distribution of Anaesthetic Agents.* McGraw-Hill 1963).

Nitrous oxide

Mechanism of action—See earlier.

Route of administration—Inhalation.

Indications—Nitrous oxide is used in the maintenance of anaesthesia (in combination with other agents), and for analgesia (50% mixture in oxygen: Entonox).

Contraindications—Pneumothorax. Nitrous oxide diffuses into air containing closed spaces resulting in an increased pressure, in the case of pneumothorax, which may compromise breathing.

Adverse effects—Nitrous oxide has been associated with bone marrow suppression if used long-term.

Therapeutic notes—Nitrous oxide cannot produce surgical anaesthesia when administered alone, because of a lack of potency. It is commonly used as a nonflammable carrier gas for volatile agents, allowing their concentration to be reduced. As a 50% mixture in oxygen, nitrous oxide is a good analgesic and is commonly prescribed during childbirth or for painful dressing changes.

Halothane

Mechanism of action—See earlier.

Route of administration—Inhalation.

Indications—Halothane is used in the maintenance of anaesthesia.

Contraindications—Halothane should not be given to people with a previous reaction to halothane or exposure to halothane in the previous 3 months.

Adverse effects—Halothane causes cardiorespiratory depression.

Respiratory depression results in elevated carbon dioxide partial pressure. Halothane also depresses cardiac muscle fibres and may cause bradycardia and ventricular arrhythmias. The result of this is a concentration-dependent hypotension.

The most significant toxic effect of halothane is severe hepatic necrosis, which occurs in 1 in 35,000 cases. Lesser degrees of liver damage may occur more frequently. The damage is caused by metabolites of the 20% of administered halothane that is biotransformed in the liver (80% of an administered dose is excreted by the lungs).

Therapeutic notes—Halothane is a halogenated hydrocarbon.

Enflurane

Mechanism of action—See earlier.

Route of administration—Inhalation.

Indications—Enflurane is used in the maintenance of anaesthesia.

Contraindications—Enflurane should not be given to people with epilepsy.

Adverse effects—Enflurane causes cardiorespiratory depression similar to that with halothane, although the incidence of arrhythmias is much lower than with halothane.

Enflurane undergoes only 2% metabolism in the liver, so it is much less likely than halothane to cause hepatotoxicity. The disadvantage of enflurane is that it may cause muscle twitching, and special caution is needed in epileptic subjects.

Therapeutic notes—Enflurane is a volatile anaesthetic similar to, but less potent than, halothane, about twice the concentration is necessary for maintenance. Induction and recovery times are faster than for halothane.

Isoflurane

Mechanism of action—See earlier.

Route of administration—Inhalation.

Indications—It is used in the maintenance of anaesthesia.

Contraindications—Susceptibility to malignant hyperthermia.

Adverse effects—Isoflurane has actions similar to those of halothane, but it has fewer effects upon the cardiorespiratory system. Hypotension is caused by a dose-related decrease in systemic vascular resistance rather than a marked fall in cardiac output. Less hepatic metabolism (0.2%) occurs than with enflurane, so hepatotoxicity is even rarer.

Therapeutic notes—Isoflurane is an isomer of enflurane. It has a potency intermediate between that of halothane and enflurane.

CLINICAL NOTE

Patients who are genetically susceptible may develop malignant hyperthermia when given a number of anaesthetics, particularly halothane and suxamethonium. Patients present with muscle rigidity, tachycardia, flushed skin, hypercapnia and a raised temperature (> 40°C).

Sevoflurane

Mechanism of action—See earlier.

Route of administration—Inhalation.

Indications—It is used both in the gas induction and in the maintenance of anaesthesia.

Contraindications—Susceptibility to malignant hyperthermia.

Adverse effects—Similar to isoflurane.

Therapeutic notes—Sevoflurane is probably the most widely used inhalation agent.

HINTS AND TIPS

Nitrous oxide is used as an adjunct to other inhaled agents because it reduces the dose required to maintain anaesthesia, thus limiting side effects and allowing more rapid recovery.

Use of neuromuscular blockers in anaesthesia

For some operations, for example, intraabdominal, complete relaxation of skeletal muscle is essential. Some general anaesthetic agents have significant neuromuscular blocking actions, but drugs that specifically block the neuromuscular junction are frequently used, for example, suxamethonium, rocuronium, vecuronium and atracurium (Chapter 2).

● **Chapter Summary**

- Pain is a subjective experience and management requires a careful assessment and use of the analgesic ladder
- Activation of nociceptors via primary afferent fibres results in pain
- Opioids are commonly prescribed analgesics but have several side effects, including respiratory depression
- Sumatriptan is used prophylactically in the management of a migraine
- Neuralgic pain is managed with low-dose antidepressants and anticonvulsants
- Potency and duration of action of local anaesthetics is dependent on lipid solubility
- Intravenous anaesthetics are used for induction and maintenance of anaesthesia
- Inhalational anaesthetics are typically used for maintenance of anaesthesia but can trigger malignant hyperthermia in susceptible individuals
  - Desflurane has a faster onset and recovery; useful for day case surgery
- Isoflurane is an irritant to the respiratory tract, causing cough and laryngospasm
  - Sevoflurane is similar to desflurane but is less of a respiratory irritant
- The speed at which induction of anaesthesia occurs is determined by two properties of the anaesthetic: its solubility in blood (blood/gas partition coefficient) and its solubility in fat (lipid solubility)

Inflammation, allergic diseases and immunosuppression 11

INFLAMMATION

Inflammation describes the changes seen in response to tissue injury or insult including pain, redness, heat, swelling and loss of function. These changes occur because of dilatation of local blood vessels, which lead to increased permeability and increased receptiveness for leucocytes. This results in the accumulation of inflammatory cells at the site of injury. The main cells seen in an acute inflammatory response are neutrophils and macrophages. Lymphocytes, basophils and eosinophils can also accumulate depending on the insult.

Inflammatory responses are produced and controlled by the interaction of a wide range of inflammatory mediators, some derived from leucocytes, some from the damaged tissues. Examples include the following.

- Histamine
- Kinins (bradykinin)
- Neuropeptides (substance-P, calcitonin gene-related peptide)
- Cytokines (e.g. interleukins [ILs])
- Arachidonic acid metabolites (eicosanoids).

Arachidonic acid metabolites: the eicosanoids

Of the inflammatory mediators mentioned previously, the eicosanoids are of special importance because they are involved in the majority of inflammatory reactions and thus most antiinflammatory therapy is based on the manipulation of their biosynthesis.

The eicosanoids are a family of polyunsaturated fatty acids formed from arachidonic acid. The biosynthetic pathway is shown in Fig. 11.1. Arachidonic acid is derived mainly from phospholipids of cell membranes, from which it is mobilized by the action of the enzyme phospholipase A_2. Arachidonic acid is then further metabolized by cyclooxygenase to produce the "classic prostaglandins", thromboxane and prostacyclin, collectively known as the proteinoids, and by lipoxygenase to produce the leukotrienes.

The actions of eicosanoids in inflammatory reactions are listed in Table 11.1.

Antiinflammatory drugs

These are the main drugs used for their broad-spectrum antiinflammatory effects.

- Nonsteroidal antiinflammatory drugs (NSAIDs).
- Steroidal antiinflammatory drugs (glucocorticoids) (Chapter 7).

Both these classes of antiinflammatory drug exert their effect by inhibiting the formation of eicosanoids (see Fig. 11.1).

In addition, there are a number of other drug classes that have more restricted antiinflammatory actions.

- Disease-modifying antirheumatic drugs (DMARDs)
- Drugs used to treat gout
- H1-receptor antagonists
- Drugs used to treat skin disorders

Nonsteroidal antiinflammatory drugs

NSAIDs all possess the ability to inhibit both forms of the enzyme cyclooxygenase (COX-1 and COX-2) (see Fig. 11.1), an action that is responsible for their pharmacological effects (Table 11.2).

The first drugs of this type were the salicylates (e.g. aspirin), extracted from the bark of the willow tree. Subsequently, many synthetic and semisynthetic NSAIDs have been created. Chemically and structurally heterogeneous, they are related through their common mechanism of action (see Table 11.3).

Mechanism of action—The main action of all the NSAIDs is inhibition of the enzyme cyclooxygenase. This enzyme is involved in the metabolism of arachidonic acid to form the prostanoids, that is, the classic prostaglandins, prostacyclin and thromboxane A_2. Inhibition of cyclooxygenase can occur by several mechanisms.

- Irreversible inhibition; for example, aspirin causes acetylation of the active site.
- Competitive inhibition; for example, ibuprofen acts as a competitive substrate.
- Reversible, noncompetitive inhibition, for example, paracetamol has a free radical trapping action that interferes with the production of hydroperoxidases, which are believed to have an essential role in cyclooxygenase activity.

Cyclooxygenase exists in two enzyme isoforms.

- COX-1: Expressed in most tissues, especially platelets, gastric mucosa and renal vasculature, and involved in physiological cell signalling. Most adverse effects of NSAIDs are caused by inhibition of COX-1.
- COX-2: Induced at sites of inflammation and produces the prostanoids involved in inflammatory responses. Analgesic and antiinflammatory effects of NSAIDs are largely caused by inhibition of COX-2.

COX-2-specific inhibitors (e.g. celecoxib) have a reduced incidence of gastric side effects. However, they are associated with an increased incidence of adverse cardiovascular events (such as myocardial infarction).

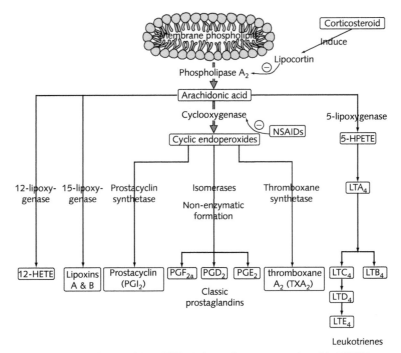

Fig. 11.1 Biosynthetic pathway of the eicosanoids. *HETE*, Hydroxyeicosatetraenoic acid; *HPETE*, hydroperoxyeicosatetraenoic acid; *LT*, leukotrienes; *NSAID*, nonsteroidal antiinflammatory drug; *PG*, prostaglandin.

Table 11.1 Actions of the eicosanoids in the inflammatory reaction

Eicosanoid	Actions in inflammation
Prostanoids	
"Classic prostaglandins" e.g. PGD_2, PGE_2, PGF_2	Produce increased vasodilatation, vascular permeability and oedema in an inflammatory reaction; prostaglandins also sensitize nociceptive fibres to stimulation by other inflammatory mediators
Thromboxane A_2 (TXA_2)	Platelet aggregation and vasoconstriction
Prostacyclin (PGI_2)	Inhibition of platelet aggregation and vasodilatation
Leukotrienes	
E.g. LTB_4, LTC_4	Increase vascular permeability, promote leucocyte chemotaxis (and cause contraction of bronchial smooth muscle)

Clinical effects—NSAIDs work by the inhibition of cyclooxygenase and resulting inhibition of prostaglandin synthesis, producing three major clinical actions of potential therapeutic benefit: analgesia, an antiinflammatory action and an antipyretic action (see Table 11.2).

Not all NSAIDs possess these three actions to exactly the same extent, an example being the lack of antiinflammatory activity possessed by paracetamol (see Table 11.3).

In addition, aspirin has a pronounced effect on inhibiting platelet aggregation, caused by reduced thromboxane synthesis. Aspirin irreversibly inhibits cyclooxygenase in platelets, and because platelets do not have a nucleus, they are unable to resynthesize a new enzyme, thus platelets are inhibited for their lifespan. Aspirin is therefore used in the primary and secondary prevention of cardiovascular and cerebrovascular events (Chapter 4).

Indications—NSAIDs are widely used for a variety of complaints. They are available on prescription and "over the counter". Their use includes musculoskeletal and joint diseases (strains, sprains, rheumatic problems, arthritis, gout, etc.), analgesia for mild to moderate pain relief and symptomatic relief of fever.

Contraindications—NSAIDs should not be given to people with gastrointestinal ulceration or bleeding or a previous hypersensitivity to any NSAID. Caution should be used in asthma and when renal function is impaired.

Adverse effects—Generalized adverse effects of NSAIDs are common, especially in the elderly and in chronic users, and mostly arise from the nonselective inhibition of COX-1 and COX-2 (Table 11.4).

Less commonly, liver disorders and bone marrow depression are seen. Other unwanted effects that are relatively specific to individual compounds are also seen (see later).

Table 11.2 Three major clinical actions of nonsteroidal antiinflammatory drugs

Clinical action	Mechanism of action
Analgesic action	The analgesic effect is largely a peripheral effect caused by the inhibition of prostaglandin synthesis at the site of pain and inflammation Prostaglandins do not produce pain directly, but sensitize nociceptive fibre nerve endings to other inflammatory mediators (bradykinin, histamine, 5-HT), amplifying the basic pain message; prostaglandins of the E and F series are implicated in this sensitizing action Thus NSAIDs are most effective against pain where there is an inflammatory component A small component of the analgesic action of NSAIDs is a consequence of a central effect in reducing prostaglandin synthesis in the CNS; paracetamol especially works in this manner
Antiinflammatory action	Prostaglandins produce increased vasodilatation, vascular permeability and oedema in an inflammatory reaction Inhibition of prostaglandin synthesis therefore reduces this part of the inflammatory reaction NSAIDs do not inhibit the numerous other mediators involved in an inflammatory reaction; thus inflammatory cell accumulation, for example, is not inhibited
Antipyretic action	During a fever, leucocytes release inflammatory pyrogens (e.g. interleukin-1) as part of the immune response; these act on the thermoregulatory centre in the hypothalamus to cause an increase in body temperature This effect is believed to be mediated by an increase in hypothalamic prostaglandins (PGEs), the generation of which is inhibited by NSAIDs NSAIDs do not affect temperature under normal circumstances or in heat stroke

5-HT, Serotonin; CNS, central nervous system; NSAIDs, nonsteroidal antiinflammatory drugs.

Table 11.3 Classes of nonsteroidal antiinflammatory drugs and comparison of their main actions

Chemical class	Examples	Analgesic	Antipyretic	Antiinflammatory
Salicylic acids	Aspirin	+	+	+
Propionic acids	Ibuprofen Fenuprofen	+	+	+
Acetic acids	Indometacin	+	+	++
Oxicams	Piroxicam	+	+	++
Pyrazolones	Phenylbutazone	+/−	+	++
Fenemates	Mefenamic acid	+	+	+/−
para-Aminophenols	Paracetamol	+	+	−

Table 11.4 General adverse effects of nonsteroidal antiinflammatory drugs

System	Adverse effect	Cause
GI	Dyspepsia, nausea, vomiting	Inhibition of the normal protective actions of prostaglandins on the gastric mucosa
	Ulcer formation and potential haemorrhage risk in chronic users	PGE_2 and PGI_2 normally inhibit gastric acid secretion, increase mucosal blood flow, and have a cytoprotective action
Renal	Renal damage/nephrotoxicity Renal failure can occur after years of chronic misuse	Inhibition of PGE_2- and PGI_2-mediated vasodilatation in the renal medulla and glomeruli
Other	Bronchospasm, skin rashes, other allergic-type reactions	Hypersensitivity reaction/allergy to drug

GI, Gastrointestinal; PG, prostaglandin.

Therapeutic notes on individual nonsteroidal antiinflammatory drugs

Salicylic acids, for example, aspirin.

- Aspirin irreversibly blocks the formation of thromboxane A_2, producing an inhibitory effect on platelet aggregation.

Its antiplatelet action is used in the management of a myocardial infarction and ischaemic stroke.

- Aspirin suppresses the production of prostaglandins because of its irreversible inactivation of cyclooxygenase enzyme. Thus it is an inexpensive drug to use in the management of mild pain despite a relatively high incidence of gastrointestinal side effects.

- Aspirin produces tinnitus in toxic doses.

Propionic acids, for example, ibuprofen.

- Ibuprofen has a lower incidence of side effects.

Acetic acids, for example, indomethacin.

- Indomethacin is a highly potent nonselective inhibitor of cyclooxygenase that is effective but associated with a high incidence of side effects.
- It may cause neurological effects such as dizziness and confusion, as well as gastrointestinal upsets.

Oxicams, for example, piroxicam.

- Piroxicam is a potent drug used for chronic inflammatory conditions, but it should only be prescribed by specialists because it causes a high incidence of severe gastrointestinal problems and skin reactions.

Fenemates, for example, mefenamic acid.

- Mefenamic acid is a moderately potent drug.
- It commonly causes gastrointestinal upset and occasionally skin rashes.

para-Aminophenols, for example, paracetamol.

- The mechanism of action of paracetamol is not completely understood, but it is not considered an antiinflammatory drug because it does not appear to inhibit the cyclooxygenase enzyme outside of the central nervous system (CNS).
- It is effective for pain, especially headaches and fever. This is probably as a result of its mechanism of action in trapping free radicals and interfering with the production of hydroperoxidases, which are believed to have an essential role in cyclooxygenase activity. In areas of inflammation, phagocytic cells produce high levels of peroxide that swamp this effect. It does appear to have some selective inhibition of cyclooxygenase within the CNS and can reduce the production of IL-1, which probably accounts for its antipyretic effect.

COX-2 specific inhibitors, for example, lumiracoxib and celecoxib.

- These preferentially inhibit the inducible COX-2 enzyme, limiting COX-1–mediated side effects observed with other, nonspecific NSAIDs.

The COX-2 inhibitors are licensed in the United Kingdom for symptomatic relief in osteoarthritis and rheumatoid arthritis. They are contraindicated in inflammatory bowel disease, ischaemic heart disease or cerebrovascular disease.

Steroidal antiinflammatory drugs (glucocorticoids)

There are two main groups of corticosteroids: the glucocorticoids and the mineralocorticoids. It is the glucocorticoids (such as cortisone and cortisol), which possess powerful antiinflammatory actions that make them useful in several diseases, for example, rheumatoid arthritis, inflammatory bowel conditions, asthma (see Chapter 3) and inflammatory conditions of the skin.

Their profound generalized inhibitory effects on inflammatory responses result from the effects of corticosteroids in altering the activity of certain corticosteroid-responsive genes.

- The antiinflammatory action results from reduced production of acute inflammatory mediators, especially the eicosanoids (see Fig. 11.1). Corticosteroids prevent the formation of arachidonic acid from membrane phospholipids by inducing the synthesis of a polypeptide called lipocortin. Lipocortin inhibits phospholipase A_2, the enzyme normally responsible for mobilising arachidonic acid from cell membrane phospholipids and thus inhibits the subsequent formation of both prostaglandins and leukotrienes.
- Corticosteroids reduce the number and activity of circulating immunocompetent cells, neutrophils and macrophages.
- Corticosteroids decrease the activity of macrophages and fibroblasts involved in the chronic stages of inflammation, leading to decreased inflammation and decreased healing. Glucocorticoids are discussed in detail in Chapter 7.

INFLAMMATORY DISEASES

Rheumatoid arthritis

Disease modifying antirheumatic drugs

DMARDs are a diverse group of agents mainly used in the treatment of rheumatoid arthritis, which is a chronic, progressive and destructive inflammatory disease of the joints (Table 11.5).

The mechanism of action of the DMARDs is often unclear; they appear to have a long-term depressive effect on the inflammatory response as well as possibly modulating other aspects of the immune system.

All DMARDs have a slow onset of action, with clinical improvement not becoming apparent until 4 to 6 months after the initiation of treatment. DMARDs have been shown

Table 11.5 Disease-modifying antirheumatic drugs

Class	Example
Gold salts	Sodium aurothiomalate, auranofin
Penicillamine	Penicillamine
Antimalarials	Chloroquine, hydroxyquinine
Sulfasalazine	Sulfasalazine
Immunosuppressants	Cytotoxic drugs: methotrexate, azathioprine, cyclosporine

to improve symptoms and reduce disease activity. They are believed to slow erosive damage at joints.

DMARDs are generally indicated for use in severe, active, progressive rheumatoid arthritis when NSAIDs alone have proved inadequate. DMARDs are frequently used in combination with an NSAID and/or low-dose glucocorticoids.

> ## HINTS AND TIPS
>
> DMARDS are also used in the management of other severe, chronic inflammatory conditions (e.g. inflammatory bowel disease or psoriasis).

Methotrexate

Mechanism of action—Acts as a competitive inhibitor of dihydrofolate reductase. Cytotoxic and immunosuppressant activity results from folic acid antagonism.

Route of administration—Oral.

Adverse effects—Potential blood dyscrasias and liver cirrhosis.

Therapeutic notes—Has a rapid onset of action and is a common first choice drug for rheumatoid arthritis. It is superior to most other DMARDS in terms of efficacy and patient tolerance.

Gold salts

Examples of gold salts include sodium aurothiomalate and auranofin.

Mechanism of action—The mechanism of action of gold salts is unknown; they may be taken up by, and inhibit, mononuclear macrophages, or may affect the production of free radicals.

Route of administration—Sodium aurothiomalate is given by intramuscular injection, and auranofin orally.

Adverse effects—Rashes, proteinuria, ulceration, diarrhoea, bone marrow suppression.

Therapeutic notes—Careful patient monitoring, including blood counts and urine analysis, is necessary. If any serious adverse effects develop, treatment must be stopped.

Penicillamine

Mechanism of action—The mechanism of action of penicillamine is unknown. It chelates metals and has immunomodulatory effects, including suppression of immunoglobulin (Ig) production and effects on immune complexes. Penicillamine may also decrease the synthesis of IL involved in the immune response associated with rheumatoid arthritis.

Route of administration—Oral.

Adverse effects—Rashes, proteinuria, ulceration, gastrointestinal upsets, fever, transient loss of taste, bone marrow suppression.

Therapeutic notes—As for gold salts.

Antimalarials

Examples of antimalarials include chloroquine and hydroxychloroquine (Chapter 12).

Mechanism of action—The mechanism of antimalarials is unclear. They interfere with a wide variety of leucocyte functions, including IL-1 production by macrophages, lymphoproliferative responses and T-cell cytotoxic responses.

Route of administration—Oral.

Adverse effects—At the low doses currently recommended for antimalarials, toxicity is rare. The major adverse effect is retinal toxicity.

Therapeutic notes—People on antimalarials should have their vision monitored.

Sulfasalazine

Mechanism of action—Sulfasalazine is broken down in the gut into its two component molecules, 5-aminosalicylate (5-ASA) and sulfapyridine. The 5-ASA moiety is believed to be a free radical scavenger and responsible for most of the antirheumatic effects of this drug.

Route of administration—Oral.

Adverse effects—Side effects of sulfasalazine are mainly caused by sulfapyridine; they are common but rarely serious. These include nausea, vomiting, headache and rashes. Rarely, blood disorders and oligospermia are reported.

Therapeutic notes—People on sulfasalazine should have their blood counts monitored.

> ## CLINICAL NOTE
>
> Mrs Arlington, a 50-year-old secretary, attends her General Practitioner (GP) with worsening pain in both her wrists and fingers, causing her increasing difficulty to type. Tender swelling is noted at those joints. A diagnosis of rheumatoid arthritis is made following an X-ray showing erosions and blood tests indicating that she is positive for IgM rheumatoid factor. Initially, she is given daily ibuprofen with omeprazole (a proton-pump inhibitor) to protect her stomach. This helps to begin with, however, 3 months later she presents with worsening symptoms. A diagnosis of progressive rheumatoid arthritis is made. She is given a short course of prednisolone (a glucocorticoid) and started on a DMARD, sulfasalazine by the rheumatology specialist.

Other Immunosuppressants

Certain drugs with immunosuppressive actions have been shown to be effective in autoimmune or inflammatory conditions (e.g. rheumatoid arthritis). These include three main groups.

- Drugs that inhibit IL-2 production or action
  - Cyclosporine is an example and is used in the management of rheumatoid arthritis as well as to suppress the rejection of transplanted organs (see later)

- Drugs that inhibit cytokine gene expression (e.g. corticosteroids) (see Chapter 7)
- Drugs that inhibit purine or pyrimidine synthesis
  - Azathioprine interferes with purine synthesis and is widely used for immunosuppression and to control autoimmune diseases. The drug is metabolized to mercaptopurine, an analogue that inhibits deoxyribonucleic acid (DNA) synthesis. The main unwanted side effect is bone marrow suppression. Other effects include nausea, vomiting, skin rashes and mild hepatotoxicity.

HINTS AND TIPS

DMARDs are prescribed by a specialist. Patients taking these agents need regular blood tests to assess their renal and liver function and to monitor their red and white blood cell counts.

Cytokine inhibitors

Cytokine inhibitors are also thought to retard destruction of joints caused by rheumatoid arthritis. They are usually used for highly active rheumatoid arthritis in those who have failed to respond to at least two standard DMARDs. The primary proinflammatory cytokines are tumour necrosis factor (TNF)-α and IL-1. Thus their inflammatory role in diseases, such as rheumatoid arthritis can be reduced via cytokine inhibitors.

Monoclonal antibodies

Examples of monoclonal antibodies include adalimumab, tocilizumab and infliximab.

Mechanism of action—The monoclonal antibodies bind TNF-α, preventing its interaction with cell surface receptors and the subsequent proinflammatory events.

Indications—Moderate to severe rheumatoid arthritis, after DMARDs have not provided an adequate response.

Contraindications—Pregnancy, breastfeeding, severe infections, heart failure.

Route of administration—Subcutaneous injection.

Adverse effects—Reemergence of tuberculosis, septicaemia, gastrointestinal disturbance, worsening heart failure, hypersensitivity reactions, blood disorders.

Interactions—Avoid concomitant use of live vaccines.

Therapeutic notes—Monitor for infections, discontinue if active tuberculosis is suspected.

Soluble tumour necrosis factor-α blocker

An example is etanercept.

Mechanism of action—Contains the ligand-binding component of the human TNF receptor. It, therefore competes with the patient's own receptors, thereby acting like a sponge to remove most of the TNF-α molecules from the joints and blood.

Indications—Moderate to severe rheumatoid arthritis after DMARDs have not provided an adequate response.

Contraindications—Pregnancy, breastfeeding, severe infections and heart failure.

Route of administration—Subcutaneous injection.

Adverse effects—Predisposition to infections, exacerbation of heart failure or demyelinating CNS disorders, blood disorders.

Interactions—Avoid concomitant use of live vaccines.

Therapeutic notes—Monitor for infections.

HINTS AND TIPS

The "-mab" of adalimumab and infliximab stands for their being monoclonal antibodies. The "-rcept" of etanercept is a useful clue to remember it is the soluble receptor for TNF-α.

Gout

Gout is a condition in which uric acid (monosodium urate) crystals are deposited in tissues, especially in the joints, provoking an inflammatory response that manifests as an extremely painful acute arthritis. Uric acid crystallizes in the tissues when plasma urate levels are high, because of either excessive production or reduced renal excretion.

There are two treatment strategies for gout: treatment of an acute attack and prophylaxis against further attacks (Table 11.6).

Treatment of an acute attack

Nonsteroidal antiinflammatory drugs

At the onset of an acute attack of gout, NSAIDs are used for their general antiinflammatory and analgesic effects.

Aspirin and other salicylates are not used in gout because they inhibit uric acid excretion in the urine, exacerbating serum concentrations. However, indomethacin can often be effective.

Table 11.6 Drugs used in the treatment of gout

Treatment of an acute attack	Example
NSAIDs	Indometacin
Immunosuppressive	Colchicine
Prophylaxis against recurrent attacks (reduction of plasma uric acid concentration)	
Agents that reduce uric acid synthesis	Allopurinol
Agents that increase uric acid excretion (uricosurics)	Sulfinpyrazone, probenecid

NSAIDs, Nonsteroidal antiinflammatory drugs

Colchicine

Mechanism of action—Colchicine helps in gouty arthritis by inhibiting the migration of leucocytes, such as neutrophils, into the inflamed joint. This effect is achieved as a result of the action of colchicine binding to tubulin, the protein monomer of microtubules, resulting in their depolymerisation. The result is that cytoskeletal movements and cell motility are severely inhibited.

The inhibition of microtubular function inhibits mitotic spindle formation, giving colchicine a cytotoxic effect on dividing cells. This cytotoxic effect is also responsible for side effects of colchicine.

Route of administration—Oral, rarely intravenously.

Adverse effects—Side effects of colchicine include gastrointestinal toxicity, with nausea, vomiting and diarrhoea, occurring in 80% of people. Rarely, bone marrow suppression and renal failure occur.

Therapeutic notes—Colchicine is rapidly effective. It is given for the first 24 hours of an attack and then for no more than 7 days. Nausea and vomiting are common side effects.

Prophylaxis against recurrent attacks

Preventative management of gout includes diet and lifestyle changes, as well as the use of drugs that reduce plasma uric acid concentration. These drugs should not be used during an acute attack because they will initially worsen symptoms. Indomethacin or colchicine should be coadministered for the first 3 months of treatment because the initiation of prophylactic treatment may precipitate an acute attack.

Agents that reduce uric acid synthesis

Allopurinol and febuxostat (xanthine oxidase inhibitors) are examples of a drug that reduces uric acid synthesis.

Mechanism of action—Allopurinol inhibits the enzyme xanthine oxidase, which converts purines (from DNA breakdown) into uric acid, thus reducing uric acid production.

Route of administration—Oral.

Adverse effects—Headaches, dyspepsia, diarrhoea, rash, drug interactions and acute exacerbation of gout initially. Rarely, life-threatening hypersensitivity occurs.

Therapeutic notes—Febuxostat is indicated in hyperuricaemia where urate deposition has occurred (in the form of tophi or arthritis).

Agents that increase uric acid excretion

Uricosurics are drugs that increase uric acid excretion. Examples of uricosurics include sulfinpyrazone and probenecid.

Mechanism of action—Uricosurics compete with uric acid for reabsorption in the proximal tubules, preventing uric acid reabsorption and resulting in uricosuria.

Route of administration—Oral.

Adverse effects—Gastrointestinal upset, deposition of uric acid crystals in the kidney, interference with excretion of certain drugs, and acute exacerbation of gout initially.

Therapeutic notes—Uricosurics should not be used during an acute attack of gout. NSAIDs or colchicine should be coadministered for the first 3 months of treatment because the initiation of treatment may precipitate an acute attack.

Skin disorders

The most common skin diseases are eczema, acne, psoriasis, skin cancer (usually managed surgically), viral warts and urticaria.

Eczema (dermatitis)

Eczema is an inflammatory disease of the skin, defined by the presence of epidermal intercellular oedema or spongiosis. It can occur because of several factors.

- Exogenous irritants and contact allergens
- Infections
- Atopy
- Drugs
- Certain environmental conditions such as low humidity and ultraviolet light

Drugs used to treat eczema and their targets are shown in Fig. 11.2.

Acne

Acne affects the pilosebaceous unit and occurs where these are numerous, such as on the face, back and chest. It is characterized by the presence of keratin plugs in the sebaceous duct openings, known as comedones. Other signs of worsening acne include inflammatory papules, pustules, nodules, cysts and scars.

Acne is stimulated by androgens, which is why it is related to puberty, and why the antiandrogen cyproterone is often used in females with acne (Chapter 7).

The drugs used to treat acne and their targets are shown in Fig. 11.3.

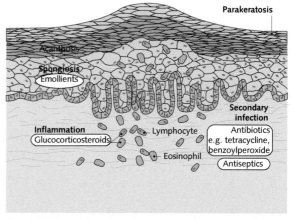

Fig. 11.2 Characteristics of eczema and point of action of its drug treatment. (Modified from Page, C., Curtis, M. Walker, M, Hoffman, B. (eds) *Integrated Pharmacology*, 3rd edn. Mosby, 2006.)

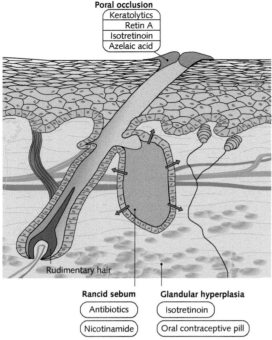

Poral occlusion
Keratolytics
Retin A
Isotretinoin
Azelaic acid

Rudimentary hair

Rancid sebum
Antibiotics
Nicotinamide

Glandular hyperplasia
Isotretinoin
Oral contraceptive pill

Fig. 11.3 Characteristics of acne and point of action of its drug treatment. (Modified from Page, C., Curtis, M. Walker, M, Hoffman, B. (eds) *Integrated Pharmacology*, 3rd edn. Mosby, 2006.)

Psoriasis

Psoriasis is a genetic skin disorder that manifests under certain conditions including stress, infection, damage from ultraviolet light, or trauma. In psoriasis, the turnover rate of skin is much greater than normal. Psoriasis is characterized by the following.

- Thickened skin plaques
- Superficial scales

- Dilated capillaries in the dermis (these might act to initiate psoriasis or as nourishment for hyperproliferating skin)
- An infiltrate of inflammatory cells, especially lymphocytes and neutrophils, in the epidermis and dermis, respectively

Drugs used to treat psoriasis and their targets are shown in Fig. 11.4.

Treatment of skin disorders

Preparations of drugs for use on skin

Drugs applied to the skin are delivered by a variety of vehicles such as ointments, creams, pastes, powders, aerosols, gels, lotions and tinctures. Factors affecting the choice of the vehicle include the following.

- The solubility of the active drug
- The ability of the drug to penetrate the skin
- The stability of the drug–vehicle complex
- The ability of the vehicle to delay evaporation, this being greatest for ointments and least for tinctures

Emollients

Emollients are used to soothe and hydrate the skin. A simple preparation is an aqueous cream, which is often as effective as more complex drugs.

Most creams are thin emollients, whereas a mixture of equal parts soft white paraffin and liquid paraffin is a thick emollient. Camphor, menthol and phenol preparations have antipruritic effects, whereas zinc-based and titanium-based emollients have mild astringent (contracting) effects.

Mechanism of action—Emollients hydrate the skin and reduce transepidermal water loss.

Route of administration—Topical. Many emollients can be added to bath water.

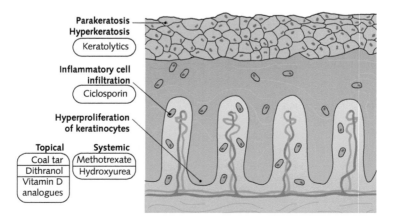

Parakeratosis
Hyperkeratosis
Keratolytics

Inflammatory cell
infiltration
Ciclosporin

Hyperproliferation
of keratinocytes

Topical
Coal tar
Dithranol
Vitamin D
analogues

Systemic
Methotrexate
Hydroxyurea

Fig. 11.4 Characteristics of psoriasis and point of action of its drug treatment. (Modified from Page, C., Curtis, M. Walker, M, Hoffman, B. (eds) *Integrated Pharmacology*, 3rd edn. Mosby, 2006.)

Indications—Emollients are used for the long-term treatment of dry scaling disorders.

Contraindications—None.

Adverse effects—Some ingredients, such as lanolin or antibacterials, may induce an allergic reaction.

Therapeutic notes—The use of emollients lessens the need for topical corticosteroids, therefore limiting potential side effects. They should be used liberally in the management of eczema and psoriasis.

Corticosteroids

Examples of corticosteroids include clobetasol propionate, betamethasone, clobetasol butyrate and hydrocortisone (Table 11.7).

Mechanism of action—Corticosteroids suppress components of the inflammatory reaction (see Chapter 7 and see Fig. 11.2).

Route of administration—Topically; orally, intradermally or intravenously in severe disease.

Indications—Corticosteroids are used for the relief of symptoms attributed by inflammatory conditions of the skin other than those caused by infection, for example, they are applied topically to affected areas in patients with eczema.

Contraindications—Rosacea, untreated skin infections.

Adverse effects—Most likely to occur with prolonged, or high dose therapy. Local: spread or worsening of infection, thinning of the skin, impaired wound healing, irreversible striae atrophicae. Systemic: immunosuppression, peptic ulceration, osteoporosis, hypertension, cataracts.

Therapeutic notes—Withdrawal of corticosteroids after high doses or prolonged use should be gradual (Chapter 7), even when used topically.

Dithranol

Dithranol is the most potent topical drug for the treatment of psoriasis.

Table 11.7 Potency of some topical steroids (UK classification and nomenclature)

Group	Approved name	Proprietary name
I (very potent)	Clobetasol propionate	Dermovate
II (potent)	Betametasone valerate 0.1%	Betnovate
	Beclometasone dipropionate	Propaderm
	Hydrocortisone 17-butyrate	Locoid
III (moderately potent)	Clobetasone butyrate	Eumovate
IV (mild)	Hydrocortisone 1%	Various
	Hydrocortisone 2%	Various

(Modified from Graham-Brown et al. Mosby's Color Atlas and Text of Dermatology, 1st edition. 1998.)

Mechanism of action—Dithranol modifies keratinisation and has an immunosuppressive effect (see Fig. 11.4).

Route of administration—Topical.

Contraindications—Dithranol should not be given to people with hypersensitivity or acute and pustular psoriasis.

Adverse effects—Local skin irritation, staining of skin and hair.

Vitamin D analogues

Calcipotriol and tacalcitol are vitamin D analogue derivatives.

Vitamin D analogues are keratolytics, although also used in vitamin D deficiency related to gastrointestinal/biliary disease and renal failure (Chapter 6).

Mechanism of action—The exact mechanism of action is still unclear, but several effects of vitamin D analogues have been observed. These include inhibition of epidermal proliferation and induction of terminal keratinocyte differentiation (see Fig. 11.4).

The antiinflammatory properties of vitamin D analogues include inhibition of T-cell proliferation and of cytokine release, decreased the capacity of monocytes to stimulate T-cell proliferation and to stimulate cytokine release from T cells, and inhibition of neutrophil accumulation in psoriatic skin.

Route of administration—Topical.

Indications—Psoriasis.

Contraindications—Vitamin D analogues should not be given to people with disorders of calcium metabolism. They should not be used on the face because irritation may occur.

Adverse effects—Side effects of vitamin D analogues include local irritation and dermatitis. High doses may affect calcium homoeostasis.

Tar preparations

Coal tar, made up of about 10,000 components, is keratolytic that is more potent than salicylic acid. It also has antiinflammatory and antipruritic properties.

Mechanism of action—Coal tar modifies keratinization, but the mechanism is unclear (see Fig. 11.4).

Route of administration—Topical.

Indications—Psoriasis and occasionally eczema.

Contraindications—Coal tar should not be given to people with acute or pustular psoriasis or in the presence of an infection. It should not be used on the face or on broken or inflamed skin.

Adverse effects—Skin irritation and acne-like eruptions, photosensitivity, staining of the skin and hair.

Salicylates

Salicylic acid is keratolytic at a concentration of 3% to 6%.

Mechanism of action—Salicylic acid causes desquamation via the solubilization of cell-surface proteins that maintain the integrity of the stratum corneum.

Route of administration—Topical.

Indications—Hyperkeratosis, eczema, psoriasis (combined with coal tar or dithranol preparations) and acne, wart and callus eradication.

Table 11.8 Other drugs used in skin disease, their indications and mechanisms of action

Drug	Indication	Mechanism of action
Benzoyl peroxide	Acne vulgaris	Antibacterial, keratolytic
Retinoids (vitamin A derivatives)	Acne vulgaris, psoriasis	Keratolytic, cytoinhibitory
Psoralen	Psoriasis	Mutates DNA/cytotoxic
Methotrexate	Psoriasis	Cytotoxic
Cyclosporine	Psoriasis	Immunosuppressant
Antibacterial, antiviral, antifungal preparations	Skin infections, warts	Antimicrobial
Antiparasite preparations	Skin/hair infestations	Parasite toxins
Tacrolimus ointment	Atopic eczema, psoriasis	Calcineurin inhibitor
Apremilast	Psoriasis	Phosphodiesterase 4 and TNF α inhibitor
Imiquimod	BCC, actinic keratosis, genital warts	Immune response modifier
Efudix (5-fluorouracil)	Benign and malignant skin lesions (e.g. BCC or SCC)	Inhibits DNA replication

BCC, Basal cell cancer; DNA, deoxyribonucleic acid; SCC, squamous cell cancer; TNF, tumour necrosis factor.
(Modified from Graham-Brown et al. Mosby's Color Atlas and Text of Dermatology, 1st edition. 1998.)

Contraindications—Sensitivity to the drug or broken or inflamed skin. High concentrations, such as those needed to treat warts, should not be given to people with diabetes mellitus or peripheral vascular disease because ulceration may be induced.

Adverse effects—Side effects of salicylic acid include anaphylactic shock in those sensitive to the drug, skin irritation and excessive drying, and systemic effects if used long-term.

Other drugs used in skin disease

Many other drugs are used in the management of skin disease. Some of the more common drugs are summarized in Table 11.8.

The future

Specific immunosuppressant drugs that selectively target interleukins (e.g. ustekinumab that targets IL-12 for psoriasis) and monoclonal antibodies used in the management of severe eczema have recently been developed and licensed for use by specialists. In addition, specialists can prescribe apremilast, an orally active phosphodiesterase 4 inhibitor, for the treatment of severe psoriasis and psoriatic arthritis. Similarly using immunotherapy for the treatment of melanoma is increasing.

ALLERGIC DISORDERS AND DRUG THERAPY

Allergic reactions occur when the immune system mounts an inappropriate response to an innocuous foreign substance.

Most common allergic disorders are caused by immunoglobulin E (IgE)-mediated type I immediate hypersensitivity reactions that occur in a previously sensitized person reexposed to the sensitising antigen. Type I immediate hypersensitivity reactions are also known as atopic disorders.

Patients with atopic diseases have an inherited predisposition to develop IgE antibodies to allergens that are normally innocuous and nonantigenic in healthy subjects. These specific IgE antibodies become bound to high-affinity IgE receptors (FcεRI) on the surface of tissue mast cells and blood basophils. The cross-linking of this cell-surface-bound IgE by antigens (allergens), on subsequent exposure, induces degranulation and release of mediators such as histamine, leukotrienes and prostaglandins (Fig. 11.5).

The released vasoactive and inflammatory mediators produce many local and systemic effects, including vasodilatation, increased vascular permeability, smooth muscle contraction, oedema, glandular hypersecretion and inflammatory cell infiltration.

Depending on the site of this reaction and release of mediators, a variety of disorders can result (Table 11.9).

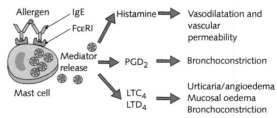

Fig. 11.5 Mechanism of type 1 hypersensitivity (allergic) reaction. *FcεRI*, Cell surface IgE receptor; *LT*, leukotriene; *PG*, prostaglandin. (Modified from Page, C., Curtis, M. Walker, M, Hoffman, B. (eds) *Integrated Pharmacology*, 3rd edn. Mosby, 2006.)

Table 11.9 Type I hypersensitivity/allergic disorders

Disorder	Site of reaction	Response	Common allergens
Anaphylaxis	Circulation	Oedema, circulatory collapse, death	Venoms, drugs
Allergic rhinitis/ hay fever	Nasal passages Conjunctiva	Irritation, oedema, mucosal hypersecretion	Pollen, dust
Asthma	Bronchioles	Bronchoconstriction, mucosal secretion, airway inflammation	Pollen, dust
Food allergy	GIT	Vomiting, diarrhoea, urticaria (hives)	Seafood, milk, etc.
Wheal and flare	Skin	Vasodilatation and oedema	Insect venom

GIT, gastrointestinal tract.

Drug therapy of allergic disorders

The most effective therapy in hypersensitivity reactions is avoidance of the offending antigen or environment. When this is not possible, drug therapy can be of use (Table 11.10).

CLINICAL NOTE

Adam, a 6-year-old boy, is rushed to A&E with a blood pressure of 65/30 mm Hg. He is clearly in distress, breathless and vomiting. Swollen lips and blisters around his mouth are also noted. His father tells the doctor that he had been fine previously and had just started having his lunch, peanut butter sandwiches. Suddenly, he became severely unwell. The doctors acted quickly to diagnose anaphylactic shock. Adam is given oxygen and 250 μg adrenaline intramuscularly. Afterwards, he is also given chlorphenamine (H1-receptor antagonist) and hydrocortisone to prevent relapse. He and his father are advised about the allergic reaction and the need to avoid peanuts. Adam is taught to carry prefilled adrenaline syringes and given a MedicAlert bracelet.

Table 11.10 Drug therapy in allergic disorders

Disorder	Drugs used	Mechanism of action
Anaphylaxis	Adrenaline Antihistamines Glucocorticoids	Vasoconstriction (α_2) Bronchodilation (β_2) Proinflammatory mediator antagonism Antiinflammatory
Allergic rhinitis/ hay fever	Antihistamines Mast-cell stabilizers Glucocorticoids Sympathomimetic vasoconstrictors	Proinflammatory mediator antagonism Inhibition of mast-cell degranulation Antiinflammatory Decongestion of nasal mucosa
Asthma	(see Ch. 3)	(see Ch. 3)
Food allergies	Antihistamines	Proinflammatory mediator antagonism
Wheal and flare	Antihistamines	Proinflammatory mediator antagonism

Histamine and H1-receptor antagonists (antihistamines)

Histamine is a basic amine that is stored in mast cells and in circulating basophils; it is also found in the stomach and CNS. The effects of histamine are mediated by three different receptor types found on target cells (Table 11.11).

As the major chemical mediator released during an allergic reaction, histamine produces a number of effects, mainly via action on H1-receptors. Therefore H1 antagonists (antihistamines) are of potential benefit in the treatment of allergic disorders.

H1-receptor antagonists: antihistamines

There are two types of H1-receptor antagonists.

- "Old" sedative types, for example, chlorphenamine and promethazine
- "New" nonsedative types, for example, cetirizine and loratadine

Mechanism of action—Antagonism of histamine H1-receptors (see Table 11.11). In the periphery, their action can inhibit allergic reactions where histamine is the main mediator involved.

The old-style antihistamines can cross the blood–brain barrier where both specific and nonspecific actions in the CNS produce sedation and antiemetic effects.

Table 11.11 Effects at histamine receptors

Histamine receptor	Effect
H1	Responsible for most of the actions of histamine in a type I hypersensitivity reaction: - capillary and venous dilatation (producing 'flare' or systemic hypotension) - increased vascular permeability (producing 'wheal' or oedema) - contraction of smooth muscle (producing bronchial and gastrointestinal contraction)
H2	Regulation of gastric acid secretion: - H2-receptors respond to histamine secreted from the enterochromaffin-like cells that are adjacent to the parietal cell
H3	Involved in neurotransmission: - the exact physiological role is not clear but there may be presynaptic inhibition of neurotransmitter release in the central and autonomic nervous system affecting itch and pain perception

Indications—The main use of H1-receptor antagonists is in the treatment of seasonal allergic rhinitis (hay fever). They are also used for the treatment and prevention of allergic skin reactions such as urticarial rashes, pruritus and insect bites, and in the emergency treatment of anaphylactic shock.

The old-style H1-receptor antagonists can also be used as mild hypnotics (Chapter 8), and to suppress nausea in motion sickness, owing to their actions on the CNS.

Route of administration—Oral, topical, transnasal. Intravenous chlorphenamine can be used in anaphylaxis.

Adverse effects—Old-style antihistamines produce quite pronounced sedation or fatigue, as well as anticholinergic effects such as dry mouth. The newer agents do not do this.

Rare hazardous arrhythmias are associated with a few H1-receptor antagonists (e.g. terfenadine), especially at high plasma levels or when in combination with imidazole antifungal agents or macrolide antibiotics (Chapter 12). Hypersensitivity reactions, especially to topically applied H1-receptor antagonists, may occur.

Mast-cell stabilizers, the antiinflammatory glucocorticoids, and sympathomimetic decongestants are all used in allergy (see Chapter 3).

IMMUNOSUPPRESSANTS

Deliberate pharmacological suppression of the immune system is used in the following three main clinical areas.

- To suppress inappropriate autoimmune responses (e.g. systemic lupus erythematosus or rheumatoid arthritis), where the host immune system is "attacking" host tissue

- To suppress host immune rejection responses to donor organ grafts or transplants
- To suppress donor immune responses against host antigens (prevention of graft-versus-host disease after bone marrow transplant [GVHD])

The main pharmacological agents used for immunosuppression are as following.

- Calcineurin inhibitors
- Antiproliferatives
- Glucocorticoids (Chapter 7).

Solid organ transplant patients require immunosuppression to prevent organ rejection. They are usually maintained on a corticosteroid combined with a calcineurin inhibitor (cyclosporine) or with an antiproliferative drug (azathioprine or mycophenolate mofetil), or with both.

> **CLINICAL NOTE**
>
> Mr Isaac, a 40-year-old man has end-stage renal failure caused by diabetic nephropathy. He fortunately receives a renal transplant. After a successful operation, he is started on cyclosporine, mycophenolate mofetil and prednisolone immunosuppression to prevent organ rejection. When he is discharged, he is also given cotrimoxazole (a mixture of the antibacterials, sulfamethoxazole and trimethoprim) and nystatin (antifungal) prophylactically. However, 2 months later, he develops an infection. Cytomegalovirus (CMV) is identified as the cause of his symptoms, chest X-ray and detection of CMV DNA by polymerase chain reaction test.
>
> Mr Isaac is treated by two methods.
>
> - A reduction in his immunosuppression (mycophenolate mofetil treatment is suspended). This is vital to allow a better immune response to clear the CMV. Close surveillance of graft function is important during this period.
> - Specific antiviral therapy (ganciclovir).
>
> Mr Isaac responds to this therapy and his symptoms resolve after 6 days.

Calcineurin inhibitors

The main drug in this class is cyclosporine.

Mechanism of action—Cyclosporine is a cyclic peptide, derived from fungi, that has powerful immunosuppressive activity. It has a selective inhibitory effect on T cells by inhibiting the T-cell receptor (TCR)-mediated signal-transduction pathway. It is believed to exert its actions after

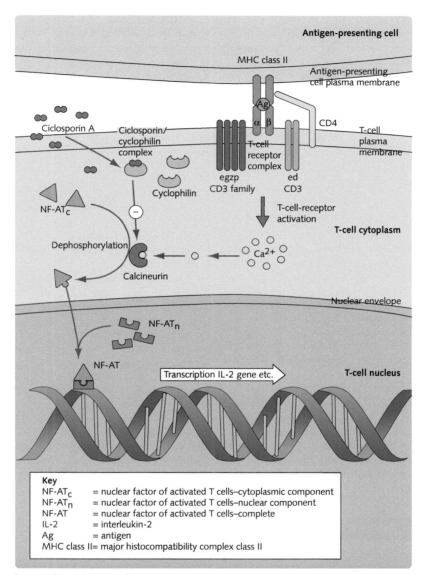

Fig. 11.6 Cyclosporine and T-cell suppression.

Key

NF-AT$_c$	= nuclear factor of activated T cells–cytoplasmic component
NF-AT$_n$	= nuclear factor of activated T cells–nuclear component
NF-AT	= nuclear factor of activated T cells–complete
IL-2	= interleukin-2
Ag	= antigen
MHC class II	= major histocompatibility complex class II

entering the T cell and preventing the transcription of specific genes (Fig. 11.6).

After entry into the T cell, cyclosporine specifically binds to its cytoplasmic binding protein, cyclophilin. This cyclosporine-cyclophilin complex then binds to a serine/threonine phosphatase called calcineurin, inhibiting its phosphatase activity. Calcineurin is normally activated when intracellular calcium ion levels rise following TCR binding to the appropriate major histocompatibility complex: antigen complex. When calcineurin is active, it dephosphorylates the cytoplasmic component of the nuclear factor of activated T cells (NF-ATc) into a form that migrates to the nucleus and induces transcription of genes such as IL-2 that are involved in T-cell activation.

Inhibition of calcineurin by the cyclosporine-cyclophilin complex therefore prevents the nuclear translocation of NF-ATc and the transcription of certain genes essential for the activation of T cells. Hence the production of IL-2 by T-helper cells, the maturation of cytotoxic T cells and the production of some other cytokines, such as interferon-γ, are all inhibited.

The overall action of cyclosporine is to suppress reversibly both cell-mediated and antibody-specific adaptive immune responses.

Indications—Cyclosporine is used for the prevention of graft and transplant rejection, and prevention of GVHD.

Route of administration—Oral, intravenous.

Adverse effects—Unlike most immunosuppressive agents, cyclosporine does not cause myelosuppression.

However, it is markedly nephrotoxic to the proximal tubule of the kidney, and renal damage almost always occurs. This may be reversible or permanent. Hypertension occurs in 50% of people.

Less serious side effects include mild hepatotoxicity, anorexia, lethargy, gastrointestinal upsets, hirsutism and gum hypertrophy.

Therapeutic notes—Cyclosporine is often used as part of a posttransplantation "triple therapy" regimen with oral corticosteroids and azathioprine.

Antiproliferatives

Azathioprine

Mechanism of action—Azathioprine is a prodrug that is converted into the active component 6-mercaptopurine in the liver. Mercaptopurine is a "fraudulent" purine nucleotide that impairs DNA synthesis and has a cytotoxic action on dividing cells.

Indications—Azathioprine is used for the prevention of graft and transplant rejection, and autoimmune conditions when corticosteroid therapy alone is inadequate.

Route of administration—Oral, intravenous.

Adverse effects—Side effects of azathioprine include bone marrow suppression, which can lead to leucopoenia, thrombocytopenia and sometimes anaemia. This is often the dose-limiting side effect.

Increased susceptibility to infections (often opportunistic pathogens), and to certain cancers (lymphomas) can occur. Common side effects include gastrointestinal disturbances, nausea, vomiting and diarrhoea. Alopecia may be partial or complete but is usually reversible.

Drug interaction with allopurinol necessitates lowering the dose of azathioprine.

Therapeutic notes—Azathioprine is used as part of a posttransplantation triple therapy regimen with oral corticosteroids.

Mycophenolate mofetil

Mechanism of action—Mycophenolate mofetil is rapidly hydrolysed to mycophenolic acid, which is the active metabolite. Mycophenolic acid is a potent, uncompetitive and reversible inhibitor of iosine monophosphate dehydrogenase, and therefore inhibits the pathway critical for T- lymphocyte and B-lymphocyte proliferation. It is selective because other cells are not solely reliant on this enzyme and so are able to maintain their rapid proliferation.

Indications—Prophylaxis of acute renal, cardiac or hepatic transplant rejection (in combination with cyclosporine and corticosteroids).

Contraindications—Pregnancy and those with hypersensitivity to the drug.

Route of administration—Oral, intravenous.

Adverse effects—Side effects of mycophenolate mofetil include bone marrow suppression, which can lead to leucopoenia, thrombocytopenia and sometimes anaemia. Increased susceptibility to infections (often opportunistic pathogens), and to certain cancers (lymphomas) can occur. Common side effects include gastrointestinal disturbances, nausea, vomiting and diarrhoea. Alopecia may be partial or complete but is usually reversible.

Glucocorticoids

The use of glucocorticoids as immunosuppressant agents involves both their antiinflammatory actions and their effects on the immune system (Chapter 7).

● Chapter Summary

- Erythema, heat, oedema and tenderness indicate inflammation
- Inflammatory mediators include histamine, bradykinin, cytokines, eicosanoids and neuropeptides
- NSAIDs inhibit cyclooxygenase and inhibit prostaglandin synthesis
- Because of the unspecific nature of NSAIDs, they have wide ranging, severe adverse effects
- DMARDS have a slow onset of action but reduce inflammation in chronic disease
- H1-receptor antagonists are used in the management of allergic reactions
- Intramuscular adrenaline is given to counteract the type I hypersensitivity reaction that occurs in anaphylactic shock
- Emollients are the mainstay of treatment of inflammatory, dry skin conditions
- Topical steroids can cause systemic side effects if used long-term and should be withdrawn slowly
- Bone marrow suppression is common with systemic immunosuppressants (e.g. azathioprine or methotrexate)
- Colchicine and NSAIDs are used to treat acute attacks of gout, allopurinol is used to prevent acute attack

Infectious diseases | 12

This chapter reviews the drugs used in the treatment of bacterial, fungal, viral and helminth infections. Malaria, tuberculosis and human immunodeficiency virus (HIV) medications are also reviewed.

ANTIBACTERIAL DRUGS

Concepts of antibacterial chemotherapy

Bacteria are prokaryotic organisms. Some bacteria are pathogenic to humans and responsible for a number of medically important diseases.

The principal treatment of infections is with antibiotics. These antibacterial agents can be:

- bacteriostatic (i.e. they inhibit bacterial growth but do not kill the bacteria), or
- bactericidal (i.e. they kill bacteria).

Note that the distinction is not clear cut because the ability of an antibacterial agent to inhibit or kill bacteria is partially dependent on its concentration and both are used frequently. Patients who are immunocompromized often require bactericidal agents because their immune system is not capable of eliminating bacteria completely.

Classification of antibiotics

There are three main ways of classifying antibiotics.

- Whether they are bactericidal or bacteriostatic
- By their site of action (Table 12.1 and Fig. 12.1)
- By their chemical structure

In this chapter, antibiotics have been described according to their site of action.

Antibiotic resistance

When an antibiotic is ineffective against a bacterium, that bacterium is said to be resistant. Resistance to antibiotics can be acquired or innate.

Innate resistance

Innate resistance is a long-standing characteristic of a particular species of bacteria. For instance, *Pseudomonas aeruginosa* has always been resistant to treatment with several antibiotics, including benzylpenicillin, vancomycin and fusidic acid.

Acquired resistance

Acquired resistance is when bacteria that were sensitive to an antibiotic become resistant. Biochemical mechanisms responsible for resistance to an antibiotic include the following.

- Production of enzymes that inactivate the drug
- Alteration of drug binding site
- Reduction in drug uptake and accumulation
- Development of altered metabolic pathways

The major stimulus for the development of acquired resistance is the over use or inappropriate use of antibiotics. Antibiotic use exerts selective pressure on bacteria to "acquire" resistance to survive. Acquired resistance to antibiotics can develop in bacterial populations in many ways, although all involve genes that code for the resistance mechanism located either on the bacterial chromosome or on plasmids. The acquisition of resistance by a bacterium can either be achieved de novo by spontaneous mutation or by being transferred from another bacterium.

The development of clinical antibiotic drug resistance is a major problem imposing serious constraints on the medical treatment of many bacterial infections. Methicillin-resistant *Staphylococcus aureus* (MRSA) and some strains of *Mycobacteria tuberculosis* are examples of multidrug-resistant bacteria.

Prescribing antibiotics

Similar to most drugs, many antibiotics have side effects. When prescribing antibiotics, there are many considerations determining which antibiotic to use, by which route, for how many days, and so on. One should consider the following points when treating an infection.

- Identify the organism responsible for, or likely to be responsible for the symptoms
- Assess the severity of illness
- Previous antibiotic therapy
- Previous adverse/allergic response to antibiotics
- Other medications being taken and their possible interactions
- Ongoing medical considerations

HINTS AND TIPS

Always try to get a sample (e.g. blood, urine or sputum) for microbial culture before starting antibiotics, unless there is a threat to life by withholding antibiotics.

Table 12.1 Sites of action of cytotoxic drugs that act on dividing cells

Site	Exploitable difference	Antibacterial drug
Peptidoglycan cell wall	Peptidoglycan cell walls are a uniquely prokaryotic feature not shared by eukaryotic (mammalian) cells. Drugs that act here are therefore very selective	Penicillins Cephalosporins Glycopeptides
Cytoplasmic membrane	Bacteria possess a plasma membrane within the wall which is a phospholipid bilayer, as in eukaryotes. However, in bacteria the plasma membrane does not contain any sterols and this results in differential chemical behaviour that can be exploited.	Polymyxins
Protein synthesis	The bacterial ribosome (50S + 30S subunits) is sufficiently different from the mammalian ribosome (60S + 40S subunits) that sites on the bacterial ribosome are good targets for drug action.	Aminoglycosides Tetracyclines Chloramphenicol Macrolides Fusidic acid
Nucleic acids	The bacterial genome is in the form of a single circular strand of DNA plus ancillary plasmids unenclosed by a nuclear envelope, in contrast to the eukaryotic chromosomal arrangement within the nucleus. Drugs may interfere directly or indirectly with microbial DNA and RNA metabolism, replication and transcription.	Antifolates Quinolones Rifampicin

DNA, Deoxyribonucleic acid; RNA, ribonucleic acid.

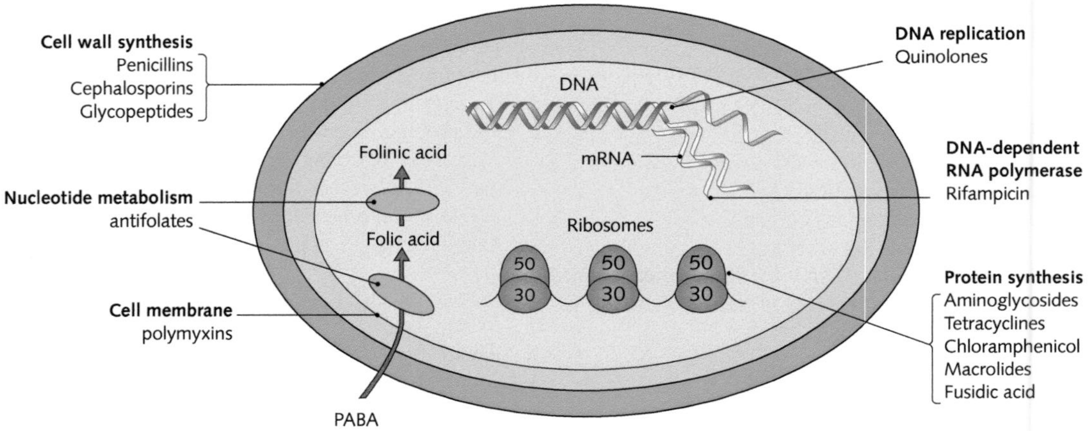

Fig. 12.1 Sites of action of different types of antibiotic agent. *DNA,* Deoxyribonucleic acid; *PABA,* para-aminobenzoic acid, *RNA,* ribonucleic acid.

Antibacterial drugs that inhibit cell wall synthesis

Penicillins

Examples of penicillins include benzylpenicillin, phenoxymethylpenicillin, flucloxacillin, amoxicillin and ampicillin.

Combinations exist to help minimize resistance; co-amoxiclav is a combination of amoxicillin and clavulanic acid, whereas tazocin is a combination of piperacillin and tazobactam.

Mechanism of action—Penicillins are bactericidal. Structurally, they possess a thiazolidine ring connected to a β-lactam ring. The side chain from the β-lactam ring determines the unique pharmacological properties of the different penicillins.

Penicillins bind to penicillin-binding proteins on susceptible microorganisms. This interaction results in inhibition of peptide cross-linking within the microbial cell wall, and indirect activation of autolytic enzymes. The combined result is lysis (see Fig. 12.1).

Spectrum of activity—Penicillins exhibit considerable diversity in their spectrum of activity (Table 12.2).

Benzylpenicillin is active against aerobic gram-positive and gram-negative cocci and many anaerobic organisms. Many staphylococci are now resistant to benzylpenicillin. Flucloxacillin is used against penicillin-resistant staphylococci because it is not inactivated by their β-lactamase. Phenoxymethylpenicillin is similar to benzylpenicillin but less active. Amoxicillin and ampicillin are broad-spectrum penicillins. The penicillins are useful for treating lung and

Table 12.2 Drugs of choice and alternatives for selected common bacterial pathogens

Bacterium	Drug(s) of choice	Alternatives	Comments
Streptococcus species	Penicillin	First-generation cephalosporins Erythromycin Clindamycin Vancomycin	A few strains are penicillin resistant, especially some S. *Pneumoniae* Erythromycin is only for mild infections Vancomycin is only for serious infections
Enterococcus species	Penicillin or ampicillin plus gentamicin	Vancomycin plus gentamicin	There are some strains for which streptomycin is synergistic but gentamicin is not Some strains are resistant to synergy with any aminoglycoside
Staphylococcus species	Antistaphylococcal penicillin, e.g. flucloxacillin	First-generation cephalosporins Vancomycin	Vancomycin is required for methicillin-resistant strains Rifampicin is occasionally used to eradicate the nasal carriage state
Neisseria meningitidis	Penicillin	Chloramphenicol Third-generation cephalosporins	Rare strains are penicillin resistant
Neisseria gonorrhoeae	Cefixime	Ciprofloxacin Third-generation cephalosporins	Some strains are fluoroquinolone resistant (especially in Asia)
Bordetella pertussis	Erythromycin	Trimethoprim with sulfamethoxazole	
Haemophilus influenzae	Aminopenicillin (ampicillin, amoxicillin)	Cefuroxime Third-generation cephalosporins Chloramphenicol	Approximately 30% are aminopenicillin-resistant: aminopenicillins should not be used empirically in serious infections until susceptibility results are available Rifampicin is used to eradicate the nasal carriage state
Enterobacteria in urine	Trimethoprim with sulfamethoxazole	Ciprofloxacin Gentamicin Nitrofurantoin	β-lactams are less effective than trimethoprim with sulfamethoxazole or fluoroquinolones for the treatment of urinary tract infection
Enterobacteria in cerebrospinal fluid	Third-generation cephalosporin	Trimethoprim with sulfamethoxazole	In neonates only, aminoglycosides are equivalent to third-generation cephalosporins Experience with trimethoprim with sulfamethoxazole in meningitis is limited
Enterobacteria elsewhere (blood, lung, etc.)	Gentamicin Third-generation cephalosporins Ciprofloxacin	Trimethoprim with sulfamethoxazole	Two-drug therapy is sometimes used in serious infection Monotherapy with a third-generation cephalosporin should be avoided if the pathogen is *E. cloacae, E. aerogenes, Serratia marcescens* or *Citrobacter freundii*
Pseudomonas aeruginosa	Antipseudomonal penicillin plus aminoglycoside	Ceftazidime Ciprofloxacin	Two-drug therapy recommended except for urinary tract infection
Bacteroides fragilis	Metronidazole or clindamycin	Imipenem Penicillin β-lactamase inhibitors	*B. fragilis* is usually involved in polymicrobial infections; therefore another antibiotic active against Enterobacteriaceae is often required
Mycoplasma penumoniae	Macrolides, e.g. erythromycin	Tetracycline	Although tetracyclines are as effective as macrolides, the latter are recommended because of better activity against *Pneumococcus*, which can mimic this infection
Chlamydia trachomatis	Tetracycline	Azithromycin Erythromycin	Azithromycin is the only therapy effective in a single dose Erythromycin is used in pregnancy

(Continued)

Table 12.2 Drugs of choice and alternatives for selected common bacterial pathogens—cont'd

Bacterium	Drug(s) of choice	Alternatives	Comments
Rickettsial species	Tetracycline	Chloramphenicol	
Listeria monocytogenes	Ampicillin plus gentamicin	Vancomycin plus gentamicin	
Legionella species	Erythromycin	Tetracycline	Rifampicin is occasionally used as a second agent in severe cases
Clostridium difficile	Metronidazole	Vancomycin (oral)	
Mycobacterium tuberculosis	Isoniazid plus rifampicin plus pyrazinamide plus ethambutol	Streptomycin Fluoroquinolones Cycloserine Clarithromycin Capreomycin	Directly observed therapy is recommended Isoniazid is used alone for preventive therapy
Mycobacterium leprae	Dapsone plus rifampicin ± clofazimine	Clarithromycin	Thalidomide is useful for erythema nodosum leprosum

skin infections. Neutropenic sepsis is commonly treated with tazocin.

Route of administration—Benzylpenicillin must be administered parenterally because it is inactivated when given orally. Phenoxymethylpenicillin, flucloxacillin, amoxicillin and ampicillin are active when given orally.

Contraindications—Known hypersensitivity to penicillins or cephalosporins.

Adverse effects—In general, very specific and safe antibiotics. Hypersensitivity reactions are the main adverse effect, including rashes (common) and anaphylaxis (rare). Neurotoxicity occurs at excessively high cerebrospinal fluid concentrations. Diarrhoea is common, owing to disturbance of normal colonic flora.

Therapeutic notes—Resistance to penicillins is often caused by the production of β-lactamase by some microorganisms, which hydrolyses the β-lactam ring. This resistance gene is located in a plasmid and is transferable. Flucloxacillin is resistant to β-lactamase.

CLINICAL NOTE

A 55-year-old male presents to the hospital to have his pacemaker upgraded. The surgery is uneventful and completed successfully. On routine observation, the wound is found to be weeping and the skin around the incision is noted to be red, swollen and tender to touch. A swab of the pus is taken and sent to microbiology for cultures and he is started on intravenous flucloxacillin and cefuroxime. The following day his temperature is noted to be 37.8°C and he reports general malaise and lethargy. The wound is still weeping with no improvement in appearance. MRSA is suspected, and he is started on intravenous vancomycin.

Cephalosporins

The cephalosporins comprise a large group of drugs. There are three main subgroups.

- First-generation drugs, for example, cefadroxil (oral) and cefradine (parenteral).
- Second-generation drugs, for example, cefuroxime (oral) and cefamandole (parenteral).
- Third-generation drugs, for example, cefixime (oral) and cefotaxime (parenteral).

Mechanism of action—Cephalosporins are bactericidal. They are β-lactam-containing antibiotics and inhibit bacterial cell wall synthesis in a manner similar to the penicillins. Structurally cephalosporins possess a dihydrothiazine ring connected to the β-lactam ring that makes them more resistant to hydrolysis by β-lactamases than are the penicillins.

Spectrum of activity—The cephalosporins are broad-spectrum antibiotics that are second-choice agents for many infections (see Table 12.2), including meningitis.

Route of administration—Oral, intravenous, intramuscular. Consult the British National Formulary (BNF).

Contraindications—Known hypersensitivity to cephalosporins or penicillins.

Adverse effects—Side effects of the cephalosporins include hypersensitivity reactions, which occur in a similar and cross-reacting fashion to the penicillins. Diarrhoea is common, owing to disturbance of normal colonic flora. Nausea and vomiting may also occur.

Therapeutic notes—The cephalosporins can be inactivated by the β-lactamase enzyme, although the later-generation drugs are more resistant to hydrolysis.

Glycopeptides

Vancomycin and teicoplanin are the classic glycopeptides.

Mechanism of action—Glycopeptides are bactericidal. They inhibit peptidoglycan synthesis, with possible effects on ribonucleic acid (RNA) synthesis (see Fig. 12.1).

Spectrum of activity—Vancomycin is active only against aerobic and anaerobic gram-positive bacteria. Glycopeptides are reserved for resistant staphylococcal infections and *Clostridium difficile* in antibiotic-associated pseudomembranous colitis (see Table 12.2).

Route of administration—Glycopeptides are usually administered intravenously as they are not well absorbed orally. Oral administration is reserved for when a local gastrointestinal tract effect is required, for example, in colitis.

Adverse effects—Side effects of glycopeptides include ototoxicity and nephrotoxicity at high plasma levels, and fever, rashes ("red man syndrome") and local phlebitis at the site of infection.

Therapeutic notes—Acquired resistance to vancomycin is rare, but reports of vancomycin-resistant enterococci are becoming more common.

Monobactam and carbapenems

Aztreonam is a monobactam antibiotic, which is less likely to cause hypersensitivity reactions in penicillin-sensitive patients. Carbapenems have the broadest spectrum of activity of all the β-lactams and include ertapenem, imipenem (used with cilastatin to increase the duration of action) and meropenem. Both groups contain β-lactam rings, although they are resistant to many β-lactamases. For indications, the spectrum of activity and adverse effects consult the *BNF*.

Antibacterial drugs that inhibit bacterial nucleic acids

Antibacterial drugs that inhibit bacterial nucleic acids (see Fig. 12.1).

- The antifolates, which affect deoxyribonucleic acid (DNA) metabolism
- The quinolones, which affect DNA replication and packaging
- Rifampicin, which affects transcription (see later)

Antifolates

Examples of antifolates include the sulphonamides (e.g. sulfadiazine) and trimethoprim.

Mechanism of action—Folate is an essential cofactor in the synthesis of purines and hence of DNA. Bacteria, unlike mammals, must synthesize their own folate from *para*-aminobenzoic acid (see Fig. 12.1). This pathway can be inhibited at two points: the sulphonamides inhibit dihydrofolate synthetase, whereas trimethoprim inhibits dihydrofolate reductase but both are bacteriostatic.

Spectrum of activity—The sulphonamides are used for "simple" urinary tract infections (UTIs). Trimethoprim and co-trimoxazole (trimethoprim and sulfamethoxazole) are used for UTIs and respiratory tract infections (see Table 12.2).

Route of administration—Oral, intravenous.

Contraindications—Pregnant women because there is a theoretic teratogenic risk with antifolates. Neonates because bilirubin displacement can damage the neonatal brain (kernicterus).

Adverse effects—Nausea, vomiting and hypersensitivity reactions, for example, rashes, fever, Stevens-Johnson syndrome. The sulphonamides are relatively insoluble and can cause crystalluria, whereas trimethoprim can cause myelosuppression/agranulocytosis.

Therapeutic notes—Antifolates are often used in combined preparations because they have synergistic effects. Resistance is common and is caused by the production of enzymes that have reduced affinity for the drugs. Resistance can be acquired on plasmids in gram-negative bacteria.

Quinolones

Ciprofloxacin and levofloxacin are quinolones.

Mechanism of action—Quinolones are bactericidal. They act by inhibiting prokaryotic DNA gyrase. This enzyme packages DNA into supercoils and is essential for DNA replication and repair (see Fig. 12.1).

Spectrum of activity—Ciprofloxacin has a broad spectrum of activity but works best against gram-negative organisms (see Table 12.2). Quinolones are typically used for pyelonephritis and atypical respiratory infections (e.g. *pseudomonas, legionella and mycoplasma*).

Route of administration—Oral, intravenous. Ciprofloxacin is so well absorbed orally that intravenous administration is rarely required unless the patient is unable to tolerate oral medication.

Contraindications—Quinolones should not be given with theophylline because theophylline toxicity may be precipitated.

Adverse effects—Gastrointestinal upset. Rarely, hypersensitivity and central nervous system (CNS) disturbances (e.g. hallucinations) occur. Quinolones can also cause tendon damage and increase the risk of *C. difficile* infection.

Antibacterial drugs that inhibit protein synthesis

Antibacterial drugs that inhibit protein synthesis include the following.

- Aminoglycosides
- Tetracyclines
- Chloramphenicol
- Macrolides
- Lincosamides
- Fusidic acid.

The site of action of these drugs is summarized in Fig. 12.2.

Aminoglycosides

Examples of aminoglycosides include gentamicin, streptomycin, and amikacin.

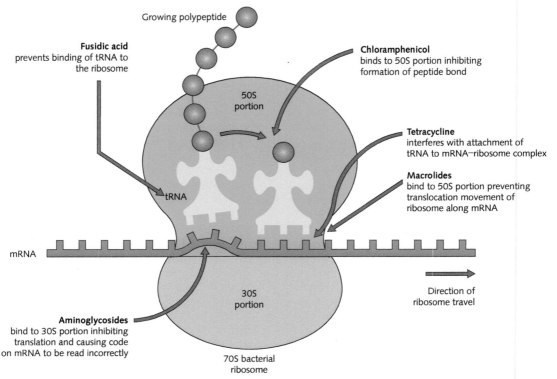

Fig. 12.2 Site of action of the antibiotics which inhibit bacterial protein synthesis. *mRNA,* Messenger ribonucleic acid; *tRNA,* transfer ribonucleic acid.

Mechanism of action—Aminoglycosides are bactericidal. They bind irreversibly to the 30S portion of the bacterial ribosome. This inhibits the translation of messenger RNA (mRNA) to protein and causes more frequent misreading of the prokaryotic genetic code (see Fig. 12.2).

Spectrum of activity—Aminoglycosides have a broad spectrum of activity but with low activity against anaerobes, gram-negative organisms, streptococci and pneumococci (see Table 12.2). Streptomycin is used against *M. tuberculosis*, whereas gentamicin is used to treat bacterial endocarditis.

Route of administration—Parenteral only.

Contraindications—Acute neuromuscular blockade can occur if an aminoglycoside is used in combination with anaesthesia or other neuromuscular blockers.

Adverse effects—Dose-related ototoxicity and nephrotoxicity at high plasma levels.

Therapeutic notes—Resistance to aminoglycosides is increasing and is primarily caused by plasmid-borne genes encoding degradative enzymes.

Tetracyclines

Examples of tetracyclines include tetracycline, minocycline, doxycycline.

Mechanism of action—Tetracyclines are bacteriostatic. They work by selective uptake into bacterial cells because of active bacterial transport systems not possessed by mammalian cells. The tetracycline then binds reversibly to the 30S subunit of the bacterial ribosome, interfering with the attachment of transfer RNA (tRNA) to the mRNA ribosome complex (see Fig. 12.2).

Spectrum of activity—Tetracyclines have broad-spectrum activity against gram-positive and gram-negative bacteria, as well as intracellular pathogens (see Table 12.2). They are typically used for atypical chest infections, acne and as malaria prophylaxis.

Route of administration—Oral, intravenous. Oral absorption is incomplete and can be impaired by calcium (e.g. milk), and magnesium or aluminium salts (e.g. antacids).

Contraindications—Tetracyclines should not be given to children or pregnant women.

Adverse effects—Gastrointestinal disturbances (especially reflux) are common after oral administration. In children, tetracyclines depress bone growth and produce permanent discolouration of teeth.

Therapeutic notes—In the majority of cases, resistance is caused by decreased uptake of the drug and is plasmid-borne.

Chloramphenicol

Mechanism of action—Chloramphenicol is both bactericidal and bacteriostatic, depending on the bacterial species.

It reversibly binds to the 50S subunit of the bacterial ribosome, inhibiting the formation of peptide bonds (see Fig. 12.2).

Spectrum of activity—Chloramphenicol has a broad spectrum of activity against many gram-positive cocci and gram-negative organisms (see Table 12.2). Despite its toxicity, it is used in the treatment of typhoid fever in the developing world, where the organism is sensitive to it. Chloramphenicol eye drops are typically used for bacterial conjunctivitis.

Route of administration—Oral, topical, intravenous.

Contraindications—Chloramphenicol should not be given to pregnant women or neonates.

Adverse effects—Myelosuppression, reversible anaemia. Neutropenia and thrombocytopenia may occur during chronic administration. Fatal aplastic anaemia is rare.

Neonates cannot metabolise chloramphenicol and "grey baby syndrome" may develop, which comprises pallor, abdominal distension, vomiting and collapse.

Therapeutic notes—Resistance to chloramphenicol is caused by a plasmid-borne gene encoding an enzyme that inactivates the drug by acetylation. Blood monitoring is necessary.

Macrolides

Erythromycin, clarithromycin and azithromycin are examples of macrolides.

Mechanism of action—Macrolides are bacteriostatic/bactericidal. They reversibly bind to the 50S subunit of the bacterial ribosome, preventing the translocation movement of the ribosome along mRNA (see Table 12.2).

Spectrum of activity—Erythromycin is effective against most gram-positive bacteria and spirochetes. Clarithromycin is active against *Haemophilus influenzae*, *Mycobacterium avium cellulare* and *Helicobacter pylori*.

Route of administration—Oral, intravenous.

Adverse effects—Side effects of erythromycin include gastrointestinal disturbance, which is common after oral administration. Liver damage and jaundice can occur after chronic administration.

Therapeutic notes—Resistance to erythromycin results from a mutation of the binding site on the 50S subunit. Erythromycin has a similar spectrum of activity to penicillin and is an effective alternative in penicillin-sensitive patients. Azithromycin can be given as a one-off dose for uncomplicated chlamydial infections of the genital tract and has been shown to be effective in reducing exacerbations of asthma and chronic obstructive pulmonary disease.

HINTS AND TIPS

Macrolides are cytochrome p450 enzyme inhibitors. Care should be taken if they are coprescribed with warfarin or statins.

Fusidic Acid

Mechanism of action—Fusidic acid is a steroid that prevents binding of tRNA to the ribosome (see Fig. 12.2).

Spectrum of activity—Fusidic acid has a narrow spectrum of activity, particularly against gram-positive bacteria (see Table 12.2). It is most useful for skin infections caused by staphylococcal infections.

Route of administration—Oral, intravenous.

Adverse effects—Gastrointestinal disturbance. Skin eruptions and jaundice may occur.

Therapeutic notes—Resistance to fusidic acid can occur via mutation or by plasmid-borne mechanisms.

Lincosamides

Clindamycin is a lincosamide.

Mechanism of action—Similar to the macrolides.

Spectrum of activity—Clindamycin is active against gram-positive cocci, including penicillin-resistant staphylococci, and many anaerobes.

Route of administration—Oral, parenteral.

Adverse effects—Antibiotic-associated (pseudomembranous) colitis; greater risk than for other antibiotics.

Therapeutic notes—Clindamycin is used for staphylococcal joint and bone infections.

Miscellaneous antibacterials

Other antibacterial drugs include the following.

- Metronidazole
- Nitrofurantoin
- Bacitracin
- Polymyxins

Metronidazole and tinidazole

Mechanism of action—Metronidazole is bactericidal. It is metabolized to an intermediate that inhibits bacterial DNA synthesis and degrades existing DNA. Its selectivity is caused by the fact that the intermediate toxic metabolite is not produced in mammalian cells.

Spectrum of activity—Metronidazole is antiprotozoal and has antibacterial activity against anaerobic bacteria (see Table 12.2). Metronidazole is particularly helpful in the treatment of intraabdominal sepsis, *C. difficile* and giardia, as well as aspiration pneumonia.

Route of administration—Oral, rectal, intravenous, topical.

Contraindications—Metronidazole should not be given to pregnant women.

Adverse effects—Mild headache, gastrointestinal disturbance. Adverse drug reactions occur with alcohol.

Therapeutic notes—Acquired resistance to metronidazole is rare. Tinidazole is similar to metronidazole but has a longer duration of action.

Nitrofurantoin

Mechanism of action—The mechanism of action of nitrofurantoin is uncertain although it possibly interferes with bacterial DNA metabolism through the inhibition of nucleic acid synthesis.

Spectrum of activity—Nitrofurantoin is active against gram-positive bacteria and *Escherichia coli* (see Table 12.2), therefore useful in the treatment of UTIs.

Route of administration—Oral; it reaches high therapeutic concentrations in the urine.

Contraindications—Third trimester of pregnancy as risk of neonatal haemolysis.

Adverse effects—Gastrointestinal disturbance. Impaired renal function, pulmonary fibrosis (if chronically used).

Therapeutic notes—Rarely, chromosomal resistance to nitrofurantoin can occur.

Polymyxins

Colistin is an example of a polymyxin, although this class is seldom prescribed because of its toxicity. Nonetheless, colistin is sometimes the last antibiotic available for patients with multidrug resistance because resistance to colistin is rare.

Mechanism of action—Polymyxins are bactericidal. They are peptides that interact with phospholipids on the outer plasma cell membranes of gram-negative bacteria, disrupting their structure. This disruption destroys the bacteria's osmotic barrier, leading to lysis (see Fig. 12.1).

Spectrum of activity—Polymyxins are active only against gram-negative bacteria including *P. aeruginosa* (see Table 12.2).

Route of administration—Intravenous, intramuscular, inhalation. Oral polymyxins are given to sterilize the bowel in neutropenic patients.

Adverse effects—Perioral and peripheral, paraesthesia, vertigo, nephrotoxicity, neurotoxicity.

Therapeutic notes—Resistance to polymyxins is rare.

Antimycobacterial drugs

The mycobacteria are slow-growing intracellular bacilli that cause tuberculosis (*M. tuberculosis*) and leprosy (*Mycobacterium leprae*) in humans.

Mycobacteria differ in their structure and lifestyle from gram-positive and gram-negative bacteria and are treated with different drugs.

Antituberculosis therapy

The first-line drugs used in the treatment of tuberculosis.

- Isoniazid: Inhibits the production of mycolic acid, a component of the cell wall unique to mycobacteria, and is bactericidal against growing organisms. Taken orally, it penetrates tuberculous lesions well. Adverse effects occur in about 5% of patients and include peripheral neuropathy, hepatotoxicity, agranulocytosis and autoimmune phenomena. Pyridoxine (vitamin B6) is given to help reduce the risk of peripheral neuritis associated with isoniazid.
- Rifampicin: Inhibits DNA-dependent RNA polymerase, causing a bactericidal effect. It is a potent drug, active

orally. Adverse effects are infrequent but can be serious, for example, hepatotoxicity and "toxic syndromes". Orange discolouration of the urine is a common side effect. There are many drug interactions because rifampicin is a cytochrome p450 enzyme inhibitor, and therefore resistance can develop rapidly.
- Ethambutol: This drug is bacteriostatic. The mechanism of action is uncertain, involving the impaired synthesis of the mycobacterial cell wall. Ethambutol is administered orally. Adverse effects are uncommon but reversible optic neuritis may occur. Resistance often develops.
- Pyrazinamide: Its mechanism of action is uncertain but may involve metabolism of the drug within *M. tuberculosis* to produce a toxic product, pyrazinoic acid, which works as a bacteriostatic agent in the low pH environment of the phagolysosome. It is active orally. Adverse effects are hepatotoxicity and raised plasma urate levels that can lead to gout. Resistance can develop rapidly.

The second-line drugs used for tuberculosis infections when first-line drugs have been discontinued owing to resistance or adverse effects include the following.

- Capreomycin: A peptide drug given intramuscularly. It can cause ototoxicity and kidney damage.
- Cycloserine: A broad-spectrum drug that inhibits peptidoglycan synthesis. This drug is administered orally and can cause CNS toxicity.
- New macrolides, for example, azithromycin and clarithromycin.
- Quinolones, for example, ciprofloxacin.

To reduce the emergence of resistant organisms, compound drug therapy is used to treat tuberculosis, involving the following phases.

- An initial phase, designed to reduce the bacterial population as quickly as possible and prevent the emergence of drug-resistance, lasts about two months and consists of three drugs: isoniazid, rifampicin and pyrazinamide. Ethambutol is added where there may be resistance to isoniazid (e.g. those who have previously been treated for tuberculosis or the immunocompromized).
- Continuation phase of four months consisting of two drugs: isoniazid and rifampicin. Longer treatment regimens may be needed for patients with meningitis or bone/joint involvement.

Antileprosy therapy
- Tuberculoid leprosy is treated with dapsone and rifampicin for 6 months.
- Lepromatous leprosy is treated with dapsone, rifampicin and clofazimine for up to 2 years.

Dapsone resembles sulphonamides chemically and may inhibit folate synthesis in a similar way. It is active orally. Adverse effects are numerous, and some fatal. Consult the *BNF*.

Clofazimine is a chemically complex dye that accumulates in macrophages, possibly acting on mycobacterial DNA. As a dye, clofazimine can discolour the skin and urine red. Other adverse effects are numerous. It is active orally.

Antiviral drugs

Concepts of viral infection

Viruses are obligate intracellular parasites that lack independent metabolism and can only replicate within the host cells they enter and infect. A virus particle, or virion, consists essentially of DNA or RNA enclosed in a protein coat (capsid). In addition, certain viruses may possess a lipoprotein envelope and replicative enzymes (Fig. 12.3).

Viruses are classified largely according to the architecture of the virion and the nature of their genetic material. Viral nucleic acid may be single stranded (ss) or double stranded (ds) (Table 12.3).

Antiviral agents

Because viruses have an intracellular replication cycle and share many of the metabolic processes of the host cell, it has proved extremely difficult to find drugs that are selectively toxic to them. In addition, by the time a viral infection becomes detectable clinically, the viral replication process tends to be very far advanced, making chemotherapeutic intervention difficult. All current antiviral agents are virustatic rather than virucidal and thus rely upon host immunocompetence for a complete clinical cure.

Nevertheless, antiviral chemotherapy is clinically effective against some viral diseases (identified with an asterisk in Table 12.3). The viruses include the following.

- Herpesviruses (herpes simplex virus [HSV], varicella-zoster virus [VZV] and cytomegalovirus [CMV])
- Influenza virus A and more recently virus B
- Respiratory syncytial virus, arenaviruses
- HIV-1

The selective inhibition of these viruses by drugs depends on either:

- Inhibition of unique steps in the viral replication pathways, such as adsorption of the virion to the cell receptor, penetration, uncoating, assembly and release.
- Preferential inhibition of steps shared with the host cell, which includes transcription and translation.

In addition to chemotherapy, immune-based therapies, such as the use of immunoglobulins and cytokines in viral infection, are also mentioned subsequently.

Inhibition of attachment to or penetration of host cells

Amantadine

Mechanism of action—Amantadine blocks a primitive ion channel in the viral membrane (named M_2) preventing fusion of a virion to host cell membranes, and inhibits the release of newly synthesized viruses from the host cell (Fig. 12.4).

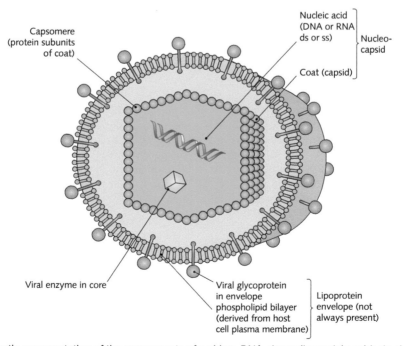

Fig. 12.3 Diagrammatic representation of the components of a virion. *DNA*, deoxyribonucleic acid*; ds*, double-stranded; *RNA*, ribonucleic acid; *ss*, single-stranded.

Table 12.3 Classification of selected medically important viruses and the diseases they cause

Family	ss/ds	Viruses	Diseases
DNA viruses			
Herpes viruses	Ds	Herpes simplex (HSV)[a] Varicella zoster (VZV)[a] Cytomegalovirus (CMV)[a] Epstein-Barr virus (EBV)[a]	Cold sores, genital herpes Chickenpox, shingles Cytomegalic disease Infectious mononucleosis
Poxviruses	Ds	Variola	Smallpox
Adenoviruses	Ds	Adenoviruses	Acute respiratory disease
Hepadnaviruses	Ds	Hepatitis B	Hepatitis
Papovaviruses	Ds	Papilloma	Warts
Parvoviruses	Ss	B19	Erythema infectiosum
RNA viruses			
Orthomyxoviruses	Ss	Influenza A[a] and B[a]	Influenza
Paramyxoviruses	Ss	Measles virus Mumps virus Parainfluenza Respiratory syncytial[a]	Measles Mumps Respiratory infection Respiratory infection
Coronaviruses	Ss	Coronavirus	Respiratory infection
Rhabdoviruses	Ss	Rabies virus	Rabies
Picornaviruses	Ss	Enteroviruses Rhinoviruses Hepatitis A	Meningitis Colds Hepatitis
Calciviruses	Ss	Norwalk virus	Gastroenteritis
Togaviruses	Ss	Alphaviruses Rubivirus	Encephalitis, haemorrhagic fevers Rubella
Reoviruses	Ds	Rotavirus	Gastroenteritis
Arenavirus	Ss	Lymphocytic choriomeningitis Lassavirus[a]	Meningitis Lassa fever
Retroviruses	Ss	HIV I, II[a]	AIDS

[a] *Viruses for which effective chemotherapy exists.*
ds, Double stranded; ss, single stranded.

Route of administration—Oral.

Indications—Amantadine is used for the prophylaxis and treatment of acute influenza A in groups at risk. It is not effective against influenza B.

Adverse effects—Some patients (5%–10%) report nonserious dizziness, slurred speech and insomnia. Neurological side effects and renal failure can occur at high concentrations.

Therapeutic notes—Resistance has been reported in 25% to 50% of patients. Amantadine is not used widely because of problems with resistance, its narrow spectrum of activity and because influenza vaccines are often preferred.

Neuraminidase inhibitors

Zanamivir belongs to the neuraminidase inhibitor class of drugs.

Mechanism of action—Zanamivir inhibits the release of newly synthesized viruses from the host cell by inhibiting the enzyme neuraminidase, which is responsible for cleaving the peptide links between virus and host.

Route of administration—Zanamivir is delivered by inhalation, although its sister drug oseltamivir may be given orally.

Indications—Treatment of influenza A or B virus within 48 hours after onset of symptoms when influenza is endemic in the community.

Contraindications—Breastfeeding.

Adverse effects—Gastrointestinal disturbances.

Immunoglobulins

Examples of immunoglobulins include human normal immunoglobulin (HNIg/gamma globulin) and specific immunoglobulins, for example, hepatitis B (HBIg), rabies (RIg), varicella zoster (VZIg) and cytomegalovirus (CMVIg) immunoglobulins.

Mechanism of action—Immunoglobulins bind specifically to antigenic determinants on the outside of virions. By specifically binding to a virus, the immunoglobulins may neutralize it by coating the virus and preventing its attachment and entry into host cells.

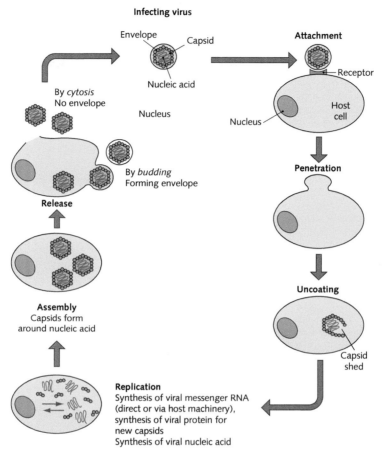

Fig. 12.4 Stages in the infection of a host's cell and replication of a virus. Several thousand virus particles may be formed from each cell. *RNA*, Ribonucleic acid. (From Mims et al. *Medical Microbiology*, 2nd edn. Mosby, 1998).

HNIg is prepared from pooled plasma of ~1000 donors and contains antibodies to measles, mumps, varicella and hepatitis A.

Specific immunoglobulins are prepared by pooling the plasma of selected donors with high levels of the antibody required.

Route of administration—Intramuscular, although immunoglobulins can be given intravenously.

Indications—HNIg is administered for the protection of susceptible contacts against hepatitis A, measles, mumps and rubella. Specific immunoglobulins may attenuate or prevent hepatitis and rabies following known exposure, and before the onset of signs and symptoms, for example, following exposure to a rabid animal. VZIg and CMVIg are indicated for prophylactic use to prevent chickenpox and cytomegalic disease in immunosuppressed patients at risk.

Contraindications—Immunoglobulins should not be given to people with a known antibody against IgA.

Adverse effects—Malaise, chills, fever and (rarely) anaphylaxis.

Therapeutic notes—Protection with immunoglobulins is immediate and lasts several weeks. HNIg may interfere with vaccinations for 3 months.

Inhibition of nucleic acid replication

Acyclovir and related drugs

Acyclovir, famciclovir and valaciclovir are all closely related antiviral drugs.

Mechanism of action—Acyclovir and related drugs are characterized by their selective phosphorylation in herpes-infected cells. This takes place by a viral thymidine kinase rather than inhibiting host kinases, as a first step.

Phosphorylation yields a triphosphate nucleotide that inhibits viral DNA polymerase and viral DNA synthesis.

These drugs are selectively toxic to infected cells because, in the absence of viral thymidine kinase, the host kinase activates only a small amount of the drug. In addition, the DNA polymerase of herpes virus has a much higher affinity for the activated drug than has cellular DNA polymerase (see Fig. 12.4).

Route of administration—Topical, oral, parenteral.

Indications—Acyclovir and related drugs are used for the prophylaxis and treatment of HSV and VZV infections, superficial and systemic, particularly in the immunocompromized.

Adverse effects—Side effects are minimal. Rarely, renal impairment and encephalopathy occur.

Therapeutic notes—The herpes genome in latent (non-replicating) cells is not affected by acyclovir therapy and so recurrence of infection after cessation of treatment is to be expected.

CMV is resistant to acyclovir because its genome does not encode thymidine kinase.

Ganciclovir

Mechanism of action—Ganciclovir is a synthetic nucleoside analogue, structurally related to acyclovir. It also requires conversion to the triphosphate nucleotide form, although by a different kinase. Ganciclovir acts as a substrate for viral DNA polymerase and as a chain terminator aborting virus replication.

Route of administration—Oral, intravenous.

Indications—Although as active as acyclovir against HSV and VZV, ganciclovir is reserved for the treatment of severe CMV infections in immunocompromized people, owing to its side effects.

Adverse effects—Reversible neutropenia in 40% of patients. There is occasional rash, nausea and encephalopathy.

Therapeutic notes—Maintenance therapy with ganciclovir at a reduced dose may be necessary to prevent recurrence of CMV.

Ribavirin (tribavirin)

Mechanism of action—Ribavirin is a nucleoside analogue that selectively interferes with viral nucleic acid synthesis in a manner similar to acyclovir.

Route of administration—For respiratory syncytial virus (RSV) by inhalation; for Lassa virus intravenously.

Indications—Severe RSV bronchiolitis in infants. Lassa fever.

Adverse effects—Reticulocytosis, respiratory depression.

Therapeutic notes—The necessity of aerosol administration for RSV limits the usefulness of this effective drug.

Nucleoside analogue reverse transcriptase inhibitors

Examples of nucleoside reverse transcriptase inhibitors (NRTI) include zidovudine (AZT), and the newer drugs, abacavir, didanosine (ddI), lamivudine (3TC), stavudine (d4T) and zalcitabine (ddC).

Mechanism of action—These nucleotide analogues all require intracellular conversion to the corresponding triphosphate nucleotide for activation. The active triphosphates competitively inhibit reverse transcriptase and cause termination of DNA chain elongation once incorporated. Affinity for viral reverse transcriptase is 100 times that for host DNA polymerase (Fig. 12.5, site 3).

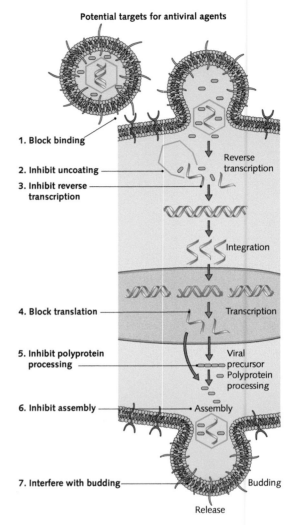

Potential targets for antiviral agents

1. Block binding
2. Inhibit uncoating
3. Inhibit reverse transcription
Reverse transcription
Integration
4. Block translation
Transcription
5. Inhibit polyprotein processing
Viral precursor
Polyprotein processing
6. Inhibit assembly
Assembly
7. Interfere with budding
Budding
Release

Fig. 12.5 The human immunodeficiency virus replicative cycle and potential sites of antiviral drug action.

Route of administration—Oral.

Indications—NRTIs are used for the management of asymptomatic and symptomatic HIV infections, and the prevention of maternal-foetal HIV transmission.

Adverse effects—Side effects of AZT are uncommon at the recommended low dosage in patients with asymptomatic or mild HIV infections, but more common in acquired immune deficiency syndrome (AIDS) patients on higher dosage regimens.

Toxicity to human myeloid and erythroid progenitor cells commonly causes anaemia and neutropenia, that is, bone marrow suppression. Other common side effects include nausea, insomnia, headaches and myalgia.

The major dose-limiting effects of ddI are pancreatitis and peripheral neuropathy, and of ddC and d4T, peripheral neuropathy.

Therapeutic notes—Drug resistance evolves to all the current NRTIs by the development of mutations in reverse transcriptase, although the kinetics of resistance development varies for the different drugs (e.g. 6–18 months for AZT). Combined therapies have a place in increasing efficacy synergistically and reducing the emergence of resistant strains.

Nonnucleoside reverse transcriptase inhibitors

Efavirenz and nevirapine are examples of drugs within this class.

Mechanism of action—Efavirenz and nevirapine both bind to reverse transcriptase near the catalytic site, leading to a conformational change that inactivates this enzyme.

Route of administration—Oral.

Contraindications—Breastfeeding.

Adverse effects—In general, well tolerated. Rash, dizziness and headache may occur.

Therapeutic notes—Resistance can develop quickly when subtherapeutic doses are used.

Inhibition of posttranslational events

Protease inhibitors

Examples of protease inhibitors include saquinavir, and the newer drugs, ritonavir, indinavir, nelfinavir and amprenavir.

Mechanism of action—Protease inhibitors prevent the virus-specific protease of HIV cleaving the inert polyprotein product of translation into various structural and functional proteins (see Fig. 12.5, site 5).

Route of administration—Oral.

Indications—Protease inhibitors are used for the management of asymptomatic and symptomatic HIV infections, in combination with NRTI.

Adverse effects—Protease inhibitors are well tolerated. Nausea, vomiting and diarrhoea are common. In addition, indinavir and ritonavir may cause taste disturbances, and saquinavir may cause buccal and mucosal ulceration.

Therapeutic notes—Combination treatment with protease inhibitors and NRTI produces additive antiviral effects and reduces the incidence of resistance. Such combination therapy is termed *highly active antiretroviral therapy* (HAART). Note that all protease inhibitors inhibit the cytochrome p450 enzyme leading to multiple drug interactions.

Immunomodulators

Interferons

Mechanism of action—Interferons (IFNs) are endogenous cytokines with antiviral activity that are normally produced by leucocytes and other cells in response to viral infection. Three major classes have been identified (α, β and γ) and have been shown to have immunoregulatory and antiproliferative effects.

The mechanism of the antiviral effect of IFNs varies for different viruses and cells. IFNs have been shown to bind to cell-surface receptors and signal a cascade of events that interfere with viral penetration, uncoating, synthesis, or methylation of mRNA, translation of viral protein, viral assembly and viral release (see Fig. 12.4). IFNs induce enzymes in the host cell that inhibit the translation of viral mRNA.

The relatively recent production of IFNs in large quantities by cell culture and recombinant DNA technology has allowed their evaluation and prescription as antiviral agents.

Route of administration—Intravenous, intramuscular.

Indications—The exact role of IFNs in the treatment of viral infections remains unclear. They have a wide spectrum of activity and have been shown to be effective in the treatment of chronic hepatitis (B and C) among others.

Adverse effects—Influenza-like syndrome with fatigue, fever, myalgia, nausea and diarrhoea is the most common side effect. Chronic administration can cause bone marrow depression and neurological effects.

Therapeutic notes—The role of IFNs remains to be clearly established. Their usefulness has been limited by the need for repeated injections and dose-limiting adverse effects.

Drugs used in human immunodeficiency virus infection

Infection with the HIV ultimately results in progression to AIDS.

There are a variety of potential sites for antiviral drug action in the HIV-1 replicative cycle (see Fig. 12.5). The four main classes of drug used in the treatment of HIV have already been discussed, but consist of the following.

- Nucleoside reverse transcriptase inhibitors, for example, zidovudine, prevent DNA chain elongation and have a competitive inhibitory effect on reverse transcriptase (see Fig. 12.5, site 3).
- Nonnucleoside reverse transcriptase inhibitors, for example, nevirapine, inactivate reverse transcriptase (see Fig. 12.5, site 3).
- Protease inhibitors, for example, ritonavir, prevent viral assembly and budding (see Fig. 12.5, site 5).
- Fusion inhibitors, for example, enfuvirtide, prevent cell infection by preventing fusion of the HIV virus with the host cell (see Fig 12.5, site 1).

Recently licensed drugs include raltegravir, an HIV-1 integrase inhibitor that may be used to treat HIV-1 which is either resistant to other drugs or to treat patients showing viral replication. Maraviroc has similar indications but blocks the interaction between HIV-1 and the chemokine receptor CCR5 on host cells.

Dr Hiroshimi, a 28-year-old man, presents with a 3-week history of persistent influenza-like symptoms. He denies any foreign travel, but he admits having unprotected sexual intercourse, last summer, with a number of homosexual men. On examination, his temperature is 39°C. He is counselled for the possibility of HIV and wishes to have an HIV test.

Two years on his CD4+ T-lymphocyte count is found to be low and his viral count raised. A decision is made to commence HAART, consisting of zidovudine, lamivudine and nevirapine.

He continued to have regular follow-ups. Then years later he is found to have a sore and painful throat. On examination, he has whitish velvety plaques on the mucous membranes of the mouth and tongue. The pattern on the tongue is distinctive of oral candidiasis. He is given nystatin (antifungal) mouthwash and a chance to rediscuss his antiretroviral therapy.

Future antihuman immunodeficiency virus drug therapy

A number of strategies are being pursued in research laboratories across the world in the quest for effective drugs to treat HIV infection.:

- Drugs which interrupt HIV binding to host cells, notably the gp120 envelope protein
- Drugs designed specifically to "smother" and prevent its entry into cells
- Antisense oligonucleotides to complement specific portions of the viral genome and inhibit transcription and replication

ANTIFUNGAL DRUGS

Concepts of fungal infection

Fungi are members of a kingdom of eukaryotic organisms that live as saprophytes or parasites. A few species of fungi are pathogenic to humans. Fungal infections are termed *mycoses* and may be superficial, affecting the skin, nails, hair, mucous membranes, or systemic, affecting deep tissues and organs.

Three main groups of fungi cause disease in humans (Table 12.4). Fungal pathogenicity results from mycotoxin production, allergenicity/inflammatory reactions and tissue invasion. Opportunistic fungal infections are important causes of disease in the immunosuppressed.

Antifungal drugs

There are four main classes of antifungal drugs.

- Polyene macrolides
- Imidazole antifungals
- Triazole antifungals
- Other antifungals

The sites of action of the antifungal drugs are summarized in Fig. 12.6.

Polyene macrolides

Examples of polyene macrolides include amphotericin B and nystatin.

Mechanism of action—Polyene macrolides bind to ergosterol in the fungal cell membrane, forming pores through which cell constituents are lost. This results in fatal damage (Fig. 12.7). These drugs are selectively toxic because in human cells, the major sterol is cholesterol, not ergosterol.

Route of administration—Amphotericin B is administered topically and intravenously. Nystatin is too toxic for intravenous use. It is not absorbed orally at all and so is applied topically as a cream or vaginal pessaries, or tablets sucked so as to deliver the drug via the oral membranes.

Indications—Amphotericin is a broad-spectrum antifungal used in potentially fatal systemic infections. Nystatin is used to suppress candidiasis (thrush) on the skin and mucous membranes (oral and vaginal).

Table 12.4 Main groups of fungi causing disease in humans

Fungal class	Form	Example	Disease caused
Moulds	Filamentous branching mycelia	Dermatophytes, e.g. *Tinea* spp. *Aspergillus fumigatus*	Athlete's foot, ringworm and other superficial mycoses Pulmonary or disseminated aspergillosis
True yeasts	Unicellular (round or oval)	*Cryptococcus neoformans*	Cryptococcal meningitis and lung infections in the immunocompromized
Yeast- like fungi	Similar to yeasts but can also form long (nonbranching) filaments	*Candida albicans*	Oral and vaginal thrush, endocarditis and septicaemias

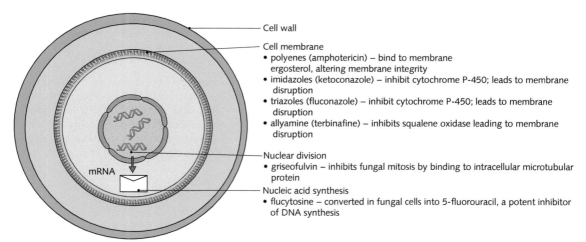

Fig. 12.6 Sites of action of antifungal drugs. *DNA*, Deoxyribonucleic acid; *mRNA*, messenger ribonucleic acid.

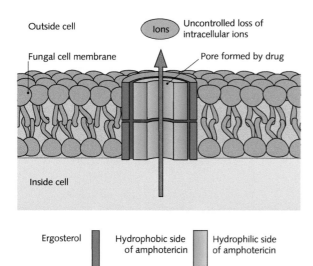

Fig. 12.7 Mechanism of action of polyene antifungal agents.

Adverse effects—Fever, chills and nausea. Long-term therapy invariably causes renal damage. Nystatin may cause oral sensitisation.

Therapeutic notes—Creatinine clearance must be monitored during amphotericin therapy to exclude renal damage. Resistance can develop in vivo to amphotericin, but not to nystatin.

Imidazoles

Examples of imidazoles include clotrimazole, miconazole and ketoconazole.

Mechanism of action—Imidazoles have a broad spectrum of activity. They inhibit fungal lipid (especially ergosterol) synthesis in cell membranes. Interference with fungal oxidative enzymes results in the accumulation of 14α-methyl sterols, which may disrupt the packing of acyl chains of phospholipids, inhibiting growth and interfering with membrane-bound enzyme systems.

Route of administration—Intravenous, topical. Ketoconazole is given orally because, unlike the other imidazoles, it is well absorbed by this route.

Indications—Candidiasis and dermatophyte mycoses. Miconazole can also be used intravenously as an alternative to amphotericin in disseminated mycoses. Ketoconazole is active orally and can be used for systemic mycoses.

Adverse effects—Topical use of imidazoles tends to be unproblematic. Intravenous miconazole is often limited by side effects of nausea, faintness and haematological disorders. Oral ketoconazole can cause serious hepatotoxicity and adrenosuppression.

Therapeutic notes—Resistance rarely develops to imidazoles.

Triazoles

Examples of triazoles include fluconazole and itraconazole.

Mechanism of action—Triazoles are similar to imidazoles (see earlier), although they have greater selectivity against fungi and cause fewer endocrinological problems.

Route of administration—Oral.

Indications—Fluconazole can be used for a wide range of systemic and superficial infections, including cryptococcal meningitis, because it reaches the cerebrospinal fluid in high concentrations. Itraconazole is similarly indicated, although unlike fluconazole, it can be used against *Aspergillus*.

Adverse effects—Nausea, diarrhoea and rashes. Itraconazole is well tolerated, although nausea, headaches and abdominal pain can occur, but should not be given to patients with liver damage.

Therapeutic notes—Resistance rarely develops to the triazoles.

Other antifungals

Allylamines

Terbinafine is an example of an allylamine.

Mechanism of action—Terbinafine prevents ergosterol synthesis by inhibiting the enzyme squalene oxidase, resulting in squalene accumulation, which leads to membrane disruption and cell death. It is lipophilic and penetrates superficial tissues well, including the nails.

Route of administration—Oral, topical.

Indications—Terbinafine has been recently introduced against dermatophyte infections including ringworm, where oral therapy is appropriate because of the site and severity of extent of infection.

Adverse effects—Mild nausea, abdominal pain, skin reactions. Loss of taste has been reported.

Therapeutic notes—Resistance rarely develops.

Flucytosine

Mechanism of action—Flucytosine is imported into fungal, but not human, cells, where it is converted into 5-fluorouracil, a potent inhibitor of DNA synthesis.

Route of administration—Intravenous.

Indications—Flucytosine is most active against yeasts and is indicated for use in systemic candidiasis and as an adjunct to amphotericin in cryptococcal meningitis.

Adverse effects—Nausea and vomiting are common. Rare side effects include hepatotoxicity, hair loss and bone-marrow suppression.

Therapeutic notes—Weekly blood counts of patients on flucytosine are necessary to monitor bone marrow suppression.

Griseofulvin

Mechanism of action—The mechanism of action of griseofulvin is not fully established, but it probably interferes with microtubule formation or nucleic acid synthesis and polymerization. It is selectively concentrated in keratin and therefore is suitable for treating dermatophyte mycoses.

Route of administration—Oral.

Indications—Griseofulvin is the drug of choice for widespread or intractable dermatophyte infections, where topical therapy has failed.

Adverse effects—Hypersensitivity reactions, headaches, rashes, photosensitivity.

Therapeutic notes—Because griseofulvin is fungistatic rather than fungicidal, treatment regimens are long, amounting to several weeks or months. Griseofulvin is more effective for skin than nail infections.

HINTS AND TIPS

Superficial mycoses (e.g. athlete's foot/thrush) are common and usually easily treated with topical drugs (e.g. terbinafine) that have few adverse effects. Deep mycoses are rare (except in the immunocompromised), serious and may be fatal despite therapy with systemic drugs, which often have adverse effects.

ANTIPROTOZOAL DRUGS

Concepts of protozoal infection

Protozoa are members of a phylum of unicellular organisms, some of which are parasitic pathogens in humans, causing several diseases of medical and global importance. Parasitic protozoa replicate within the host's body and are usually divided into four subphyla according to their type of locomotion (Table 12.5).

Malaria

Malaria is responsible for 2 million deaths per year and 200 million people worldwide are infected. Malaria is caused by four species of plasmodial parasites that are transmitted by female anopheline mosquitoes.

Antimalarial drugs target different phases of the life cycle of the malarial parasite (Fig. 12.8). This life cycle proceeds as follows.

- When an infected mosquito feeds on a human, it injects sporozoites into the bloodstream from its salivary glands.
- The sporozoites rapidly penetrate the liver where they transform and grow into tissue schizonts containing large numbers of merozoites. In the case of *Plasmodium vivax* and *Plasmodium ovale,* some schizonts remain dormant in the liver for years (hypnozoites), before rupturing to cause a relapse.
- The large tissue schizonts rupture after 5 to 20 days, releasing thousands of merozoites that invade circulating red blood cells (RBCs), and multiply inside the cell.
- The host's RBCs rupture, leading to the release of more merozoites. These then invade and destroy more RBCs. This cycle of invasion/destruction causes the episodic chills and fever that characterize malaria.
- Some merozoites develop into gametocytes. If these are taken up by a feeding mosquito, the insect becomes infected, thus completing the cycle.

The clinical features and severity of malaria depend upon the species of parasite and the immunological status of the person infected. Clinically significant malaria is less common in adults who have always lived in endemic areas, as partial immunity develops.

There are four types of plasmodium causing malaria.

- *Plasmodium falciparum:* Widespread and causes malignant tertian (fever every third day) malaria. There is no exoerythrocytic stage, so that, if the erythrocytic forms are eradicated, relapses do not occur.
- *P. vivax:* Widespread and causes benign, tertian relapsing malaria. Exoerythrocytic forms may persist in the liver for years and cause relapses.
- *Plasmodium malariae:* Rare and causes benign quartan (fever every fourth day) malaria. There is no

Table 12.5 Classification of medically important protozoan species causing disease in humans

Subphyla	Defining characteristics	Medically important species	Disease
Amoebae (sarcodina)	Amoeboid movement with pseudopods	*Entamoeba histolytica*	Amoebiasis (amoebic dysentery)
Flagellates (mastigophora)	Flagella that produces a whip-like movement	*Giardia lamblia* *Trichomonas vaginalis* *Leishmania* spp. *Trypanosoma* spp.	Giardiasis Trichomonal vaginitis Leishmaniasis Trypanosomiasis (sleeping sickness and Chagas disease)
Ciliates (ciliophora)	Cilia beat to produce movement	—	—
Sporozoans (sporozoa)	No locomotor organs in adult stage	*Plasmodium* spp.	Malaria

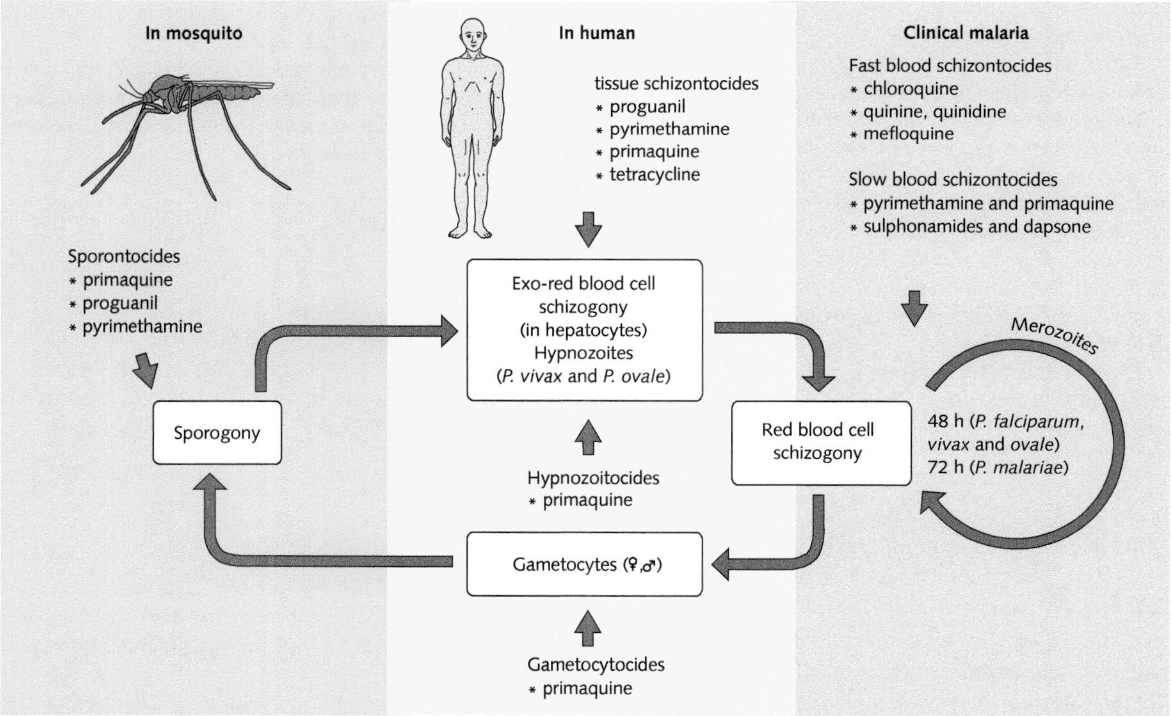

Fig. 12.8 Life cycle of the malarial parasite and point of action of chemotherapeutic agents.

exoerythrocytic stage, so that, if the erythrocytic forms are eradicated, relapses do not occur.

- *P. ovale*: Mainly African and causes a rare form of benign relapsing malaria. Exoerythrocytic forms may persist in the liver for years and cause relapses.

Approaches to antimalarial chemotherapy

Antimalarial drugs are usually classified in terms of their action against different stages of the parasite (see Fig. 12.8).

They are used to protect against or cure malaria or to prevent transmission.

Prophylactic use

The aim of prophylactic use is to prevent the occurrence of infection in a previously healthy individual who is at potential exposure risk.

Suppressive prophylaxis involves the use of blood schizonticides to prevent acute attacks; causal prophylaxis involves the use of tissue schizonticides or drugs against the sporozoite to prevent the parasite becoming established in the liver.

Curative (therapeutic use)

Antimalarial drugs can be used curatively (therapeutically) against an established infection.

Suppressive treatment aims to control acute attacks, usually with blood schizonticides; radical treatment aims to kill dormant liver forms, usually with a hypnozonticide, to prevent relapsing malaria.

Antimalarial drugs

4-aminoquinolines

Chloroquine is an example of a 4-aminoquinoline.

Mechanism of action—Chloroquine is a rapidly acting blood schizonticide (see Fig. 12.8). It is concentrated 100-fold in erythrocytes that contain plasmodial parasites; this occurs because of ferriprotoporphyrin IX, a degradation product of haemoglobin digestion by the parasites, acts as a chloroquine receptor. It is unclear how the high chloroquine concentrations kill the parasites; possibly, the digestion of haemoglobin is inhibited.

Route of administration—Oral. In severe falciparum malaria infections, injections or infusions can be used.

Indications—Suppressive chemoprophylaxis and treatment of susceptible strains of plasmodium.

Adverse effects—Nausea, vomiting, headache, rashes and, rarely, neurological effects and blurred vision.

Therapeutic notes—Chloroquine is considered safe for use in pregnant women. It rapidly controls fever (24–48 hours) but cannot produce a lasting radical cure in *P. vivax* and *P. ovale* strain infections, because it does not affect hypnozoites.

In most areas, *P. falciparum* is resistant to chloroquine, necessitating combination chemoprophylaxis with antifolates (see later).

HINTS AND TIPS

Chloroquine is the drug of choice for the treatment of all nonfalciparum malaria. It is highly effective against *P. Malariae*, *P. Ovale* and *P. Vivax*. Quinine, artemether with lumefantrine can be used as second line. Primaquine is used to destroy liver stage parasites and prevent relapse.

Quinoline-methanols

Examples of quinoline-methanols include quinine and mefloquine.

Mechanism of action—Quinoline-methanols are rapidly acting blood schizonticides (see Fig. 12.8). It is not precisely known how the quinoline-methanols work but, similar to chloroquine, they are known to bind to a product of haemoglobin digestion. It has no effect on exoerythrocytic forms or on the gametocytes of *P. falciparum*.

Route of administration—Quinine is administered orally or by rate-controlled infusion in severe cases. Mefloquine is only given orally.

Indications—Quinine is the drug of choice for treating the acute clinical attack of falciparum malaria resistant to chloroquine. Mefloquine is effective against all malarial species including multidrug-resistant *P. falciparum* and can also be used for chemoprophylaxis.

Adverse effects—Quinine may cause tinnitus, headache, nausea, blurring of vision, hypoglycaemia and, rarely, blood disorders. Overdose results in profound hypotension because of peripheral vasodilatation and myocardial depression (see Chapter 4). Quinine is safe in pregnancy.

Mefloquine may cause nausea, vomiting, gastrointestinal disturbance and postural hypotension. Rarely, acute neuropathic conditions may occur. Mefloquine may cause foetal abnormalities.

Therapeutic notes—The quinoline-methanols are used in combination therapy with other agents such as the sulphonamides or tetracyclines.

Monitoring for hypoglycaemia should occur in patients with malaria because the malarial parasite consumes glucose and quinine can stimulate insulin release, causing a reduction in blood glucose levels.

HINTS AND TIPS

Quinine is usually given orally as a 7-day course but can be given intravenously for severe *P. Falciparum* malaria or in patients who are vomiting. In some areas of the tropics, quinine was incorporated into tonic waters to help protect against malaria, giving the water a bitter taste.

Antifolates

Examples of antifolates include type 1 drugs, for example, sulphonamides and dapsone, and type 2 drugs, for example, pyrimethamine and proguanil. Both types are useful.

Mechanism of action—Antifolates are slow-acting (in comparison with chloroquine, quinine and mefloquine) blood schizonticides, tissue schizonticides and sporonticides. These drugs inhibit the formation of folate compounds and thus inhibit DNA synthesis and cell division. All growing stages of the malarial parasite are affected.

The sulphonamides and dapsone are known as type 1 antifolate drugs. They compete with *para*-aminobenzoic acid for the enzyme dihydropteroate synthetase, which is found only in the parasites.

Proguanil and pyrimethamine are known as type 2 antifolate drugs. They selectively inhibit malarial dihydrofolate reductase.

These two groups of drugs act on the same pathway but at different points; they are used in combination as their synergistic blockade is more powerful than any one drug acting alone.

Route of administration—Oral.

Indications—Antifolates are used in combination for the causal chemoprophylaxis of malaria, or in combination with quinine for the treatment of acute chloroquine-resistant malaria.

Adverse effects—Antifolates have almost no side effects if used in therapeutic doses. In toxic doses, type 2 antifolates can inhibit mammalian dihydrofolate reductase and cause a megaloblastic anaemia. Skin rashes occasionally occur.

Therapeutic notes—Common chemoprophylactic combinations include chloroquine plus pyrimethamine with a sulphonamide or dapsone.

Monitoring of a patient's full blood count is key when taking antifolate medication.

8-aminoquinolines

Primaquine is an example of an 8-aminoquinoline.

Mechanism of action—Primaquine is an hypnozonicide and gametocide. It is unclear how the drug works, but it may cause oxidative damage to the parasite. It is effective against the nongrowing stages of malaria, that is, hypnozoites and gametocytes (see Fig. 12.8).

Route of administration—Oral.

Indications—Primaquine is used for the radical cure of relapsing malarias (*P. ovale* and *P. vivax)* and prevention of transmission of *P. falciparum.*

Contraindications—Pregnancy.

Adverse effects—Nausea, vomiting, bone marrow depression. Intravenous haemolysis can occur in people with glucose 6-phosphate deficiency.

Therapeutic notes—Primaquine is usually used in combination with chloroquine. Resistance is rare.

Artemisinin

Artemisinin is given with the antimalarial lumefantrine because together they are much more effective than either drug given individually. There is a synergistic effect. This medication is effective at treating resistant *P. Falciparum* cerebral malaria.

Mechanism of action—A peroxide (trioxane) structure is responsible for its blood schizontocide activity against plasmodium, including multiresistant strains of *P. falciparum.*

Route of administration—Oral.

Indications—Treatment of uncomplicated falciparum malaria.

Contraindications—Breastfeeding, congestive heart failure, congenital Q-T interval prolongation, arrhythmias.

Adverse effects—Nausea, vomiting, abdominal pain, diarrhoea, dizziness, arthralgia, myalgia.

CLINICAL NOTE

A 25-year-old student, presents with a 4-day history of high fever (40°C), general malaise, feeling intensely cold and shaky followed by profuse sweating. He denies any homosexual contacts, unprotected sexual intercourse or intravenous drug use. He returned from Nigeria 3 weeks ago and was completing his proguanil with atovaquone malarial prophylaxis treatment. On examination, he looked unwell. His pulse was 98 beats per minutes with a blood pressure of 132/72 mm Hg. There are no heart murmurs. There are no enlarged lymph nodes.

Blood tests reveal raised bilirubin with normal liver enzymes, mild anaemia and a low platelet count. Light microscopy of a Giemsa-stained blood smear shows approximately 1% of red blood cells are infected with *Plasmodium* parasite.

He is kept well hydrated and treated with oral quinine for 7 days, after which his fever resolves, and he starts to improve.

Treatment of other protozoal infections

Amoebiasis

Amoebic dysentery is caused by infection with *Entamoeba histolytica,* which is ingested in a cystic form. Dysentery results from invasion of the intestinal wall by the parasite. Occasionally, the organism encysts in the liver, forming abscesses.

Metronidazole is the drug of choice for acute invasive amoebic dysentery, it kills the trophozoites although has no activity against the cyst forms. Diloxanide and tinidazole are also used to treat amoebiasis.

Giardiasis

Giardiasis is a bowel infection caused by the flagellate *Giardia lamblia.* Infection follows ingestion of contaminated water or food and involves flatulence and diarrhoea.

Metronidazole is the drug of choice for giardiasis.

Trichomonas vaginitis

Trichomonas vaginitis is caused by the flagellate *Trichomonas vaginalis.* It is a sexually transmitted inflammatory condition of the female vagina and, occasionally, male urethra.

Metronidazole is the drug of choice for trichomonas vaginitis.

Trypanosomiasis and leishmaniasis

Trypanosomiasis

African trypanosomiasis (sleeping sickness) and South American trypanosomiasis (Chagas disease) are caused by species of flagellate trypanosome.

Insect vectors introduce the parasites into the human host, where they reproduce, causing bouts of parasitaemia and fever. Toxins released cause damage to organs. The CNS is affected in sleeping sickness and the heart, liver, spleen, bone and intestine in Chagas disease.

The drug suramin kills the African trypanosomiasis parasite, possibly related to an ability to reversibly inhibit a number of enzymes (in the host and parasite). However, it does not penetrate into the CNS and thus its use is restricted to early trypanosomiasis.

Melarsoprol is used to treat the late CNS form of African trypanosomiasis. It may act by inactivating pyruvate kinase, a critical enzyme in the metabolism of trypanosomes.

Nifurtimox and benznidazole are used to treat acute American trypanosomiasis.

Leishmaniasis

Leishmania species are flagellated parasites that are transmitted by a sandfly vector, assuming a nonflagellated intracellular form that resides within macrophages on infecting humans. Clinical infections range from simple, resolving cutaneous infections to systemic "visceral" forms with hepatomegaly, splenomegaly, anaemia and fever.

Leishmaniasis can usually be treated with stibogluconate, a trivalent antimonial compound that reacts with thiol groups and reduces adenosine triphosphate (ATP) production in the parasite.

Pneumocystis pneumonia

Pneumocystis pneumonia is most often associated with HIV infection and is now considered an AIDS-defining illness. The infective agent *Pneumocystis jiroveci* (previously called *Pneumocystis carinii)* is not truly a protozoa, although it has similarities with both protozoa and fungi, and remains difficult to classify.

Signs and symptoms of *P. jiroveci* pneumonia are similar to other pneumonias, but culture is not possible, and the microorganism must be visualized on direct microscopy.

High-dose oral or parenteral co-trimoxazole (trimethoprim and sulfamethoxazole) is the drug of choice. Dapsone with trimethoprim is given as an alternative treatment.

ANTHELMINTIC DRUGS

Concepts of helminthic infection

Helminth is derived from the Greek *helmins,* meaning worm. Anthelmintic drugs are therefore medicines acting against parasitic worms.

There are three groups of helminths that parasitize humans.

- Cestoda (tapeworms)
- Nematoda (roundworms)
- Trematoda (flukes).

Table 12.6 lists medically important helminth infections and the main drugs used in their treatment.

The anthelmintic drugs

To be effective, an anthelmintic drug must be able to penetrate the cuticle of the worm, or gain access to its alimentary tract, so that it may exert its pharmacological effect on the physiology of the worm.

Anthelmintic drugs act on parasitic worms by a number of mechanisms. These include the following.

- Damaging or killing the worm directly
- Paralysing the worm
- Damaging the cuticle of the worm so that host defences, such as digestion and immune rejection, can affect the worm
- Interfering with worm metabolism

Because there is great diversity across the different helminth classes, drugs highly effective against one species of worm are often ineffectual against another species.

Mechanism of action—Niclosamide, a salicylamide derivative, is the most used drug for tapeworm infestations. It blocks glucose uptake at high concentrations, irreversibly damaging the scolex (attachment end) of the tapeworm, leading to the release and expulsion of the tapeworm. It is a safe, selective drug because very little is absorbed from the gastrointestinal tract.

Route of administration—Oral.

Indications—Tapeworm infestation (see Table 12.6).

Adverse effects—Mild gastrointestinal disturbance.

Therapeutic notes—Patients fast before treatment with niclosamide. Purgatives to expel the dead worm segments (proglottides) can be used, but are probably unnecessary because the worm may be digested after the effects of the drug.

Praziquantel

Mechanism of action—Praziquantel increases the permeability of the helminth plasma membrane to calcium. At low concentrations, this causes contraction and spastic paralysis and, at higher concentrations, vesiculation and vacuolization damage is caused to the tegument of the worm.

Route of administration—Oral.

Indications—Praziquantel is the drug of choice for all schistosome infections (see Table 12.6), and for cysticercosis (a rare cestode condition caused by encystation of larvae of the tapeworm *Taenia solium* in human organs).

Adverse effects—Mild gastrointestinal disturbance, headache and dizziness may occur shortly after administration.

Therapeutic notes—Praziquantel should be taken after meals 3 times a day for 2 days only.

Table 12.6 Classification of medically important helminth infections and the main drugs in their treatment

	Helminth species	Drugs used in treatment
Cestodes		
Beef tapeworm	Taenia saginata	Niclosamide, praziquantel
Pork tapeworm	Taenia solium	Niclosamide, praziquantel
Fish tapeworm	Diphyllobothrium latum	Niclosamide, praziquantel
Hydatid tapeworm	Echinococcus granulosus	Albendazole
Nematodes		
Intestinal species		
Common round worms	Ascaris lumbricoides	Mebendazole, piperazine
Threadworms/pin worms	Enterobius vermicularis	Mebendazole, piperazine
Threadworms (USA)	Strongyloides stercoralis	Thiabendazole, albendazole
Whipworms	Trichuris trichiura	Mebandazole
Hookworms	Necator americanus	Mebendazole
	Ankylostoma duodenale	Mebendazole
Tissue species		
Trichinella	Trichinella spiralis	Thiabendazole
Guinea worm	Dracunculus medinesis	Metronidazole
Filarioidea	Wuchereria bancrofti	Diethylcarbamazine
	Loa loa	Diethylcarbamazine
	Brugia malayi	Diethylcarbamazine
	Onchocerca volvulus	Ivermectin
Trematodes		
Blood flukes/schistosomes	Schistosoma japonicum	Praziquantel
	Schistosoma mansoni	Praziquantel
	Schistosoma haematobium	Praziquantel

Piperazine

Mechanism of action—Piperazine is a reversible neuro-muscular blocker that causes a flaccid paralysis in worms, leading to their expulsion by gastrointestinal peristalsis. It has very little effect on the host.

Route of administration—Oral.

Indications—Piperazine is used for roundworm and threadworm gastrointestinal infestation.

Adverse effects—Gastrointestinal disturbance and neuro-toxic effects (dizziness) may occur.

Therapeutic notes—A single dose of piperazine is usually effective for treating roundworm infection; threadworm in-festation may require a longer course (7 days).

Benzimidazoles

Examples of benzimidazoles include mebendazole, thiaben-dazole and albendazole.

Mechanism of action—Benzimidazoles bind with high affinity to a site on tubulin dimers, thus preventing the polymerisation of microtubules. Subsequent depolymerisa-tion leads to complete breakdown of the microtubule.

The selectivity of benzimidazoles arises because they are 250 to 400 times more potent in helminth than in mamma-lian tissue. The process takes time to have an effect, and the worm may not be expelled for days.

Route of administration—Oral.

Indications—Benzimidazoles are used in the treatment of hydatid disease, and many nematode infestations (see Table 12.6).

Contraindications—Benzimidazoles should not be given to pregnant women because they are teratogenic and embryotoxic.

Adverse effects—Occasional gastrointestinal disturbance. Thiabendazole causes more frequent gastrointestinal dis-turbance, headache and dizziness. Serious hepatotoxicity rarely occurs.

Therapeutic notes—Dosage regimens of benzimidazoles range from a single dose for pinworm infestation to multi-ple doses for up to 5 days for trichinosis.

Diethylcarbamazine

Mechanism of action—it is not clear exatly how diethylcarbamazine exerts its filaricidal effect. It has been suggested that it damages or modifies the parasites in such a way as to make them more susceptible to host immune defences. Diethylcarbamazine kills both microfilariae in the peripheral circulation and adult worms in the lymphatics

Route of administration—oral

Indications—diethylcarbamazine is the drug of choice for lymphatic filariasis caused by Wucheria Bancrofti, Loa Loa and Brugia malayia. See Table 12.6

Adverse effects—gastrointestinal disturbance, headache, lassitude. Material from the damaged and dead worms causes allergic side effects, including skin reactions, lymph gland enlargement, dizziness and tachycardia, lasting from 3 to 7 days.

Therapeutic notes—to minimise the dangerous sudden release of dead worm material, the initial dose of diethylcarbamazine is started low and then increased and then maintained for 21 days.

Ivermectin

Mechanism of action—Ivermectin immobilizes the tapeworm *Onchocerca volvulus* by causing tonic paralysis of the peripheral muscle system. It does this by potentiating the effect of γ-aminobutyric acid at the worm's neuromuscular junction.

Route of administration—Oral.

Indications—Ivermectin is the drug of choice for *O. volvulus,* which causes river blindness and may be the most effective drug for chronic *Strongyloides* infection (see Table 12.6).

Adverse effects—Ocular irritation, transient electrocardiographic changes and somnolence. An immediate immune reaction to dead microfilariae (Mazzotti reaction) can be severe.

Levamisole

Mechanism of action—Levamisole stimulates nicotinic receptors at the neuromuscular junction and results in a spastic paralysis, which causes faecal worm expulsion.

Route of administration—Oral.

Indications—Treatment of choice for *Ascaris lumbricoides* roundworm infection (see Table 12.6).

Adverse effects—Mild nausea and vomiting.

VACCINATIONS

Artificial immunity is achieved by giving a vaccine (active immunisation) or immunoglobulin (passive immunisation).

Active immunity is the stimulation of the immune mechanism to produce antibodies by giving an antigen as a vaccine.

- Live attenuated viruses (e.g. rubella, measles, mumps, oral polio)
- Inactivated viruses (e.g. parenteral polio, hepatitis A)
- Inactivated bacterial toxins (e.g. diphtheria and tetanus)
- Genetically engineered (e.g. hepatitis B)

The body is then able to generate an immune response (either humoral or cell-mediated) and have protection against the bacteria/virus that they are inoculated against.

Precautions before vaccination

Avoid giving vaccinations to patients with allergies or previous reactions. Similarly, patients with an acute febrile illness should not be given a vaccine. Live vaccines should not be given to patients on chemotherapy and immunosuppressive medications (including corticosteroids). Likewise, they should not be given to patients who have had a recent bone marrow transplant.

● Chapter Summary

- Bactericidal (kill bacteria) antibiotics often have to be used in immunocompromized individuals
- Acquired resistance occurs when bacteria produce enzymes that inactive the antibiotic
- Broad-spectrum antibiotics include penicillins, tetracyclines and cephalosporins
- Antibiotics are either protein synthesis inhibitors (e.g. tetracyclines), cell wall synthesis inhibitors (e.g. glycopeptides) or nucleic acid synthesis (e.g. quinolones)
- Treatment of tuberculosis involves four drugs for two months (rifampicin, isoniazid, pyrazinamide and ethambutol) and then two drugs for four months (rifampicin and isoniazid)
- Treatment of HIV involves four main classes of drug; nucleoside reverse transcriptase inhibitors, nonnucleoside reverse transcriptase inhibitors, protease inhibitors and fusion inhibitors
- Vaccines can be live attenuated viruses, inactivated viruses, inactivated bacterial toxins or genetically engineered

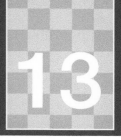

Cancer 13

Cancers are malignant neoplasms (new growths) occurring when cells no longer differentiate in an orderly fashion but multiply in a haphazard way. Despite their variability, cancers share these characteristics.

- Uncontrolled proliferation
- Local invasiveness
- Tendency to spread (metastasis)
- Changes in some aspects of original cell morphology/retention of other characteristics

Cancer accounts for 20% to 25% of deaths in the Western world. Management options include surgery, radiotherapy and chemotherapy. These methods are not mutually exclusive, often being used in combination, for example, adjuvant chemotherapy after surgical removal of a tumour.

CONCEPTS OF CANCER CHEMOTHERAPY

Chemotherapy

Cancer chemotherapy is the use of drugs to inhibit the rate of growth of or to kill cancerous cells. The ideal anticancer drugs target malignant cells in preference to nonmalignant cells. This is achieved by exploiting the molecular differences between them.

CLINICAL NOTE

A 60-year-old man presents with a 6-week history of the passage of fresh blood from his rectum and looser stool. He also admits to low appetite, significant weight loss and feeling fatigued. He is referred for investigative colonoscopy, which reveals an abnormal growth in the descending colon. A biopsy confirms an adenocarcinoma. Staging computed tomography scans show no other areas of disease. He is managed by surgical resection of the tumour. Following this, he undergoes adjuvant chemotherapy.

The most striking difference between cancerous and noncancerous cells is their accelerated rate of cell division. This remains a common target for therapeutic intervention.

The chemotherapeutic techniques currently used include the following.

- Cytotoxic therapy (which is the main approach)
- Endocrine therapy
- Immunotherapy

Cancers differ in their sensitivity to chemotherapy, from the very sensitive (e.g. lymphomas, testicular carcinomas) where complete clinical cures can be achieved, to the resistant (generally solid tumours, e.g. colorectal, squamous cell bronchial carcinoma).

A diagnosis of cancer carries a significant social and emotional impact. Hair loss and sickness are more often the initial concern for patients, rather than other potentially serious side effects of chemotherapy. Nausea and vomiting should be taken seriously in cancer management, as these can have a devastating impact on quality of life; antiemetic drugs are discussed in Chapter 6.

HINTS AND TIPS

Adjuvant chemotherapy is given after successful treatment of cancer, where no remaining disease is found, or for prophylaxis against reoccurrence.

CYTOTOXIC CHEMOTHERAPY

Mechanisms of action

Most cytotoxic drugs affect deoxyribonucleic acid (DNA) synthesis and thus cell division. They can be classified according to their site of action affecting the process of DNA synthesis within the cancer cell (Fig. 13.1). Cytotoxic drugs are therefore most effective against actively cycling/proliferating cells, both normal and malignant, and least effective against nondividing cells.

Some drugs are only effective at killing cycling cells during specific parts of the cell cycle. These are known as phase-specific drugs (Fig. 13.2). Other drugs are cytotoxic towards cycling cells throughout the cell cycle (e.g. alkylating agents) and are known as cycle-specific drugs.

Selectivity

Cytotoxic drugs are not specifically toxic to cancer cells, and the selectivity they show is marginal at best.

Cytotoxic drugs affect all dividing tissues, both normal and malignant, and thus are likely to have a wide range of toxic side effects (Table 13.1), most often related to the inhibition of division of noncancerous host cells, namely in

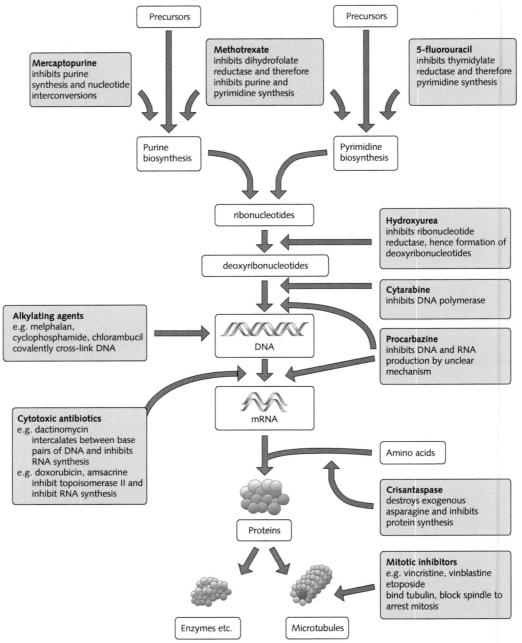

Fig. 13.1 Sites of action of cytotoxic drugs that act on dividing cells. *DNA*, Deoxyribonucleic acid; *mRNA*, messenger ribonucleic acid; *RNA*, ribonucleic acid.

the gut, in the bone marrow and in the reproductive and immune systems.

Relative selectivity can occur with some cancers.

- In malignant tumours, a higher proportion of cells are undergoing proliferation than in normal proliferating tissues.

- Normal cells seem to recover from chemotherapeutic inhibition faster than some cancer cells.
- Knowledge of these principles and knowing that cytotoxic drugs kill a constant fraction, not a constant number, of cells, lays down the foundation for chemotherapeutic dosing schedules (Fig. 13.3).

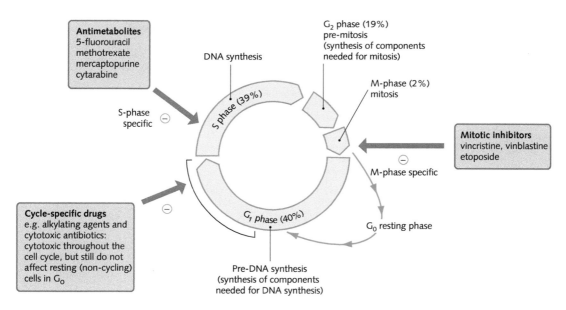

Fig. 13.2 Cell cycle and point of action of phase-specific drugs. *DNA*, Deoxyribonucleic acid.

Table 13.1 General adverse effects of cytotoxic drugs

Site	Effects
Bone marrow	Myelosuppression can lead to leucopoenia, thrombocytopenia and sometimes anaemia, this is often the dose-limiting side effect; there is a high risk of haemorrhage, immunosuppression and infection as a result
Gastrointestinal tract	Inhibition of mucosal cell division may produce anorexia, ulceration or diarrhoea; nausea and vomiting are common, especially with alkylating agents and cisplatin
Skin	Loss of hair (alopecia) may be partial or complete but is usually reversible
Wounds	Impaired wound healing results from cell reproduction inhibition
Reproductive system	Sterility, teratogenesis and mutagenicity are all possible
Secondary cancers	Many cytotoxic drugs are carcinogenic, additionally the immunosuppression resulting from myelosuppression may reduce immune surveillance of emerging dysplastic cells, leading to an increased risk of development of some cancers after chemotherapy

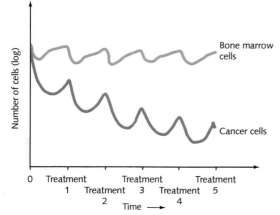

Fig. 13.3 Theoretical anticancer cytotoxic dosing schedule, allowing recovery of normal tissues.

Resistance to cytotoxic drugs

Genetic resistance to cytotoxic drugs can be inherent to the cancer cell line or acquired during the course of chemotherapy, as a result of selection induced by the chemotherapeutic agent.

Mechanisms of genetic resistance to cytotoxic drugs

The mechanisms of genetic resistance to cytotoxic drugs.

- Abnormal transport
- Decreased cellular retention/active transport out of cells
- Increased cellular inactivation (binding/metabolism)
- Altered target protein

Table 13.2 Summary of cancer therapies

Class of drug	Drug	Mechanism of action	Use	Important side effects
Alkylating agent	Cyclophosphamide	Pronounced effect on lymphocytes Immunosuppressant Intrastrand cross-linking of DNA	Haematological malignancy	N&V Bone marrow depression Haemorrhagic cystitis
Alkylating agent	Procarbazine	Inhibits DNA and RNA synthesis Interferes with mitosis	Hodgkin disease	Hypertension Flushing reaction
Platinum compound	Cisplatin	Intrastrand cross-linking of DNA	Solid tumours (especially testes and ovary)	Nephrotoxic Severe N&V
Antimetabolite	Fluorouracil	Inhibition of DNA synthesis	Basal cell carcinoma	Gastrointestinal upset Myelotoxicity
Antimetabolite	Cytarabine	Pyramidine analogue— inhibits DNA polymerase	Acute myeloid leukaemia	Gastrointestinal upset Myelotoxicity
Cytotoxic antibiotic	Doxorubicin	Inhibits DNA and RNA synthesis, through interference with topoisomerase II	Bladder cancer	N&V Myelosuppression Hair loss Cardiotoxic in high doses
Vinca alkaloids (mitotic inhibitor)	Vincristine	Bind to tubulin and inhibit its polymerisation, causing arrest at metaphase inhibiting mitosis	Haematological malignancy	Mild myelosuppression Neurotoxic → paraesthesia and weakness Abdominal pain
Mitotic inhibitor	Etoposide	Inhibits DNA synthesis by action on topoisomerase II Inhibits mitochondrial function	Haematological malignancy	Vomiting Alopecia Myelosuppression
Monoclonal antibody	Rituximab	It binds to CD20 protein → lyses B lymphocytes	Lymphoma	Hypotension Chills and fever Hypersensitivity reaction
Monoclonal antibody	Trastuzumab (Herceptin)	Binds to oncogenic protein HER2	Breast cancer that overexpress HER2	
Protein kinase inhibitor	Imatinib	Inhibits oncogenic cytoplasmic kinase (BCR/ABL) & platelet-derived growth factor	Chronic myeloid leukaemia	Gastrointestinal upset Headaches Rashes (can get resistance)

DNA, Deoxyribonucleic acid; N nausea and vomiting; RNA, ribonucleic acid.

- Enhanced repair of DNA
- Altered processing

Some tumours are relatively resistant to chemotherapy because they exist in so-called "pharmacological sanctuaries". These occur when a tumour is in a privileged compartment, for example, inside the blood–brain barrier, or in large solid tumours when poor blood supply and diffusion limit the penetration of the drug.

In clinical practice, cancers may be treated more successfully with combinations of cytotoxic drugs simultaneously.

The theory is that multiple attacks with cytotoxic agents acting at different biochemical sites will increase efficacy while reducing the likelihood of resistance.

Cytotoxic agents

Cytotoxic agents, the major group of anticancer drugs, include the following (see Table 13.2).

- Alkylating agents
- Antimetabolites

- Cytotoxic antibiotics
- Mitotic inhibitors
- Platinum compounds
- Miscellaneous agents

CLINICAL NOTE

A 58-year-old female presents to her General Practitioner (GP) following increasing vague abdominal pain and discomfort for the past 4 months and abdominal distension for the past 1 month. She is referred to A&E and admitted. A CT scan is done and an ascitic drain inserted, from which a sample of the fluid is sent for cytology. CT shows ovarian and omental masses. Cytological examination of ascitic fluid indicates adenocarcinoma.

Laparotomy is done allowing peritoneal biopsy, which shows ovarian malignancy. The management includes removal of her uterus, ovaries and omentum. After surgery, she is started on a 6-month course of carboplatin.

Alkylating agents

Examples of alkylating agents include melphalan, cyclophosphamide and chlorambucil.

Mechanism of action—Alkylating agents act via a reactive alkyl group that reacts to form covalent bonds with nucleic acids. There follows either cross-linking of the two strands of DNA, preventing replication, or DNA strand breakage (see Fig. 13.1).

Route of administration
- Melphalan and cyclophosphamide orally and intravenously.
- Chlorambucil orally.

Indications
- Melphalan is used in myeloma and in some solid tumours.
- Cyclophosphamide is used to treat a variety of leukaemias, and lymphomas, and some solid tumours.
- Chlorambucil is used for leukaemias, lymphomas and ovarian cancers.

Adverse effects—Generalized cytotoxicity is common with alkylating agents (see Table 13.1). A urinary metabolite of cyclophosphamide, acrolein, may cause serious haemorrhagic cystitis. This effect may be reduced by high fluid intake (4 L/day).

Damage to gametogenesis and the development of secondary acute nonlymphocytic leukaemias is a particular problem with these alkylating agents. Alopecia is also common.

Antimetabolites

Examples of antimetabolites include the folic acid antagonists (e.g. methotrexate), antipyrimidines (e.g. fluorouracil and cytarabine) and antipurines (e.g. mercaptopurine).

Mechanism of action—Antimetabolites are analogues of normal metabolites and act by competition, replacing the natural metabolite and then subverting cellular processes (see Fig. 13.1).

- Methotrexate competitively antagonizes dihydrofolate reductase and prevents the regeneration of intermediates (tetrahydrofolate) essential for the synthesis of purine and thymidylate, thus inhibiting the synthesis of DNA. Methotrexate should therefore be prescribed with folic acid.
- Fluorouracil is converted into a fraudulent pyrimidine nucleotide, fluorodeoxyuridine monophosphate, that inhibits thymidylate synthetase, impairing DNA synthesis.
- Cytarabine is converted intracellularly to a triphosphate form that inhibits DNA polymerase.
- Mercaptopurine is converted into a fraudulent purine nucleotide that impairs DNA synthesis.

Route of administration
- Methotrexate is administered orally, intravenously, intramuscularly and intrathecally.
- Fluorouracil is usually given intravenously, although it can be given orally and topically.
- Cytarabine is given subcutaneously intravenously and intrathecally.
- Mercaptopurine is given orally.

Indications—Methotrexate is used for acute lymphoblastic leukaemia and non-Hodgkin lymphoma. It is also used in the treatment of psoriasis and rheumatoid arthritis (see Chapter 11).

Fluorouracil is used for the treatment of solid tumours and some malignant skin conditions.

Cytarabine is used for the treatment of acute myeloblastic leukaemia.

Mercaptopurine is used as maintenance therapy for acute leukaemias.

Adverse effects—A common side effect of antimetabolites is generalized cytotoxicity (see Table 13.1).

Methotrexate can cause liver cirrhosis, pulmonary fibrosis and bone marrow suppression.

Contraindications—Methotrexate is contraindicated in acute infections and in pregnancy because it is a teratogenic.

Therapeutic notes—Methotrexate should not be given to people with significant hepatic or renal impairment. Folic acid should be prescribed alongside methotrexate.

Cytotoxic antibiotics

Dactinomycin (actinomycin D), bleomycin and doxorubicin are examples of cytotoxic antibiotics.

Mechanism of action—Cytotoxic antibiotics work mainly by preventing cell division either through direct action on DNA itself or by blocking the enzymes involved in DNA replication.

Dactinomycin prevents transcription by interfering with ribonucleic acid (RNA) polymerase.

Doxorubicin inhibits transcription and DNA replication by inhibiting topoisomerase II. Bleomycin acts to fragment DNA chains.

Route of administration—Intravenous. Doxorubicin can be given intravesically for bladder cancer.

Indications—Dactinomycin is principally used in paediatric cancers. Doxorubicin is used for acute leukaemias, lymphomas and a variety of solid tumours. Bleomycin is used for lymphomas and certain solid tumours.

Adverse effects—Generalized cytotoxicity (see Table 13.1). Doxorubicin produces dose-dependent cardiotoxicity, because of irreversible free radical damage to the myocardium. Bleomycin may cause pulmonary fibrosis, but has virtually no myelosuppression, unlike doxorubicin and dactinomycin.

Mitotic inhibitors

Examples of mitotic inhibitors include the vinca alkaloids, vincristine, vinblastine and vinorelbine, ixabepilone and etoposide.

Mechanism of action—Mitotic inhibitors act by binding tubulin and inhibiting the polymerization of microtubules, which is necessary to form the mitotic spindle. This prevents mitosis and arrests dividing cells at metaphase (see Fig. 13.1).

Route of administration—The vinca alkaloids are administered intravenously, and etoposide orally or intravenously.

Indications—Mitotic inhibitors are used for acute leukaemias, lymphomas and some solid tumours.

Adverse effects—Side effects of mitotic inhibitors result from the fact that tubulin polymerization is relatively indiscriminate, inhibiting other cellular processes that involve microtubules, as well as cell division.

Generalized cytotoxicity occurs (see Table 13.1), except that vincristine is unusual in producing little or no bone marrow suppression.

Neurological and neuromuscular effects occur, especially with vincristine, and include peripheral neuropathy leading to paraesthesia, loss of reflexes and weakness. Recovery from these effects occurs but is slow.

Therapeutic notes—Intrathecal administration of vinca alkaloids is contraindicated as it is usually fatal. Vinorelbine is used for the treatment of advanced breast cancer when other treatments have failed, and for advanced nonsmall cell lung cancer.

Platinum compounds

Cisplatin (first-generation drug), carboplatin (second generation), and lastly oxaliplatin (third generation).

Mechanism of action—Cross-linking of DNA subunits, thus inhibiting DNA synthesis, transcription and function. They can act in any cell cycle.

Indications

- Cisplatin is mainly used for lung, cervical, bladder, testicular and ovarian cancers (although carboplatin is preferred for ovarian cancer).
- Carboplatin is mainly used for advanced ovarian and lung cancer (particularly small cell type).
- Oxaliplatin is used in combination with 5-fluorouracil and folinic acid to treat metastatic colorectal cancer and as colon cancer adjuvant treatment.

Contraindications—Pregnancy, breastfeeding.

Route of administration—Intravenous.

Adverse effects—Cisplatin may cause nausea, vomiting, nephrotoxicity, ototoxicity, peripheral neuropathy, hypomagnesaemia, myelosuppression.

Carboplatin has the same adverse effects as cisplatin, but all to a lesser extent, with the exception of greater myelosuppression.

Oxaliplatin may cause neurotoxicity, gastrointestinal disturbances, myelosuppression.

Therapeutic note—Ondansetron (5-HT3 antagonist) is effective against severe nausea and vomiting associated with platinum salts.

Multikinase inhibitors

Multikinase inhibitors (pazopanib, sunitinib, sorafenib, imatinib) are used, for example, in advanced renal cell carcinoma. They inhibit cell signalling induced by the growth factors; vascular endothelial growth factor and platelet-derived growth factor. Imatinib is commonly used in the treatment of chronic myeloid leukaemia and acute lymphoblastic leukaemia that is Philadelphia chromosome positive. If in advanced renal cell carcinoma multikinase inhibitors are not affective, mTOR (mammalian target of rapamycin) kinase inhibitors (e.g. everolimus, temsirolimus) can be considered.

Miscellaneous agents

Several chemotherapeutic cytotoxic agents do not fall into any of the aforementioned groups.

Procarbazine

Mechanism of action—Procarbazine is a methylhydrazine derivative with monoamine oxidase inhibitor actions and cytotoxicity. It inhibits DNA and RNA synthesis by a mechanism that is unclear (see Fig. 13.1).

Route of administration—Oral.

Indication—Procarbazine is used in Hodgkin lymphoma.

Adverse effects—Generalized cytotoxicity (see Table 13.1). It causes an adverse reaction in combination with alcohol.

Therapeutic notes—Procarbazine forms part of MOPP (mechlorethamine [chlormethine], vincristine, procarbazine and prednisone) therapy for Hodgkin lymphoma.

Hydroxyurea

Mechanism of action—Hydroxyurea causes the inhibition of ribonucleotide reductase and hence the formation of deoxyribonucleotides (Fig. 13.1).

Route of administration—Oral.

Indications—Hydroxyurea is used for chronic myeloid leukaemia. Polycythemia rubra vera.

Adverse effects—Generalized cytotoxicity (see Table 13.1).

Crisantaspase

Mechanism of action—Some tumour cells lose the ability to synthesize asparagine, requiring an exogenous source of the substance to grow; normal host cells can synthesize their own. Crisantaspase is a preparation of bacterial asparaginase that breaks down any circulating asparagine, hence inhibiting the growth of some cancers, namely acute lymphoblastic leukaemia (see Fig. 13.1).

Route of administration—Intramuscular, subcutaneous.

Indication—Acute lymphoblastic leukaemia.

Adverse effects—The most serious side effects of crisantaspase include severe toxicity to the liver and pancreas. Central nervous system (CNS) depression and anaphylaxis are also risks.

Therapeutic notes—Regular testing of patients given crisantaspase is necessary to monitor organ functions.

Many other anticancer agents are used in the management of malignant tumours, including mTOR kinase inhibitors (temsirolimus, everolimus), amsacrine, altretamine, dacarbazine, mitotane, pentostatin, taxanes, thalidomide, topoisomerase I inhibitors, and tretinoin. Detailed information on these can be gained from the British National Formulary or specialist textbooks.

ENDOCRINE THERAPY

Hormones and antihormones

The growth of some cancers is hormone dependent and can be inhibited by surgical removal of the source of the driving hormone, such as the gonads, adrenals or pituitary. Increasingly, however, administration of hormones or antihormones is preferred.

Endocrine therapy can cause side effects, the nature of which can normally be deduced from the physiological effects of the hormone being given or antagonized. Endocrine therapy generally has the advantage that it has far fewer serious adverse effects than cytotoxic therapy.

Hormones used in endocrine therapy include the following.

- Adrenocortic steroids (Chapter 7), for example, prednisolone, which inhibit the growth of cancers of the lymphoid tissues and blood. In addition, they are used to treat some of the complications of cancer (e.g. oedema). They are also useful in the palliative care of end-stage malignant disease because they elevate mood and stimulate appetite.
- Oestrogens (Chapter 7), for example, diethylstilbestrol, which has an antiandrogenic effect and can be used to suppress androgen-dependent prostatic cancers.
- Progesterones (Chapter 7), which inhibit endometrial cancer and carcinomas of the prostate and breast.

Hormone antagonists

Oestrogen antagonists

Mechanism of action—Tamoxifen and toremifene are competitive inhibitors at oestrogen receptors. Inhibition of the stimulatory effects of oestrogen suppresses the division of breast cancer cells.

Route of administration—Oral.

Indication—Treatment of oestrogen receptor-positive breast cancer with metastatic disease.

Prevention of recurrences among women with early oestrogen receptor-positive breast cancer.

Adverse effects—Nausea, flushing, bone pain, oedema. Increased risk of endometrial cancer, thromboembolism

Contraindications—Pregnancy and breastfeeding.

Therapeutic notes—Tamoxifen increases the anticoagulant effect of warfarin.

Aromatase inhibitors

Mechanism of action—Letrozole and anastrozole are nonsteroidal aromatase inhibitors.

Exemestane is a steroidal aromatase inhibitor.

Aromatase inhibitors inhibit the action of the enzyme aromatase, which converts androgens into oestrogens. Oestrogen stimulates breast tissue and subsequently cancer growth.

Indications

- Treatment of oestrogen receptor-positive breast cancer in postmenopausal women.
- Treatment of advanced breast cancer in postmenopausal women.

Adverse effects—Hot flushes, vaginal dryness, anorexia, gastrointestinal upset, bone fractures.

Contraindications—Premenopausal women. When used in premenopausal women, the decrease in oestrogen peripherally increases gonadotrophin secretion, which in turn stimulates the ovary to increase androgen production. This increases the total amount of oestrogen, stimulating breast tissue and cancer growth.

CLINICAL NOTE

In premenopausal women, the ovaries produce the majority of oestrogen whereas, in postmenopausal women, oestrogen is produced in the peripheral tissue through the conversion of androgens by the aromatase enzyme. Therefore aromatase inhibitors should only be prescribed in postmenopausal women

---

Androgen antagonists

Androgen antagonists, for example, flutamide, bicalutamide, cyproterone acetate inhibit androgen-dependent prostatic cancers. Side effects include gynaecomastia, weight loss and decreased libido.

Gonadotrophin-releasing hormone (GnRH) (e.g. gonadorelin, goserelin, buserelin) analogues stimulate the production of oestrogen and testosterone in a nonphysiological manner, resulting in the disruption of endogenous hormonal feedback systems and in the downregulation of testosterone and oestrogen production. They are used in the treatment of prostate and breast cancer. Side effects include gynaecomastia.

- Degarelix is a GnRH antagonist, which competes with endogenous GnRH and reversibly binds to the GnRH receptors in the pituitary gland. This blocks the release of luteinising hormone (LH) and follicle stimulating hormone (FSH), suppressing the release of testosterone from the testes and subsequently reduces the growth of prostate cancer.

IMMUNOTHERAPY

Immunotherapy treatment for cancer is derived from the fact that bacterial infections sometimes provoked the regression of cancer, that is, indirect immunostimulation. Immunotherapy involves using treatments that use the body's immune system to stimulate a response to cancer (i.e. the drug's target is certain cells involved in the immune system: CD20 cells or interleukins).

Approaches of immunotherapy include the following.

- The use of vaccines for example, bacille Calmette Guérin (BCG) to provide nonspecific immunostimulation (e.g. in the treatment of bladder cancer).
- The human papilloma virus (HPV) has been found to be a causative factor in most cases of cervical cancer. HPV strains 6, 11, 16 and 18 have been implicated in cervical cancer and therefore have been incorporated into cervical cancer vaccines (Gardasil and Cervarix), which have recently been introduced into a national vaccination scheme and given to girls age 12 to 13 years.
- The use of specific vaccines prepared using tumour cells from similar cancers, in an attempt to raise an adaptive immune response against cancer. An example of autologous cellular immunotherapy is sipuleucel-T, the first approved "cancer vaccine" for the treatment of metastatic prostate cancer.
- Immunostimulation using drugs, for example, levamisole.
- The use of cytokines to regulate the immune response so as to favourably target cancer. Cytokines used include interferon α, interleukin (IL)-2, and tumour necrosis factor. Aldesleukin is an IL-2 drug used in the treatment of metastatic renal cell carcinoma, via subcutaneous injection.

- The use of recombinant colony-stimulating factors to reduce the level and duration of neutropenia after cytotoxic chemotherapy.
- Recombinant human granulocyte colony-stimulating factor (rh-G-CSF; filgrastim) and granulocyte-macrophage colony-stimulating factor (GM-CSF; molgramostim) promote the development of their respective haemopoietic stem cells in the marrow. Their use to raise white blood cell counts after cytotoxic chemotherapy is effective, although this has not been shown to alter overall survival rates.
- The use of tumour-specific monoclonal antibodies (MAbs) to target drugs specifically to cancerous cells; the so-called "magic-bullet" approach (see later).

Monoclonal antibodies

Examples are: rituximab, alemtuzumab, cetuximab, trastuzumab, ofatumumab.

Mechanism of action—MAbs recognize specific proteins found on the surface of the cancer cell and lock onto them. It can then either trigger the body's immune system to destroy the cell or it may be attached to a cancer drug or radioactive substance, which can target the selected cells. The development of MAbs targeting ligands overexpressed on certain tumour types is a rapidly expanding area. By targeting factors overexpressed on tumour cells, the therapy becomes more personalized for the patient and improves the chances of effective treatment with less unwanted effects, unlike most of the other cytotoxic drugs that have been more commonly used. This is because the biologics should only be used in patients whose tumours are expressing the particular target protein the antibody recognizes.

Antibody directed enzyme prodrug therapy (ADEPT) uses MAbs to carry enzymes directly to the cancer cells. A cytotoxic prodrug is then administered, which is only activated in cells with the enzyme, thus resulting in treatment targeting cancer cells but not normal cells.

Indications
- Trastuzumab (herceptin) is licensed for metastatic breast cancer in patients with tumours overexpressing human epidermal growth factor (EGFR) 2 (HER2) receptor.
- Cetuximab (targets EGFR) in combination with irinotecan, is licensed for metastatic colorectal cancers overexpressing epidermal growth factor receptors.
- Nonsmall cell lung cancer. Some overexpress EGFR and mutations of this receptor have been found and the MAb gefinitib is now used instead of chemotherapy in patients with these mutations.

- Basiliximab and daclizumab are both MAbs directed against T lymphocytes, preventing them from proliferating.
- Rituximab targets B lymphocytes and is used in the treatment of diffuse large B non-Hodgkin lymphoma
- Rituximab lyses B lymphocyte by its effect on CD20 protein and also sensitizes resistant cells to other chemotherapeutic drugs. It is given via an infusion for the treatment of lymphoma.
- Bevacizumab neutralizes vascular endothelial growth factor and therefore prevents angiogenesis that is crucial to tumour survival. It is used for the treatment of colorectal cancer.
  Contraindications—Severe dyspnoea at rest, breastfeeding.
  Route of administration—Intravenous.
  Adverse effects—Hypersensitivity reactions, chills, fevers, cardiotoxicity, hypotension, gastrointestinal symptoms, airway obstruction, aches and pains.

THE FUTURE AND PERSONALIZED MEDICINE

Newer therapeutics that target certain oncogene and disease pathways seem to be the future. Patients diagnosed with common cancers today can have further testing of their cancer tissue receptors. Drug therapies that can target certain cancer receptor types present in the cancerous tissue can then be used rather than generic cytotoxic medication used previously, reducing the side-effect profile and improving cure rates and survival. These include noncytotoxic therapies (e.g. inhibitors of tyrosine kinase, MAbs to cell surface proteins and activating the patient's own immunity to target cancer cells).

For example, patients with oestrogen-dependent breast cancer respond better than nonoestrogen-dependent breast cancer if treated with tamoxifen and aromatase inhibitors. Patients with HER2 receptor-positive breast cancer can be treated with trastuzumab, which is a form of immune targeting. Similarly, patients with lung cancer that have the EGFR mutation can be given erlotinib rather than treatment with generic chemotherapy and the wide range of side effects this causes. Most recently, nivolumab, an anti-programmed death ligand 1 (PDL1) antibody, has been approved for the treatment of advanced melanoma.

These new immunotherapies are extremely promising in the treatment of various cancers, particularly because they are less toxic than current cytotoxic therapy. However, they are expensive, which limits their use.

Chapter Summary

- Cancer therapy intervention is aimed at inhibiting or reducing the accelerated growth of cell division that leads to malignancy
- Cytotoxic chemotherapy causes side effects because of the inhibition of noncancerous host cell division (especially gut, bone marrow and immune system)
- Cytotoxic antibiotics include doxorubicin and bleomycin
- Mercaptopurine is converted into a fraudulent purine nucleotide that impairs DNA synthesis
- Endocrine therapy is generally less toxic than chemotherapy
- Patients with certain receptors expressed within their cancer tissue can receive targeted drug therapy

SELF-ASSESSMENT

Single best answer (SBA) questions

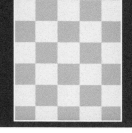

Chapter 1 Introduction to Pharmacology

1. A 30-year-old man is diagnosed with tuberculosis and is started on rifampicin and isoniazid treatment for 2 months.

   Which of the following medications will be affected by the enzyme induction associated with this treatment?
   A. Allopurinol.
   B. Cyclosporine.
   C. Phenytoin.
   D. Salbutamol.
   E. Warfarin.

2. An 80-year-old woman presents with severe sepsis secondary to a chest infection. She requires antibiotics. Which is the most direct route of drug administration?
   A. Intramuscular.
   B. Intravenous.
   C. Per oral.
   D. Per rectum.
   E. Subcutaneous.

3. A healthy male volunteer is keen to be involved in the development of a novel drug. In which phase of the drug development process will he be recruited into?
   A. Preclinical.
   B. Phase 1.
   C. Phase 2.
   D. Phase 3.
   E. Phase 4.

4. Which one of the following drugs is an agonist at β receptors?
   A. Isoprenaline.
   B. N-acetyl-P-aminophenol.
   C. Paracetamol.
   D. Proguanil hydrochloride.
   E. Syntometrine.

5. Which one of these is an example of a G-protein-coupled receptor?
   A. B2 adrenergic receptor.
   B. Insulin receptor.
   C. Nicotinic acetylcholine receptor.
   D. Platelet derived growth factor (PDGF) receptor.
   E. Steroid receptor.

Chapter 2 Peripheral nervous system

1. A 60-year-old man presents with dysuria, frequency, loin pain and fever. He is diagnosed with pyelonephritis and is started on antibiotics. However, he develops septic shock and has to be intubated and taken to intensive care unit. Unfortunately, after intubation with a neuromuscular blocker he remains paralysed. Which drug is responsible for this adverse effect occurring?
   A. Ciprofloxacin.
   B. Co amoxiclav.
   C. Gentamicin.
   D. Paracetamol.
   E. Trimethoprim.

2. A 52-year-old man is admitted for a routine surgical procedure. The anaesthetist gives him anaesthesia to ensure his muscles are paralysed for the surgery.

   Which of the following medication is a depolarising neuromuscular blocking agent that is often used during induction of anaesthesia?
   A. Atracurium.
   B. Botulinum.
   C. Hemicholinium.
   D. Suxamethonium.
   E. Vecuronium.

3. A 35-year-old female presents with a 2-month history of muscle weakness and early fatigue particularly at the end of the day. She gets tired when brushing her teeth in the evenings. Investigations so far have been inconclusive. Which drug can be used to help aid the diagnosis?
   A. Alcuronium.
   B. Edrophonium.
   C. Neostigmine.
   D. Pancuronium.
   E. Suxamethonium.

4. A 25-year-old woman presents with episodes of anxiety, sweating, tremor and palpitations associated with severe hypertension. Currently her blood pressure is 190/90 mm Hg and her heart rate is 110 beats per minute. You suspect a phaeochromocytoma. What is the most appropriate way of managing her hypertension acutely?
   A. Oral propranolol.
   B. Intravenous (IV) labetalol.

C. IV phentolamine.

D. Oral phenoxybenzamine.

E. IV atropine.

5. A 60-year-old man is prescribed medication for his benign prostatic hyperplasia and his General Practitioner notes show an improvement in his blood pressure. Which antihypertensive drug acts as an α1-adrenoreceptor antagonist?

A. Clonidine.

B. Labetalol.

C. Phenylephrine.

D. Prazosin.

E. Propranolol.

6. A 24-year old female with asthma has recently been started on an inhaler containing ipratropium bromide. Which of the following symptoms or signs can be related to the mechanism of action of ipratropium bromide?

A. Blurred vision.

B. Bradycardia.

C. Increase salivation.

D. Pin point pupils.

E. Urinary frequency.

Chapter 3 Respiratory system

1. A 40-year-old woman presents to the emergency department with a 2-day history of worsening breathlessness. She normally has an average peak expiratory flow rate of 450 L per minute, is on regular salmeterol and fluticasone inhalers but she ran out of all her medications a few days ago. On examination, she is alert with a respiratory rate of 30 breaths per minute. She has widespread bilateral polyphonic wheeze and her peak expiratory flow is 140 L per minute. She has already received nebulizers of salbutamol and ipratropium in the emergency department with minimal response.

Which of the following is most appropriate next step in this patient's management?

A. Inhaled budesonide and ipratropium.

B. Inhaled budesonide and intravenous (IV) magnesium.

C. Inhaled budesonide, IV magnesium and IV theophylline.

D. Continue with nebulizers, add IV hydrocortisone and IV magnesium.

E. Inhaled salmeterol and ipratropium, IV methylprednisolone and IV theophylline.

2. A 30-year-old man with asthma presents to his General Practitioner (GP) because he is worried that he has been coughing at night at least 3 times per week over the past few months. Recently, he has also been wheezy and breathless when playing football,

despite regular use of his salbutamol inhaler. He has been well otherwise. His regular medications include salbutamol 100 mcg inhaler 2 puffs when he needs it and beclomethasone 200 mcg inhaler 2 puffs twice a day. On examination, his vital signs are within normal limits and his chest is clear.

Which of the following is the most appropriate next step in the patient's management?

A. Continue salbutamol inhaler and add in a fixed dose combination inhaler with budesonide and formoterol and add in a short course of oral antibiotics.

B. Continue salbutamol and beclometasone inhaler.

C. Continue current inhalers and start antibiotics for a chest infection.

D. Continue salbutamol inhaler and increase dose of beclometasone inhaler.

E. Continue salbutamol inhaler and add in a fixed dose combination inhaler with fluticasone propionate and salmeterol.

3. A 59-year-old woman who has been smoking approximately 15 cigarettes a day for the past 40 years presents with intermittent breathlessness and a 3-month history of a cough, which is productive of sputum. A diagnosis of COPD is made based on her history, examination and lung function tests. She is commenced on ipratropium. Over winter she has several exacerbations and presents to her GP with persistent breathlessness. Her FEV1 is 55%.

Which of the following would not be an appropriate option?

A. Advice smoking cessation.

B. Offer a pneumococcal vaccination.

C. Add in a long-acting muscarinic antagonist (LAMA).

D. Add in a long-acting B2 agonist (LABA).

E. Add in short-acting B2 agonist (SABA).

4. A 60-year-old woman is admitted with a cough productive of green sputum, breathless and wheeze. She is a current smoker and her regular medications include ipratropium inhaler, fluticasone propionate and salmeterol inhaler. She has had several admissions to hospital with exacerbations and type II respiratory failure. Her GP has given her a dose of oral clarithromycin.

On examination, she looks breathless, heart rate is 120 beats per minute, respiratory rate is 35 breaths per minute, oxygen saturation 85%, temperature 37.2 °C, blood pressure 135/80 mm Hg. Crackles are heard on the right base.

Which of the following is appropriate in the immediate management?

A. 15 L of oxygen, continue oral clarithromycin, add in oral prednisolone and nebulized ipratropium.
B. Controlled oxygen, continue oral clarithromycin, add in oral prednisolone, nebulized ipratropium and intravenous (IV) theophylline.
C. Controlled oxygen, continue oral clarithromycin, add in oral prednisolone and nebulized ipratropium.
D. 15 L of oxygen, continue oral clarithromycin, add in oral prednisolone, nebulized ipratropium and IV theophylline.
E. Continue oral clarithromycin, add in oral prednisolone, nebulized ipratropium and IV theophylline.

5. A 40-year-old male presents to the GP complaining of itchy eyes, overproduction of nasal mucus and a blocked nose every time he visits his girlfriend who owns a dog and has been a problem for the past month. His medical history includes type 2 diabetes, hypertension and asthma.
What medication would be inappropriate to prescribe for this patient's symptoms?
A. Oral cetirizine.
B. Oral chlorphenamine.
C. Oral ephedrine.
D. Nasal ephedrine.
E. Nasal glucocorticosteroid.

Chapter 4 Cardiovascular system

1. A 29-year-old female presents in her second trimester of pregnancy. She presents to the General Practioner (GP) with high blood pressure.
Which medication can be given to treat her hypertension?
A. Bisoprolol.
B. Furosemide.
C. Losartan.
D. Methyldopa.
E. Ramipril.

2. A 75-year-old female presents acutely short of breath. She has a cough productive of pink frothy sputum. On examination, she has peripheral oedema and a raised jugular venous pressure (JVP). She had a myocardial infarction two weeks ago. She is diagnosed with acute pulmonary oedema secondary to right-sided heart failure.
Which of the following medications will off load the fluid most effectively?
A. Bendroflumethiazide.
B. Bumetanide.
C. Furosemide.
D. Glyceryl trinitrate.
E. Morphine.

3. A 60-year-old man presents to the emergency department with central, heavy chest pain, which radiates down his left arm and started suddenly an hour ago. He feels nauseous and breathless and grades the severity as 10/10. Medical history includes angina, hypertension and high cholesterol. He is not known to have any allergies. The patient is diagnosed with a myocardial infarction (MI) and prescribed the following medications.
Which of the following medications' mechanism of action is inhibition of ADP?
A. Aspirin.
B. Clopidogrel.
C. Fondaparinux.
D. Morphine sulphate.
E. Unfractionated heparin.

4. A 48-year-old Afro-Caribbean man attends his GP for a routine medical examination for his work insurance and is noted to have a blood pressure (BP) measurement of 152/92 mm Hg. On subsequent measurements of his BP, it remains over 140/90 mm Hg. He has mild asthma.
Which of the following medications would be appropriate to start as management of his hypertension?
A. ACE inhibitor.
B. ß-Blocker.
C. Calcium channel blocker.
D. Loop diuretic.
E. Thiazide diuretic.

5. A 48-year-old man is commenced on lisinopril for hypertension. Which of the following statements are true about ACE inhibitors?
A. There is a risk of hypokalaemia.
B. Cough is an uncommon side effect.
C. Precaution needs to be taken if the patient develops diarrhoea and vomiting.
D. ACE inhibitors cause liver failure.
E. Blood tests are required every 6 months.

6. A 65-year-old man presents to a hospital complaining of general lethargy and weakness. He has hypertension and takes regular ramipril and amlodipine. He recently had a flare of his osteoarthritis and has been taking regular ibuprofen for the last week. He attends his GP for a general review, and blood tests reveal he has raised potassium and an acute kidney injury. His blood results a month ago were normal.
What should the GP advise the patient to do?
A. Stop amlodipine.
B. Stop ibuprofen.
C. Stop Ramipril.
D. Stop ibuprofen and amlodipine.
E. Stop ibuprofen and Ramipril.

7. A 55-year-old woman who takes bisoprolol and warfarin for atrial fibrillation has a routine blood test to check her international normalized ratio (INR). The INR result is 6.5 (target range 2–3). She denies any bleeding and is well. However, she does admit that she drank more alcohol than normal over the weekend.
What is the most appropriate next step?
   A. Stop bisoprolol and recheck INR.
   B. Give vitamin K and recheck INR.
   C. Reduce dose of warfarin to 2 mg daily and recheck INR.
   D. Increase warfarin to 5 mg daily and recheck INR.
   E. Omit warfarin for at least 2 days and recheck INR.

8. A 60-year-old female presents with swollen ankles and feeling constipated. She takes ramipril for hypertension, verapamil for rate control and rivaroxaban for anticoagulation as she has atrial fibrillation and has recently been started on furosemide for suspected heart failure, but her echocardiogram is normal. She is also on simvastatin for hypercholesterolaemia.
Which medication could be responsible for her symptoms?
   A. Furosemide.
   B. Ramipril.
   C. Rivaroxaban.
   D. Simvastatin.
   E. Verapamil.

9. A 65-year-old female is noted to have high cholesterol and a 10-year cardiovascular disease risk of greater than 20%. The GP would like to start her on simvastatin. Which one of the following parameters would be the most important to monitor before prescribing simvastatin?
   A. Blood pressure.
   B. Creatinine kinase.
   C. Muscle biopsy.
   D. Serum liver transaminases (alanine aminotransferase/aspartate aminotransferase).
   E. Weight.

10. An 82-year-old female with a history of atrial fibrillation is prescribed warfarin and presents to A&E with an episode of epistaxis. Her INR is 7.2. A week earlier she had commenced on a course of oral antibiotics for a treatment of a chest infection. Which one of the following antibiotics do you suspect is most likely to have been prescribed?
   A. Amoxicillin.
   B. Augmentin.
   C. Clarithromycin.
   D. Co-amoxiclav.
   E. Trimethoprim.

11. A 70-year-old woman presents with heart failure and would like to know which medications have a proven mortality benefit.
Which of the following medications have this benefit in patients with heart failure?
   A. ACE inhibitors.
   B. Angiotensin-receptor blockers.
   C. Cardiac glycosides.
   D. Calcium-channel blockers.
   E. Loop diuretics.

Chapter 5 Kidney and urinary system

1. Which part of the nephron is the main site of potassium secretion?
   A. Distal convoluted tubule.
   B. Glomerulus.
   C. Juxtaglomerular apparatus.
   D. Loop of Henle.
   E. Proximal tubule.

2. A 60-year-old man with hypertension is seen by his General Practitioner (GP) for review. He is currently taking amlodipine, but his blood pressure remains elevated. He is unable to tolerate an ACE inhibitor, so his GP starts him on Bendroflumethiazide. Of which of the following complications should the GP be aware?
   A. Hyperkalaemia.
   B. Hypernatraemia.
   C. Hyperuricaemia.
   D. Hypocalcaemia.
   E. Hypomagnesaemia.

3. A 60-year-old patient is admitted with worsening breathlessness, orthopnoea and leg swelling for the last 3 days. She has no medical history and is taking no regular medications. She has crepitations to both midzones with a raised jugular venous pressure and pitting oedema in both legs. Her blood results are normal. Which of the following diuretics is the most appropriate to administer in the initial management?
   A. Amiloride.
   B. Indapamide.
   C. Bumetanide.
   D. Furosemide.
   E. Spironolactone.

4. A 74-year-old patient is recovering from an ischaemic stroke one week ago. He has hypertension and takes amlodipine. He also has heart failure for which he takes furosemide and spironolactone. He has been started on aspirin and simvastatin as secondary management.
His blood results are the following:
Na   140   (135–145 mmol/L)

K   6.2   (3.5–5 mmol/L)
Urea   3.2   (3–7 mmol/L)
Creatinine   78   (60–125 umol/L)

Which is the most likely medication responsible for his hyperkalaemia?

A. Amlodipine.
B. Aspirin.
C. Furosemide.
D. Spironolactone.
E. Simvastatin.

5. A 66-year-old man comes to the clinic complaining of dizziness and unsteadiness on standing up in the mornings. He has recently been started on treatment for BPH after he reported poor urinary flow and hesitancy associated with a normal prostate specific antigen. A digital rectal examination identified a smooth enlarged prostate. Which of the following medications is most likely to be responsible for his current symptoms?

A. Bethanechol.
B. Doxazosin.
C. Duloxetine.
D. Finasteride.
E. Oxybutynin.

6. A 55-year-old female presents to clinic with symptoms of urge incontinence. Her GP discusses starting oxybutynin and informs her of the side effects. Which of the following is a side effect of oxybutynin?

A. Loose stool.
B. Hypoglycaemia.
C. Blurred vision.
D. Hypotension.
E. Excess saliva.

7. A 45-year-old diabetic presents with erectile dysfunction and requests treatment. Which of the following is the most appropriate?

A. Intracavernous sildenafil.
B. Oral alprostadil.
C. Oral papaverine.
D. Oral sildenafil.
E. Topical papaverine.

8. A 62-year-old female with a history of a myocardial infarction is diagnosed with mild heart failure and commenced on furosemide.

Which one of the following parameters is the most important to monitor in the community?

A. Blood pressure.
B. Full blood count.
C. Heart rate.
D. Serum electrolytes.
E. Urinary sodium.

Chapter 6 Gastrointestinal system

1. A 29-year-old man presents to his GP with epigastric abdominal pain and reflux with occasional vomiting. He has a 2-month history of loose stool with up to 5 episodes a day. He reports fatigue and a one-half stone weight loss over the past month. He drinks 15 to 20 units socially at the weekend and infrequently smokes with friends. He recently took ibuprofen for a week for left ankle pain following a football injury. A year ago, he took triple therapy for a small peptic ulcer in his stomach. When seen by a gastroenterologist, he is found to have several various sized ulcers in his stomach, duodenum and jejunum.

What is the underlying diagnosis?

A. Alcohol induced peptic ulceration.
B. Gastrinoma induced peptic ulceration.
C. H. pylori induced peptic ulceration.
D. NSAID induced peptic ulceration.
E. Smoking induced peptic ulceration.

2. A 65-year-old man is seen by his GP for a routine check-up. On examination, he is noted to have enlarged breast tissue. He denies drinking alcohol and is not known to have any liver problems. He has been taking regular medication for dyspepsia for many years. Which medication is most likely to be responsible?

A. Aluminium hydroxychloride.
B. Amoxicillin.
C. Ranitidine.
D. Misoprostol.
E. Omeprazole.

3. A 67-year-old woman is seen in A&E with epistaxis. A week ago, she saw her GP who started her on some additional medication for treatment of her longstanding GORD. She is known to have atrial fibrillation and takes warfarin.

Which medication is her GP likely to have started to cause this complication?

A. Bismuth chelate.
B. Cimetidine.
C. Magnesium carbonate.
D. Misoprostol.
E. Omeprazole.

4. A 65-year-old male who is undergoing treatment for pancreatic carcinoma presents with nausea and vomiting. He vomits undigested food and feels full very quickly. Which of the following treatments is most useful for gastric outlet obstruction related emesis?

A. Cyclizine.
B. Dexamethasone.
C. Levomepromazine.
D. Metoclopramide.
E. Ondansetron.

5. In acute chemotherapy induced nausea and vomiting, which of the following is the most useful antiemetic in addition to dexamethasone?
   A. Cyclizine.
   B. Domperidone.
   C. Metoclopramide.
   D. Ondansetron.
   E. Prochlorperazine.

6. A 62-year-old man with Parkinson disease is seen by his GP with nausea and vomiting associated with vertigo. He is prescribed an antiemetic. A few days later, his wife phones the surgery concerned that her husband is stiffer than normal and less mobile and has fallen twice.
   Which of the following medications is contraindicated in this patient?
   A. Cimetidine.
   B. Chlorpromazine.
   C. Cyclizine.
   D. Dexamethasone.
   E. Ondansetron.

7. A 25-year-old girl presents to her GP with a 4-week history of frequent, bloody diarrhoea associated with colicky abdominal pain and general malaise. She is a nonsmoker. She denies any recent travel. Her maternal aunt is known to have ulcerative colitis. On examination, she appears pale and unwell with generalized abdominal tenderness. She is referred to hospital. A faecal calprotectin result is positive. A colonoscopy confirms involvement of the bowel mucosa only. She is started on oral corticosteroids. Which of the following medications is used to maintain remission?
   A. Azathioprine.
   B. Cyclosporine.
   C. Ispaghula husk.
   D. Infliximab.
   E. Mesalazine.

8. A 50-year-old patient who develops pain arising from metastases is placed on opiate pain relief and subsequently develops constipation. Which of the following medications is a stimulant laxative?
   A. Ispaghula husk.
   B. Lactulose.
   C. Methylcellulose.
   D. Peppermint oil.
   E. Senna.

Chapter 7 Endocrine and reproductive

1. A 35-year-old woman presents to her GP feeling generally unwell with a sore throat. On examination, she has a red throat but otherwise appears well.

She has recently started taking medication for an overactive thyroid.
Which of the following investigations is most important to check?
   A. Electrocardiogram (EKG).
   B. Full blood count.
   C. Glucose.
   D. Liver function test.
   E. Thyroid function test.

2. A 62-year-old man presents to his GP feeling generally unwell. On direct questioning, he reports a new tremor, feeling hot and sweaty and thinks he may have lost some weight. He has recently been started on treatment by the cardiologists for atrial fibrillation. He has known structural heart disease. Which of the following medications is he most likely to have been started on which could account for his symptoms?
   A. Amiodarone.
   B. Carbimazole.
   C. Iodide.
   D. Levothyroxine.
   E. Propanalol.

3. A 55-year-old male is seen in the GP surgery. He has type 2 diabetes and already takes maximum dose metformin but his HbA1c remains above 58 mmol/L. He is commenced on gliclazide 40 mg once daily, in addition to metformin.
   Which of the following statements should be conveyed to the patient regarding gliclazide?
   A. Hypoglycaemia is not a risk when taking gliclazide.
   B. Drinking alcohol while on gliclazide should not cause any problems.
   C. Gliclazide can cause weight loss.
   D. β-Blocker medication may mask the hypoglycaemic symptoms associated with gliclazide.
   E. If a dose is missed then a double dose should be taken the next day.

4. A mother brings her 14-year-old son to the GP clinic because she is concerned that he has been passing urine more often than normal, over the past 2 to 3 weeks. He reports feeling thirsty all the time and feels really tired. On direct questioning, he thinks he has lost weight. A random venous glucose is 12 mmol/L and he has glucose in his urine. Which of the following options is the most appropriate management?
   A. Acarbose.
   B. Dietary modification
   C. Gliclazide.
   D. Insulin.
   E. Metformin.

5. A 58-year-old male who is a known type 2 diabetic is seen in the endocrine clinic because his glucose levels remain high despite dual therapy with metformin and gliclazide. He is started on pioglitazone. Which of the following statements is true regarding pioglitazone?
   A. Pioglitazone causes weight loss.
   B. Pioglitazone can reduce the need for exogenous insulin by 30%.
   C. Pioglitazone can be given to patients with a history of bladder cancer.
   D. Pioglitazone can protect against bone fractures.
   E. Pioglitazone is safe to use in patients with heart failure.

6. A 48-year-old man with type 2 diabetes attends his GP with dysuria and offensive penile discharge. He was recently reviewed by the diabetes clinic and commenced on an additional medication, as his glycaemic control remains poor despite therapy started by his GP.
   Which of the following antidiabetic medications could be responsible for his symptoms?
   A. Acarbose.
   B. Dapagliflozin.
   C. Linagliptin.
   D. Liraglutide.
   E. Pioglitazone.

7. A 32-year-old female attends her GP surgery complaining of general fatigue and weakness. She also reports some abdominal pain and muscle cramps. Her GP notes that she has a postural drop in her blood pressure and appears slightly tanned. She is diagnosed with primary adrenal insufficiency by the endocrinologist.
   Which medication is she most likely to be started on?
   A. Beclometasone.
   B. Dexamethasone.
   C. Fludrocortisone.
   D. Prednisolone.
   E. Triamcinolone.

8. A 40-year-old male with inflammatory bowel disease presents to the clinic. He requires long-term steroids.
   Which of the following symptoms or signs are side effects of glucocorticosteroids?
   A. Hypoglycaemia.
   B. Muscle bulk.
   C. Osteoporosis.
   D. Thickened skin.
   E. Weight loss.

9. A 21-year-old female sees her GP regarding contraception. Which of the following contraindicates the prescription of the combined oral contraceptive pill?
   A. Asthma.
   B. Hypotension.
   C. Migraine.
   D. Previous pregnancy.
   E. Renal disease.

10. Which of the following medications reduce the effectiveness of the progestogen-only pill?
    A. Amiodarone.
    B. Ciprofloxacin.
    C. Erythromycin.
    D. Phenytoin.
    E. Sodium valproate.

11. An 80-year-old female presents with pain in her left thigh with no history of trauma. She is known to have osteoporosis and hypertension but is otherwise well. An X-ray indicates an incomplete fracture of the femur shaft.
    Which of these drugs for osteoporosis can cause this complication?
    A. Alendronate.
    B. Ergocalciferol.
    C. Raloxifene.
    D. Strontium ranelate.
    E. Teriparatide.

12. Mr. Simpson, a 65-year-old male visits his GP because he feels more lethargic and thirsty compared with normal. His GP notes he has glycosuria and a random blood glucose of 12. Mr. Simpson had normal blood sugars 3 months ago and has a normal body mass index. However, he has been started on several drugs for blood pressure and cholesterol control over the past year. He also takes medication for gout and osteoarthritis.
    Which of the following medications is associated with inducing hyperglycaemia?
    A. Allopurinol.
    B. Bendroflumethiazide.
    C. Celecoxib.
    D. Paracetamol.
    E. Ramipril.

Chapter 8 Central nervous system

1. Mr. Jeffers, a 56-year-old male attends his GP surgery after noticing that his left-hand shakes when he is watching television. His wife notes that he is unsteady when standing in the morning. On examination, Mr. Jeffers appears to have a fixed facial expression

with infrequent blinking and bradykinesia while walking. His medical history includes hypertension only. He is referred to a neurologist and started on new medication. Which of the following medications inhibits dopa carboxylase in the periphery?

A. Carbidopa.
B. Domperidone.
C. Entacapone.
D. Levodopa.
E. Selegiline.

2. A 29-year-old female with acute anxiety is prescribed a short course of diazepam. Which of the following statements is correct regarding benzodiazepines?

A. She is safe to drive while taking diazepam.
B. She is safe to drink alcohol while taking diazepam.
C. She may experience drowsiness while taking diazepam.
D. If she were to overdose on diazepam, there is no reversal agent.
E. She can continue to take the diazepam for more than 4 weeks and then stop taking them.

3. A 26-year-old female with known anxiety presents to her GP. She is due to give a presentation at work to an important crowd of people and is worried about sweating, flushing and shaking publically, and has asked for some medication. She is not known to have any medical history and has no drug allergies.

Which of the following medication can provide the most appropriate symptomatic control of her performance related anxiety?

A. Buspirone.
B. Midazolam.
C. Pentobarbital.
D. Propranolol.
E. Zolpidem.

4. A 29-year-old female presents to her GP with low mood over the past 8 weeks, almost every day associated with a loss of energy. On direct questioning, she has a reduced ability to think and is easily irritated by her colleagues at work. She also admits to feelings of hopelessness and problems sleeping. The GP notes she has recently started cognitive behavioural therapy. Her past medical history includes hypertension. Which of the following medications should she be commenced on?

A. Amitriptyline.
B. Citalopram.
C. Mirtazapine.
D. Moclobemide.
E. Venlafaxine.

5. A psychiatrist wishes to prescribe lithium as second-line treatment for a patient with bipolar disorder. Which blood test, if any, is the most important to arrange, other than renal function?

A. Full blood count.
B. Liver function tests.
C. No blood test required.
D. Parathyroid hormone.
E. Thyroid function tests.

6. Which of the following medications is the most appropriate antihypertensive for a patient who is taking lithium for their bipolar disorder?

A. Amlodipine.
B. Bendroflumethiazide.
C. Furosemide.
D. Losartan.
E. Ramipril.

7. A 24-year-old girl with depression is reviewed by her GP. Despite taking fluoxetine for the past 2 months, she remains low in mood with biological symptoms of depression. Her GP wishes to start her on moclobemide. Which of the following statements is true regarding this medication?

A. Fluoxetine can safely be prescribed alongside this antidepressant.
B. This antidepressant can lower the seizure threshold.
C. This antidepressant can safely be taken with cough mixtures.
D. This antidepressant can be prescribed to patients who have had a recent myocardial infarction.
E. This antidepressant can cause weight gain and teary red eyes.

8. A 21-year-old female presents to the neurologist after having had two seizures (involving her body becoming rigid, followed by her limbs jerking) over the past 3 months. Her CT head scan is normal. Which of the following medication causes the use-dependent blockade of voltage-gated sodium channels and is used first line in the treatment of epilepsy?

A. Ethosuximide.
B. Lamotrigine.
C. Phenytoin.
D. Sodium valproate.
E. Vigabatrin.

Chapter 9 Drug misuse

1. A 21-year-old male asks his friend who is a trainee doctor what the effects of cannabis are. Which of the following is true regarding cannabis?

A. Cannabis reduces heart rate and constricts pupils.
B. Cannabis reduces appetite.

C. Cannabis causes an apparent sharpening of sensory experience.

D. Cannabis is used clinically as an analgesic.

E. Injecting cannabis enhances its effects.

2. A 24-year-old female regularly takes heroin. However, she presents to A&E after being unable to buy any more. Which of the following symptoms are consistent with the opioid withdrawal syndrome?

A. Euphoria.

B. Increased appetite.

C. Hypothermia.

D. Pupillary constriction.

E. Yawning.

3. A 35-year old female who has been a heavy smoker for the past 15 years attends her GP and would like to try a nicotine replacement product. Her medical history includes epilepsy and hay fever. She is currently receiving psychological support from the smoking cessation specialist nurse.

Which of the following medications should she be prescribed?

A. Bupropion.

B. Disulfiram.

C. Flumazenil.

D. Methanol.

E. Varenicline.

Chapter 10 Pain and anaesthesia

1. A 45-year-old man with lower back pain is seen by his General Practitioner (GP) for a review. Sinister causes for his back pain have been excluded but he has extensive osteoarthritis. He is currently taking paracetamol and ibuprofen, but the pain is persisting. His examination is normal, and his blood results are unremarkable. He has no allergies.

Which of the following analgesia should he be prescribed next?

A. Ibuprofen, paracetamol and aspirin.

B. Ibuprofen paracetamol and morphine.

C. Ibuprofen, paracetamol and codeine.

D. Paracetamol and morphine.

E. Ibuprofen and codeine.

2. Mr Jones, a 60-year-old male with a history of prostate cancer, is admitted with a short history of back pain. He is in severe pain, particularly when moving and it comes on very quickly. He is already taking regular paracetamol and codeine phosphate 60 mg six hourly. A pelvic X-ray indicates a possible metastatic deposit. His urea and electrolytes reveal a creatinine of 200 (one month previously 85) and his full blood count and liver function tests are normal. An isotope bone scan and oncology review are arranged.

Which one of the following options is the most appropriate analgesic for "as required" use?

A. Diamorphine subcutaneously.

B. Fentanyl lozenges.

C. Methadone orally.

D. Morphine sulphate orally.

E. Oxycodone orally.

3. A 30-year-old male is brought to A&E with femur and tibia fracture and multiple rib fractures, following a motorbike accident. He is given regular morphine to control the pain.

Which of the following adverse effects are associated with opioids?

A. Cough.

B. Diarrhoea.

C. Dilated pupils.

D. Fast respiratory rate.

E. Flushing.

4. Miss Joules is reviewed by her GP. She has been having episodes of unilateral, severe headaches associated with photophobia and vomiting for the past 6 weeks. She has a family history of migraine. Despite treatment for her acute attacks, Miss Joules is concerned that her migraines are impacting negatively on her ability to work effectively. She has come to discuss sumatriptan.

What is the mechanism of action of sumatriptan?

A. 5-HT1 receptor agonist.

B. 5-HT1 receptor antagonist.

C. β-Receptor antagonist.

D. Nonsteroidal anti-inflammatory.

E. Serotonin-noradrenaline reuptake inhibitor.

5. A 45-year old female requires a general anaesthetic for an appendectomy. Her past medical history includes hypertension, epilepsy and hay fever. She is given propofol during the induction stage of anaesthesia.

Which of the following medication should she be given to maintain her anaesthesia during the surgery?

A. Enflurane.

B. Isoflurane.

C. Halothane.

D. Etomidate.

E. Ketamine.

Chapter 11 Inflammation, allergic diseases and immunosuppression

1. A 65-year-old male attends his GP practice with a sprained ankle and informs his doctor that he has been taking ibuprofen over the counter but is

concerned about what he has read in the patient leaflet. Which of the following statements is correct regarding ibuprofen?

Ibuprofen can be given to patients with:

A. Renal impairment.
B. Asthma.
C. Gastrointestinal ulceration.
D. Joint inflammation.
E. Liver failure.

2. A patient with severe rheumatoid arthritis who has been taking regular ibuprofen and short courses of prednisolone is commenced on hydroxychloroquine.

Which of the following side effects is most associated with hydroxychloroquine?

A. Diarrhoea.
B. Oligospermia.
C. Thinning of the skin.
D. Transient loss of taste.
E. Visual loss.

3. Before commencing adalimumab, a history of which of the following should be excluded?

A. Chronic obstructive pulmonary disease.
B. Hypertension.
C. Ischaemic heart disease.
D. Recurrent urinary tract infections.
E. Tuberculosis.

4. A 30-year-old female has been referred to a dermatologist by her GP. She has several thickened skin plaques on her elbows, knees and scalp with superficial scales. Her GP notes that she has hyperlipidemia on her blood tests.

Which of the following statements is true?

A. Clobetasone butyrate is a very potent topical steroid used on affected areas.
B. Methotrexate is used first-line in the treatment of psoriasis.
C. Dithranol can be safely applied to pustular psoriasis.
D. Calcipotriol can be used in patients with disorders of calcium metabolism.
E. Coal tar causes an acne like eruption and photosensitivity

5. A 20-year-old female with a chest infection is prescribed oral co-amoxiclav. Within a few minutes, she experiences chest tightness, lip tingling and an urticarial rash on her arms.

Which of the following statements is true?

A. The release of histamine causes bronchoconstriction.
B. This reaction is mediated by IgA and is a type II hypersensitivity reaction.

C. Adrenaline acts at α2-receptors to cause vasoconstriction and β2-receptors to cause bronchodilation.
D. Promethazine is a new nonsedative H2 receptor antagonist.
E. Intravenous adrenaline is required to treat this reaction.

Chapter 12 Infectious diseases

1. Which of the following antibiotics acts as a protein synthesis inhibitor?

A. Co-amoxiclav.
B. Gentamicin.
C. Meropenem.
D. Metronidazole.
E. Trimethoprim.

2. Which of the following antibiotics are known to cause ototoxicity, nephrotoxicity and red man syndrome?

A. Erythromycin.
B. Levofloxacin.
C. Metronidazole.
D. Trimethoprim.
E. Vancomycin.

3. A 19-year-old man attends the walk-in sexual health clinic complaining of a painful, white discharge from his urethra and dysuria. He has a positive swab for a gram-negative organism.

Which antibiotic can be given as a one-off dose to treat his symptoms?

A. Azithromycin.
B. Ciprofloxacin.
C. Co-amoxiclav.
D. Meropenem.
E. Trimethoprim.

4. A 65-year-old man attends A&E with a productive cough, fever and chest tightness. Past medical history: atrial fibrillation. DH: Warfarin (international normalized ratio [INR] yesterday 2.6). Allergy: penicillin.

He is started on an antibiotic for a presumed lower respiratory tract infection. His repeat bloods show an INR of 1.

Which of the following antibiotics was likely to have been prescribed?

A. Amoxicillin.
B. Clarithromycin.
C. Co-amoxiclav.
D. Co-trimoxazole.
E. Levofloxacin.

5. A 34-year-old 16/40 pregnant female is found to have asymptomatic bacteriuria of E. coli on screening. Which of the following is the most appropriate action?

A. None.
B. Trimethoprim.
C. Doxycycline.
D. Nitrofurantoin.
E. Ciprofloxacin.

6. A 48-year-old male patient receiving treatment for tuberculosis attends his General Practitioner complaining of orange tears and urine. Which of the following antituberculosis medications is responsible for these side effects?
   A. Ethambutol.
   B. Isoniazid.
   C. Pyrazinamide.
   D. Pyridoxine.
   E. Rifampicin.

7. A 45-year old male is referred to the infectious diseases team because he has recently been diagnosed with HIV. He is commenced on antiretroviral therapy. Which of the following antiretroviral agents is classed as a nonnucleoside reverse transcriptase inhibitor?
   A. Didanosine.
   B. Lamivudine.
   C. Nevirapine.
   D. Ritonavir.
   E. Zidovudine.

8. A 28-year-old female attends a travel clinic for vaccinations. She would like to know which of the following vaccines include a live attenuated virus?
   A. Diphtheria.
   B. Hepatitis A.
   C. Hepatitis B.
   D. Parenteral polio.
   E. Rubella.

9. Which of the following antihelminth medications is most appropriately used in the treatment of pinworm?
   A. Ivermectin.
   B. Levamisole.
   C. Mebendazole.
   D. Niclosamide.
   E. Praziquantel.

10. Which of the following antimalarial medications is safe to use in pregnancy for treatment of malaria?
    A. Chloroquine.
    B. Dapsone.
    C. Mefloquine.

D. Primaquine.
E. Sulphonamide.

Chapter 13 Cancer

1. Which cytotoxic drug is an alkylating agent?
   A. Cisplatin.
   B. Dactinomycin.
   C. Melphalan.
   D. Methotrexate.
   E. Vinblastine.

2. Which of the following cytotoxic medication is known to cause haemorrhagic cystitis?
   A. Chlorambucil.
   B. Cyclophosphamide.
   C. Doxorubicin.
   D. Melphalan.
   E. Methotrexate.

3. A patient with lymphoma is started on chemotherapy, given intravenously and complains of weakness and loss of sensation in his hands and feet. On examination, it is apparent that his power is reduced, and he has reduced reflexes. Which of the following chemotherapy agents is likely to be responsible?
   A. Bleomycin.
   B. Methotrexate.
   C. Mercaptopurine.
   D. Rituximab.
   E. Vincristine.

4. A patient is recently diagnosed with acute lymphoblastic leukaemia that is Philadelphia chromosome positive. Which of the following chemotherapy agents is the most appropriate treatment given its underlying mechanism of action?
   A. Everolimus.
   B. Hydroxyurea.
   C. Imatinib.
   D. Oxaplatin.
   E. Procarbazine.

5. A patient with lymphoma is given a MAb that targets the CD20 protein found on the surface of white blood cells. Which of the following MAb acts in this way?
   A. Cetuximab.
   B. Erlotinib.
   C. Nivolumab.
   D. Rituximab.
   E. Trastuzumab.

Extended-matching questions (EMQs)

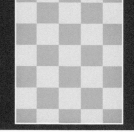

Each option may be used once, more than once or not at all.

Chapter 1 Introduction to Pharmacology

Receptor interactions and pharmacokinetics

A. Absorption of drug
B. Activation of receptor linked to ion channel
C. Activation of adenylyl cyclase
D. Adherence
E. Administration of drug
F. Agonist
G. Antagonist (competitive)
H. Antagonist (noncompetitive)
I. Distribution of drug
J. Excretion of drug
K. Inactivation of receptor linked to ion channel
L. Inactivation of
M. Partial agonist
N. Pharmacodynamics interaction
O. Pharmacokinetic interaction
P. Phase 1 metabolic reaction
Q. Phase 2 metabolic reaction

For each subsequent scenario choose the most likely corresponding option from the list given earlier.

1. A patient presents with watery diarrhoea and is diagnosed with cholera and the underlying mechanism of the disease is this.
2. A patient should not be given lidocaine orally because of this pharmacokinetic property.
3. A patient has taken a heroin overdose and is given naloxone. Through this action at the opiate receptor, the symptoms of respiratory depression are reversed.
4. A patient who has taken a paracetamol overdose requires N-acetyl cysteine because this process is saturated.
5. A patient presents with a persistent whooping cough because of this.
6. An anaesthetist must consider this pharmacokinetic property before giving a highly lipid soluble medication to a patient.
7. A patient should be given morphine by injection or delayed release capsules because of this pharmacokinetic property.

8. A patient has been on the oral contraceptive pill and is started on phenytoin to control her seizures. Two months later she finds that she is pregnant because of the pharmacokinetics of the two drugs.
9. A patient is currently taking ibuprofen (a nonsteroidal antiinflammatory) and despite being given a diuretic, their blood pressure remains high.
10. An elderly patient with kidney disease should have their medication doses reviewed and perhaps altered because of this pharmacokinetic property.
11. A patient is taking their antibiotics at different times on different days and is not getting better.

Chapter 2 Peripheral nervous system

Medications – their actions and side effects

A. Atracurium
B. Atropine
C. Botulinum toxin A
D. Clonidine
E. Carbidopa
F. Labetalol
G. Lidocaine
H. Methyldopa
I. Neostigmine
J. Phentolamine
K. Phenelzine
L. Phenylephrine
M. Phenoxybenzamine
N. Physostigmine
O. Pyridostigmine
P. Reserpine
Q. Salbutamol
R. Suxamethonium

For each subsequent scenario, choose the most likely corresponding option from the list given earlier.

1. A local anaesthetic is required to allow excision of a small mole.
2. This drug can be used in the treatment of dystonia and spasticity.
3. A patient with asthma develops bronchospasm after receiving this medication.
4. An α2-adrenoreceptor agonist used in the treatment of hypertensive migraine.

5. An α1-adrenoreceptor agonist used in the treatment of nasal decongestion.
6. A medication used intravenously to reverse the effects of nondepolarising blockers.
7. A medication given to prevent bradycardia associated with muscarinic receptor activation caused by depolarising blocking agents.
8. A medication used topically in the treatment of glaucoma.
9. A reversible nonselective α-adrenoreceptor antagonist that can be prescribed for the treatment of hypertension.
10. This medication is given to patients with Parkinson disease and increases dopamine levels.
11. This drug acts presynaptically by preventing the accumulation of noradrenaline in vesicles.
12. This drug acts presynaptically to inhibit the breakdown of leaked noradrenaline stores.

Chapter 3 Respiratory system

Respiratory system drugs and their side effects and contraindications

A. Aminophylline
B. Chlorphenamine
C. Ipratropium
D. Montelukast
E. Naloxone
F. Oxygen
G. Prednisolone
H. Salbutamol
I. Salmeterol
J. Magnesium sulphate

For each subsequent scenario, choose the most likely corresponding option from the list given earlier.

1. A 19-year-old girl seen in the emergency department is treated acutely. After 30 minutes of treatment, she develops a bilateral tremor.
2. A 20-year-old man with asthma complains of a dry mouth, headache and gastrointestinal disturbance after taking this medication.
3. A 60-year-old man with benign prostatic hypertrophy and glaucoma cannot be prescribed this medication for treatment of his obstructive airways disease.
4. A 20-year-old girl requires treatment after being admitted with a low respiratory rate and reduced Glasgow Coma Scale following attendance at a party.
5. A 15-year-old boy admitted with life-threatening asthma is given this medication, and levels need to be checked to ensure the dose is within range.

Chapter 4 Cardiovascular system

Mechanism of action of antiarrhythmics

A. Adenosine
B. Amiodarone
C. Amlodipine
D. Bumetanide
E. Digoxin
F. Flecainide
G. Furosemide
H. Lidocaine
I. Metoprolol
J. Procainamide
K. Spironolactone
L. Verapamil

For each subsequent scenario, choose the most likely corresponding option from the list given earlier.

1. An antiarrhythmic drug that blocks voltage-gated sodium channels which slows phase 0 of the cardiac action potential and therefore increases the effective refractory period.
2. An antiarrhythmic drug that slows phases 0 to 3 of the cardiac action potential, prolonging the cardiac action potential duration and effective refractory period.
3. An antiarrhythmic drug that shortens phase 2 of the cardiac action potential by calcium antagonism.
4. An antiarrhythmic and cardiac glycoside with positive inotropic action that shifts the frank starling ventricular function curve upward.
5. An antiarrhythmic drug that blocks voltage-dependent sodium channels in their open (activated) or refractory state. Their effects are to slow phase 0 and phase 4 and to prolong action potential duration.
6. An antiarrhythmic that reduces the excitability of the myocardium and inhibits conduction through the His Purkinje fibres, used in treatment of paroxysmal AF without left ventricular dysfunction.
7. An antiarrhythmic that increases the refractory period of the AV node and is used in the treatment of atrial fibrillation where there is sympathetic activation.
8. An antiarrhythmic that acts at A1 receptors to slow the action potential rising and thus delays conduction

Side effects and contraindications of cardiovascular medications

A. Adenosine
B. Amiodarone
C. Amlodipine
D. Bumetanide

E. Digoxin

F. Enoxaparin

G. Flecainide

H. Furosemide

I. Glyceryl trinitrate

J. Lidocaine

K. Losartan

L. Metoprolol

M. Procainamide

N. Spironolactone

O. Verapamil

For each subsequent scenario, choose the most likely corresponding option from the list given earlier.

1. This antiarrhythmic causes transient flushing, chest pain and bronchospasm for approximately 30 seconds after administration.

2. This antiarrhythmic is contraindicated in patients with systemic lupus erythematous.

3. This antiarrhythmic can cause deranged thyroid function tests and slate grey discolouration of skin.

4. This antiarrhythmic is contraindicated in patients with Wolff-Parkinson-White syndrome.

5. This antihypertensive can cause hyperkalaemia.

6. A patient with profound hypertension associated with their myocardial infarction cannot be given this medication.

7. This medication can reduce the glucose tolerance of patients with diabetes.

8. A patient is started on a medication to slow their heart rate and develops hypokalaemia while on a loop diuretic.

9. A patient with severe heart failure is prescribed an additional potassium-sparing diuretic.

10. A patient is initiated on treatment for a deep vein thrombosis. He develops hyperkalaemia and thrombocytopenia.

Appropriate management

A. Adrenaline 1:10,000 intravenously

B. Adrenaline 1:1000 intramuscularly

C. Bisoprolol

D. Clopidogrel

E. Dipyridamole

F. Digoxin

G. Ezetimibe

H. Fish oils

I. Fondaparinux

J. Nicotinic acid

K. Phenoxybenzamine

L. Rivaroxaban

M. Verapamil

For each subsequent scenario, choose the most likely corresponding option from the list given earlier.

1. In a cardiac arrest situation, this medication via this route should be administered.

2. In managing a patient with an acute myocardial infarction, this indirect factor Xa inhibitor should be prescribed.

3. A 65-year-old female is admitted with fast ventricular rate atrial fibrillation and has asthma. She is allergic to calcium channel blockers.

4. A patient presents with facial flushing, sweating, tachycardia and paroxysmal hypertension and requires immediate treatment.

5. A patient presents with a 20-minute history of facial droop and arm weakness, consistent with a transient ischaemic stroke. Aspirin and an additional medication is started.

6. A patient has ongoing raised cholesterol despite changes to his diet and on maximum dose statins.

Chapter 5   Kidney and urinary system

Mechanism of action and adverse effects of medications

A. Alprostadil

B. Amiloride

C. Amlodipine

D. Desmopressin

E. Doxazosin

F. Duloxetine

G. Eplerenone

H. Finasteride

I. Furosemide

J. Ibuprofen

K. Indapamide

L. Lithium

M. Mannitol

N. Mirabegron

O. Paracetamol

P. Sildenafil

Q. Sodium Valproate

R. Solifenacin

For each subsequent scenario, choose the most likely corresponding option from the list given earlier.

1. A patient with heart failure who takes isosorbide mononitrate presents with erectile dysfunction. This medication is contraindicated.

2. This medication is a potassium-sparing diuretic which acts through sodium-channel blockade and is used in the treatment of heart failure in combination with other diuretics.

3. This medication is used in the treatment of bipolar disorder. The patient may complain of excreting large volumes of urine because of this drug's action on the kidney.

4. This diuretic acts on the early distal tubule and can increase serum calcium levels.

5. This medication used in the treatment of urge incontinence is contraindicated in patients with glaucoma.

6. This diuretic is used intravenously in the treatment of raised intracranial pressure.

7. Coadministration of this medication can exacerbate salt and water retention in patients with heart failure and precipitate heart failure.

8. Hypotension, flushing and headache are common side effects associated with this medication.

9. The combination of this aldosterone antagonist with Ramipril (an ACE inhibitor) can result in hyperkalaemia.

10. A diuretic that can result in hyponatraemia, hypokalaemia, hypomagnesaemia and hypocalcaemia.

11. This medication is an inhibitor of the enzyme 5α-reductase used in the treatment of benign prostate hyperplasia.

12. This medication is a selective β-agonist that can be used in urge incontinence.

Chapter 6 Gastrointestinal system

A. Aluminium hydroxide
B. Azathioprine
C. Biscodyl
D. Cholestyramine
E. Cyclosporine
F. Cinnarizine
G. Cyclizine
H. Docusate sodium
I. Domperidone
J. Enterochromaffin-like paracrine cells
K. Hyoscine
L. Ispaghula Husk
M. Lactulose
N. Loperamide
O. Magnesium salts
P. Mebeverine
Q. Metoclopramide
R. Methylcellulose
S. Orlistat
T. Parietal cells
U. Peptic cells
V. Pantoprazole
W. W.Propantheline

X. Sulfasalazine
Y. Terlipressin
Z. Ursodeoxycholic acid

For each subsequent scenario, choose the most likely corresponding option from the list given earlier.

1. Gastrin exerts its acid secretory effect indirectly by stimulating these cells.

2. This medication is commonly prescribed for the dissolution of gallstones and causes diarrhoea as a side effect.

3. This medication increases the volume of the nonabsorbable solid residue in the gut.

4. This medication irreversibly inhibits H+/K+-ATPase that is responsible for H+ secretion from parietal cells.

5. An 18-year-old girl is admitted with nausea and vomiting associated with gastroparesis. She develops involuntary upward eye movements and involuntary twisting of the neck.

6. A 40-year-old male is seen by his GP because of worsening constipation. During the last few months, he has been taking large amounts of an antacid preparation to help relieve his dyspepsia.

7. This medication is a direct relaxant of smooth muscle and can be used in the management of irritable bowel syndrome.

8. This medication causes the vasoconstriction of dilated splanchnic blood vessels and is used in patients with raised portal hypertension.

9. This medication increases gastrointestinal peristalsis and can be given via a suppository before a procedure.

10. This medication is a pancreatic lipase inhibitor used in the management of obesity.

11. This immunosuppressant medication is a purine analogue that is deactivated by TPMT.

12. This medication increases the water content of the bowel and can be used in the prevention of hepatic encephalopathy in patients with liver disease.

13. A male patient with ulcerative colitis needs to be counselled about the possibility of infertility before being prescribed this medication.

Chapter 7 Endocrine and reproductive systems

Adverse effects of endocrine drugs

A. Alendronate
B. Calcitonin
C. Carbimazole
D. Clomifene

E. Denosumab
F. Iodide
G. Levothyroxine
H. Metformin
I. Octreotide
J. Prednisolone
K. Tamoxifen

For each subsequent scenario, choose the most likely corresponding option from the list given earlier.

1. A 50-year-old man presents with right upper quadrant abdominal pain and jaundice. His ultrasound scan shows multiple gallstones and a dilated bile duct. He is noted to have an enlarged tongue, hands and feet.
2. A 27-year-old woman presents to the emergency department with severe acute lower abdominal pain and her ultrasound shows massive cystic enlargement of both ovaries. She has recently started treatment for infertility.
3. A 55-year-old woman presents to her GP with retrosternal pain having started treatment for osteoporosis. Gastroscopy reveals severe oesophageal erosions and ulceration.
4. This medication can cause depression, insomnia and impotence if used long-term in the treatment of hyperthyroidism.

Chapter 8 Central nervous system

Medications used in the treatment of Parkinson disease, dementia and the eye

A. Buspirone
B. Carbegoline
C. Domperidone
D. Donepezil
E. Entacapone
F. Latanoprost
G. Levodopa
H. Memantine
I. Melatonin
J. Pilocarpine
K. Procyclidine
L. Selegiline
M. Timolol

For each subsequent scenario, choose the most likely corresponding option from the list given earlier.

1. Patients with Parkinson disease taking this medication are at risk of cardiac arrhythmias.

2. This medication is a dopamine agonist selective for the D2 receptor and is used in combination with L-dopa to reduce the on-off effect for patients with Parkinson disease.
3. A patient, recently prescribed a medication to help reduce his disabling tremor, presents to his GP complaining of a dry mouth and blurred vision.
4. A patient with moderate Alzheimer dementia is prescribed a selective NMDA receptor inhibitor.
5. On routine optician review, a patient is noticed to have raised intraocular pressure. He is warned of the risk of his iris developing brown pigmentation.
6. A patient presents to A&E with a red, painful eye with blurred vision. He is given a medication that causes pupillary constriction.

Medications used in the treatment of mood disorders and insomnia

A. Buspirone
B. Chlordiazepoxide
C. Clozapine
D. Flumazenil
E. Fluoxetine
F. Melatonin
G. Mirtazapine
H. Olanzapine
I. Reboxetine
J. Risperidone
K. Sertraline
L. Zopiclone

For each subsequent scenario, choose the most likely corresponding option from the list given earlier.

1. A patient with depression is prescribed an α2-adrenoceptor antagonist and advised to have an urgent blood test if they develop a sore throat and feel unwell.
2. This medication is thought to reduce 5-HT transmission by acting as a partial agonist at 5-HT1A receptors and is used for the short-term relief of generalized anxiety.
3. The doctor explains the risk of gynaecomastia, weight gain, tremor and risk of developing involuntary movements of the face before prescribing medication to a patient with schizophrenia.
4. This medication is prescribed in refractory cases of schizophrenia, given the risk of fatal neutropenia.
5. This medication binds to a site on GABAA receptors and potentiates the action of GABA and is used in the treatment of acute alcohol withdrawal.
6. A patient with severe insomnia is prescribed a MT1 receptor agonist.

7. This medication is an atypical neuroleptic that has a high affinity for D1 and D4 receptors and low affinity for D2 receptors and is used first line in the treatment of schizrenia.

8. A patient presents with respiratory depression. He is known to have severe social anxiety and takes medication. He requires an antidote to this medication.

Medications used in the treatment of epilepsy

A. Carbamazepine
B. Clonazepam
C. Diazepam
D. Ethosuximide
E. Lamotrigine
F. Phenobarbital
G. Phenytoin
H. Sodium Valproate
I. Vigabatrin

For each subsequent scenario, choose the most likely corresponding option from the list given earlier.

1. A patient on warfarin attends his GP practice for a routine international normalized ratio check. The practice nurse reports that it is lower than normal and not within the target range. He is known to have epilepsy and informs the nurse that his anticonvulsant dose has recently been increased.

2. Paramedics on route to hospital give a patient with prolonged seizures this medication.

3. This medication is a GABA agonist and can cause diplopia, nausea and agranulocytosis.

4. This medication inhibits T-type low-threshold calcium current channels and dampens thalamocortical oscillations and is used in the treatment of absence seizures.

5. This medication acts via sodium channels to inhibit the release of glutamate and is used in the monotherapy of partial seizures.

Chapter 9 Drug misuse

Drugs of misuse

A. Clonidine
B. Cocaine
C. Delta-9-tetrahydrocannabinol (THC)
D. Diazepam
E. Disulfiram
F. Ethanol
G. Flumazenil
H. Hashish
I. Ketamine
J. LSD
K. MDMA
L. Methadone
M. Methanol
N. Naloxone

For each subsequent scenario, choose the most likely corresponding option from the list given earlier.

1. This drug of abuse can cause an altered state of perception with euphoric sensations.

2. The psychoactive constituent of cannabis.

3. This α2-adrenoceptor agonist drug is sometimes prescribed to suppress the effects of opioid withdrawal.

4. A patient presents confused, with shallow and slow breathing, constricted pupils and has a flushed face. He requires treatment for his drug overdose.

5. This commonly prescribed drug potentiates inhibitory GABA transmission.

6. This drug, if taken in excess, can cause confusion, ataxia and ophthalmoplegia, as well as memory impairment and confabulation.

7. This drug causes a throbbing headache, flushed face and palpitations.

8. This drug causes bladder dysfunction and problems passing urine.

9. This drug inhibits the reuptake of catecholamines at noradrenergic neurones, enhancing sympathetic activity.

Chapter 10 Pain and anaesthesia

Analgesia and anaesthesia

A. δ Receptors
B. κ Receptors
C. μ Receptors
D. Adrenaline
E. Amitriptyline
F. Atropine
G. Etomidate
H. Halothane
I. Ketamine
J. Lidocaine
K. Midazolam
L. Morphine
M. Naloxone
N. Naltrexone
O. Nitric oxide
P. Thiopental

For each subsequent scenario, choose the most likely corresponding option from the list given earlier.

1. A local anaesthetic (LA) used to aid the removal of a mole.
2. This inhaled anaesthetic is contraindicated in patients with a pneumothorax.
3. Activation of these receptors account for the analgesic effects of opioids.
4. A lady presents with a shooting pain down her leg associated with tingling in her foot. She requires analgesia.
5. Activation of these opioid receptors accounts for the dysphoria associated with opioids.
6. This medication is given to relieve apprehension before anaesthesia.
7. This induction anaesthetic can cause extraneous muscle movement.
8. This long-acting opioid receptor antagonist can be used to reverse opioid toxicity.
9. This anaesthetic acting at NMDA-type receptors results in amnesia and insensitivity to pain.
10. This medication is given with LA to prevent the spread of the anaesthetic into the systemic circulation.
11. This inhaled anaesthetic has a high blood solubility and has a much slower induction time.

Chapter 11 Inflammation, allergic diseases and immunosuppression

Medications used in the treatment of inflammation and immunosuppression

A. Aspirin
B. Azathioprine
C. Benzoyl peroxide
D. Cyclosporine
E. Celecoxib
F. Colchicine
G. COX-1
H. COX -2
I. Efudix
J. Etanercept
K. Febuxostat
L. H1-receptor
M. H2-receptor
N. Methotrexate
O. Penicillamine
P. Prostacyclin
Q. Prostaglandin
R. Thromboxane A2

For each subsequent scenario, choose the most likely corresponding option from the list given previously.

1. This eicosanoid is involved in platelet aggregation and vasoconstriction.
2. This antiinflammatory medication is a folic acid antagonist.
3. This isoform of cyclooxygenase is expressed on platelets, gastric mucosa and renal vasculature.
4. This antiinflammatory medication inhibits platelet aggregation.
5. This medication is a TNF-α blocker that competes with the patient's own receptors.
6. This medication is a xanthine oxidase inhibitor.
7. This medication is used in the treatment of basal cell carcinomas and inhibits DNA replication.
8. Histamine acting at this receptor results in a type 1 hypersensitivity reaction.
9. This immunosuppressant inhibits calcineurin reducing IL-2 levels.
10. This immunosuppressant is converted to 6-mercaptopurine in the liver and impairs DNA synthesis.

Chapter 12 Infectious diseases

Medications used in the treatment of inflammation and immunosuppression

A. Acyclovir
B. Amantadine
C. Benzylpenicillin
D. Ceftriaxone
E. Ciprofloxacin
F. Clindamycin
G. Co-amoxiclav
H. Doxycycline
I. Enfuvirtide
J. Flucloxacillin
K. Ganciclovir
L. Indinavir
M. Metronidazole
N. Nevirapine
O. Nitrofurantoin
P. Nystatin
Q. Tazocin
R. Trimethoprim
S. Zanamivir
T. Ziduvidine

For each subsequent scenario, choose the most likely corresponding option from the list given earlier.

1. This is the antibiotic combination of piperacillin and tazobactam.
2. This antibiotic is not inactivated by the β-lactamase produced by penicillin resistant staphylococci and is commonly used in the treatment of skin infections.
3. This antibiotic has cross-reactivity with penicillin and is used in the treatment of meningitis.
4. This antibiotic should be avoided in children because of the effects on bone and teeth.
5. A commonly used antibiotic for the treatment of a urinary tract infection that is teratogenic in the first trimester and can cause kernicterus in neonates.
6. This bactericidal antibiotic is used in the treatment of atypical respiratory infections but increase the risk of C. difficile infections.
7. This protein synthesis inhibitor is used in the treatment of severe cellulitis but has a high risk of causing C. difficile infections.
8. This antibiotic is useful in the treatment of giardia.
9. This antiviral medication inhibits the release of newly synthesized viruses from the host cell by inhibiting the enzyme neuraminidase.
10. This antiviral medication selectively phosphorylates viral thymidine kinase and inhibits viral DNA synthesis.
11. This antiretroviral agent prevents DNA chain elongation and has a competitive inhibitory effect to reverse transcriptase.
12. This antiretroviral agent prevents viral assembly and budding.
13. This polyene macrolide is used in the treatment of candidiasis on the skin and mucous membranes.

Chapter 13 Cancer

Medications used in the treatment of cancer

A. Aldesleukin
B. Bicalutamide
C. Bleomycin
D. Cisplatin
E. Crisantaspase
F. Degarelix
G. Doxorubicin
H. Filgastrin
I. Fluorouracil
J. Gardasil
K. Gonadorelin
L. Methotrexate
M. Prednisolone
N. Sipuleucel T
O. Tamoxifen

For each subsequent scenario, choose the most likely corresponding option from the list given earlier.

1. This cytotoxic medication inhibits thymidylate synthetase impairing DNA synthesis.
2. This cytotoxic antibiotic inhibits topoisomerase II and causes significant myelosuppression.
3. This cytotoxic medication can cause severe nausea and vomiting in association with acute kidney injury and myelosuppression.
4. This cytotoxic medication contains bacterial asparaginase and inhibits the growth of acute lymphoblastic leukaemia.
5. This medication can be used to elevate mood and stimulate appetite in a patient with cancer.
6. This medication is used in the treatment of oestrogen receptor-positive breast cancer.
7. This medication competes with endogenous GnRH.
8. This vaccine is given against the HPV.
9. This medication is used to stimulate haematopoeitic stem cells in the bone marrow.
10. This medication is a GnRH agonist used in the treatment of prostate cancer.

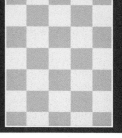

Chapter 1 Introduction to Pharmacology

1. E. Rifampicin is an enzyme inducer and will affect the metabolism of Warfarin. Rifampicin induces the hepatic P450 system, therefore increasing the metabolism of several drugs, including warfarin. Therefore levels may be subtherapeutic, rendering them ineffective. Drugs that inhibit enzymes affect the other medications in the options list.

2. B. The intravenous route is the most direct route of administering a drug because it avoids the need for absorption, which is the rate limiting step.

3. B. Preclinical phase involves laboratory animals or is in vitro. Phase 1 looks at drug metabolism and bioavailability as well as evaluating the safety of the drug and requires healthy individuals and/or patients. Phases 2-4 involves patients.

4. A. Isoprenaline is a nonselective β-receptor agonist. Salbutamol and Salmeterol are other β-receptor agonists. Answers B and C are incorrect because N-acetyl-P-aminophenol is the nontrade name for paracetamol. Paracetamol is thought to be a weak inhibitor of the synthesis of prostaglandins (PGs) and has some COX 2 inhibition. Proguanil hydrochloride is involved in the biosynthesis of pyrimidines required for nucleic acid replication and thus answer D is incorrect. Answer E is incorrect because syntometrine is a synthetic combination of oxytocin (hormone) and ergometrine, an alpha-adrenergic, dopaminergic and serotonin (5-HT2) receptor agonist.

5. A. B2 adrenergic receptors are an example of G-protein-coupled receptor. Insulin receptor and PDGF receptors are tyrosine linked receptors and steroid receptor is a DNA-linked receptor.

Chapter 2 Peripheral nervous system

1. C. When aminoglycoside antibiotics (e.g., gentamicin, streptomycin) are given concurrently with neuromuscular blocking agents, a rare but serious toxic reaction resulting in paralysis can occur. It results from the aminoglycoside inhibiting calcium uptake necessary for the exocytotic release of acetylcholine. It can be reversed by the administration of calcium salts (refer to p. 22).

2. D. Suxamethonium is the main depolarising neuromuscular blocking agent used as an adjunct to general anaesthesia to permit intubation of the airway. Most other neuromuscular blocking agents used during anaesthesia are nondepolarising

(answers A & E) and can be reversed by anticholinesterases (unlike depolarising blocking agents). Answer C (hemicholinium) blocks choline uptake but is not used clinically. Answer B (botulinum) blocks acetylcholine release and is not used during anaesthesia (refer to p. 22).

3. B. A young female presenting with muscle weakness and early fatigue at the end of the day or with repetitive activities should raise the possibility of myasthenia gravis. This is a disorder of neuromuscular transmission because of autoantibodies to the acetylcholine receptors at the neuromuscular junction, leading to "fatigability" and muscle weakness that worsens with exercises but improves with rest. Edrophonium is a short-acting anticholinesterase, which is selective for the neuromuscular junction. It is sometimes administered intravenously to patients with suspected myasthenia gravis. There should be a transient improvement in muscle strength. However, it is rarely done because it can result in life-threatening bradycardia and requires resuscitation facilities. Usually, the diagnosis is made if the patient is found to have positive acetylcholine receptor antibodies (refer to p. 24). Answer C (neostigmine) is incorrect because it is used in the treatment of myasthenia gravis. Answers A & D are incorrect because pancuronium and alcuronium are anaesthetic agents (nondepolarising neuromuscular blocking agents) and answer E (suxamethonium) is a depolarising neuromuscular blocking agent that has little effect in patients with myasthenia gravis (see Box 2.2).

4. C. Medical management of phaeochromocytoma-induced hypertension relies on the powerful α-adrenoceptor antagonist phentolamine. α-Adrenoceptor blockade reduces peripheral vascular resistance and lowers blood pressure. The use of β-adrenoceptor antagonists is dangerous (i.e., answers A and B are incorrect) because tumour-secreted sympathomimetics act unopposed on α-adrenoceptors, increasing both peripheral vascular resistance and blood pressure. Once the patient is stabilized with IV phentolamine (which will reduce the blood pressure safely) the patient can be given oral phenoxybenzamine (answer D). Then answer A (oral propanolol) can be added in. Answer E is incorrect because atropine is a muscarinic antagonist (refer to p. 30).

5. D. Prazosin acts as an α1-adrenoreceptor antagonist and is used in the treatment of benign prostatic hyperplasia and hypertension. Side effects include

hypotension, tachycardia and nasal congestion (refer to Box. 2.12). Answer A is incorrect: Clonidine is an α2-adrenoreceptor agonist used in the treatment of resistant hypertension and migraine (refer to Box 2.11). Answers B and E are incorrect because they are antihypertensives that work at β receptors in the main. Answer C is incorrect because phenylephrine is an α1 agonist that can be used in the treatment of hypotension but is more commonly used as a nasal decongestant.

6. A. Ipratropium bromide acts as a muscarinic antagonist. Muscarinic antagonists can cause the following side effects: blurred vision, dry mouth and skin, dilated pupils, and urinary retention. Therefore, answers B to E are incorrect (refer to pp. 30–31).

Chapter 3 Respiratory system

1. D. In the "rescue" of a patient with an acute exacerbation of asthma, only a few medications are helpful. The single most effective therapy in an acute exacerbation of asthma is systemic steroids. Inhaled steroids are less effective in an acute exacerbation of asthma. Inhaled salmeterol is for long-term management. If this patient does not respond to oral/IV steroids and IV magnesium, the next step in management is theophylline infusion. Steroids can be given as oral or IV (there is no clear benefit of IV therapy over oral therapy if the patient can take pills). Systemic steroids take 4 to 6 hours to start to work by either route.

2. E. This patient's asthma symptoms are not controlled on his current level of treatment. He is currently on stage 2 of the chronic asthma management guideline (see Table 3.1). Continuing only with his salbutamol and beclometasone inhaler is not adequately controlling his symptoms and therefore he needs his treatment to be escalated to level 3. This would entail prescribing an inhaled short-acting β2 agonist (e.g., salbutamol), plus a long-acting β2 agonist (LABA) and a low-dose inhaled corticosteroid (can be given as a fixed dose combination inhaler of either fluticasone propionate and salmeterol or budesonide and formoterol). In this patient, you would need to stop the beclometasone inhaler. If the patient continued to have symptoms and had limited response to the LABA, then stop it and increase the dose of inhaled corticosteroid. If he had some benefit from the LABA but his control remained inadequate, continue the LABA and increase the inhaled corticosteroid to a moderate dose. Because there is no evidence of a chest infection in the case (e.g., no productive cough, no pyrexia, no crackles on the chest, normal vital signs), we can assume that his asthma is poorly controlled rather than him having an infective trigger of his symptoms; therefore antibiotics are not required.

3. C. This woman's symptoms are poorly controlled and therefore she requires a step up in her treatment. Because her FEV1 is above 50%, in line with NICE guidance, she needs to be given either a LABA or a LAMA, but the LAMA is not appropriate unless the SAMA is stopped, which is not an option in the answer list. She could have been started on a SABA initially as an alternative to ipratropium (SAMA) and then tiotropium (LAMA) would have been appropriate at the next stage. A LABA plus an inhaled corticosteroid would be appropriate if her symptoms are still inadequately controlled or her FEV1 falls below 50%.

4. B. This case illustrates a woman who is likely to have an exacerbation of COPD with an infective component. She requires oxygen because her saturations are low, but with COPD patients, caution needs to be exercised with regards to the amount of oxygen administered in case the patient relies on a hypoxic drive to breathe and if they are chronic retainers of carbon dioxide (CO2). The patient's saturations should be above 90% and should be given enough oxygen to ensure this via a controlled venturi oxygen mask. Because she is a chronic retainer of CO2, her target saturations should be 88% to 92%. There is evidence to suggest that giving 15 L of high-flow oxygen to patients with COPD can cause significant harm and should be avoided, provided that the patient's saturations are within the target range. If this patient required IV theophylline, the clarithromycin would have to be switched to something other than a macrolide. Theophylline plasma concentrations would increase enzymes involved in theophylline breakdown occupied by macrolide antibiotics and there is a significant risk of toxicity.

5. C. This patient has presented with allergic rhinitis. The management of allergic rhinitis is with oral or nasal antihistamines (e.g., cetirizine and chlorphenamine) and nasal glucocorticosteroids. Nasal decongestants (e.g., ephedrine) are available for the treatment of allergic rhinitis. However, they can only be used for 2 to 3 days a time and therefore are not recommended for long-term management. Oral ephedrine is not used and would be contraindicated in this patient because he has diabetes and hypertension. Leukotriene modifiers may be used for patients with asthma or who cannot tolerate nasal sprays.

Chapter 4 Cardiovascular system

1. D. Methyldopa is an α2-adrenoceptor agonist that is safe to use in pregnancy. It should be avoided in patients with liver disease or depression (refer to pp. 57–58). Bisoprolol is a β-adrenoceptor antagonist and it may cause intrauterine growth restriction and neonatal bradycardia and thus is avoided in

pregnancy. Labetalol can, however, be used in maternal hypertension if required. Furosemide, a loop diuretic, is not commonly used as an antihypertensive agent. It is more commonly prescribed in the management of acute and chronic heart failure. Losartan (angiotensin II receptor antagonist) and ramipril (ACE inhibitor) are contraindicated because they adversely affect foetal blood pressure control and renal function. They can also cause oligohydramnios.

2. C. Furosemide (a loop diuretic) is the mainstay of treatment in acute heart failure and should be given intravenously. Bumetanide is also a loop diuretic but is given as a second-line treatment. Bendroflumethiazide is a thiazide diuretic used in the treatment of hypertension and uncommonly to manage chronic heart failure. Glyceryl trinitrate is a nitrate and can be helpful in the management of heart failure (dilates systemic veins, decreasing preload and thus the oxygen demand of the heart) but does not directly off load fluid (refer to p. 52). Morphine is an opiate which can help alleviate the uncomfortable feeling of breathlessness associated with acute pulmonary oedema, but again does nothing to remove the fluid.

3. B. Clopidogrel inhibits ADP-induced platelet aggregation by irreversible inhibition of P2Y receptors (refer to p. 66). It is used in the acute treatment of an MI. Aspirin is an antiplatelet like clopidogrel but aspirin inhibits the synthesis of thromboxane A2 and cyclooxygenase 1 (refer to p. 65). Fondaparinux is a low-molecular-weight heparin and they increase the action of antithrombin III on factor Xa, thus limiting the formation of blood clots. Fondaparinux is often used in the acute treatment of an MI (refer to p. 65). Morphine is an opiate used in the management of the acute pain associated with an MI. Unfractionated heparin activates antithrombin III which inhibits thrombin and factor Xa and thus limits blood clotting. It is used in the acute treatment of an MI if renal function is impaired (refer to p. 65).

4. C. NICE guidance and evidence indicate that patients aged over 55 years or who are Afro-Caribbean respond better to calcium channel blockers as first-line treatment of hypertension. Those younger than 55 years of age who are not of Afro-Caribbean origin should be started on an ACE inhibitor (provided they do not have contraindications – refer to p. 55). If second-line treatment is required, then a combination of an ACE inhibitor and a calcium-channel blocker can be used. Then third-line treatment is a thiazide diuretic (e.g., bendroflumethiazide). Therefore answer E would be correct if the patient was already on an ACE inhibitor and calcium channel blocker. Answer B is incorrect because ß-blockers are not commonly used as first-line treatment of hypertension and importantly, the patient is known to have asthma and ß-blockers are contraindicated (refer to p. 52). Answer D is

incorrect because loop diuretics (e.g., furosemide) are not typically used in the management of hypertension.

5. C. ACE inhibitors reduce angiotensin II and aldosterone levels and thus cause vasodilation and a reduction in blood pressure. They also cause an increase in bradykinin levels. Answer C is correct because ACE inhibitors are excreted renally and thus if a patient is dehydrated secondary to diarrhoea and vomiting, there is an increased risk of acute kidney injury and they need to be stopped. Answer A is incorrect because ACE inhibitors can increase potassium levels, causing hyperkalaemia as an adverse effect. Answer B is incorrect because a cough is a common side effect secondary to the increased levels of bradykinin. Answer D is incorrect because ACE inhibitors are not known to commonly cause liver failure but there is an increased risk that they cause acute renal failure, especially if there is underlying renal artery stenosis. Blood tests (including urea and electrolytes) should be monitored following initiation of ACE inhibitors and after any dose change (refer to p. 55).

6. E. Answer A is incorrect because amlodipine (calcium-channel blocker) has no effect on electrolyte levels nor renal function so can continue. Answers B and C are partially correct because both ibuprofen (a nonsteroidal antiinflammatory) and ramipril (ACE inhibitor) need to be stopped. The issue in this scenario is the combination of these two medications resulting in hyperkalaemia and acute kidney injury. Ibuprofen decreases renal blood flow by inhibiting prostaglandins that normally dilate blood vessels flowing to the kidney. Reduced blood flow to the kidney can result in prerenal failure and, if prolonged, causes intrarenal failure with raised urea, creatinine and potassium. Adding ibuprofen to a medication that already increases the risk of hyperkalaemia and renal failure is dangerous if left unmonitored. ACE inhibitors may cause hyperkalaemia directly through reduced aldosterone production caused by the inhibition of the ACE. Renal failure can occur because efferent vessels leaving the kidney rely on angiotensin II to constrict. Thus ACE inhibitors which decrease angiotensin II production, reduce blood pressure and can cause renal damage, particularly if there is underlying renal artery stenosis, as is likely in this case (refer to p. 55). Answer D is incorrect because amlodipine can be continued (refer to p. 52).

7. E. Answer A is incorrect because bisoprolol, a ß-adrenoceptor antagonist, is used as rate control in atrial fibrillation. It has no effect on clotting and thus the INR will be unaffected. In addition, she has been taking this without any problems until now and it should be continued to ensure rate control. Answer B is incorrect because there is no evidence of bleeding and the INR is not over 8. Vitamin K reverses the

effect of warfarin by allowing synthesis of factors II, VII, IX and X. Vitamin K is indicated and given intravenously if there is bleeding with any INR or orally if the INR exceeds 8 without bleeding. Answer C is incorrect because reducing the dose would only be appropriate if the INR was less than 6. Answer D is incorrect as increasing the dose would risk the INR to go up even further and the patient may start bleeding, thus this option is dangerous. Answer E is correct because the INR is greater than 6 and there is no evidence of bleeding. It is likely that the acute alcohol consumption over the weekend has affected the metabolism of the warfarin. Acute alcohol intake is an enzyme inhibitor and thus the warfarin is not broken down and its anticoagulant effects are potentiated, increasing the INR and risk of bleeding. Note that chronic alcohol consumption acts as an enzyme inducer.

8. E. Answer E is correct because verapamil, a calcium channel antagonist can cause peripheral oedema and constipation as side effects (refer to pp. 51–53). Answer A is incorrect bcause furosemide (loop diuretic) is used in the treatment of heart failure and should reduce the peripheral oedema. Answer B is incorrect. Ramipril is an ACE inhibitor and common side effects include a cough, muscle cramps and hyperkalaemia (refer to p. 55). Answer C is incorrect. Rivaroxaban is a direct oral anticoagulant and its major side effect is haemorrhage. Answer D is incorrect. Simvastatin is a HMG-COA reductase inhibitor and common side effects include gastrointestinal upset and myalgia (refer to p. 61).

9. D. Statins are contraindicated in patients with liver disease because they are metabolized by the liver. An increased level of serum transaminases (indicating hepatic impairment) increases the risk of side effects, importantly myopathy and myositis. These blood tests should be checked before starting statins, after starting and at 12 months. If at any point the transaminases are raised more than three times the normal range, then statins should be stopped (refer to p. 61).

Answer A, blood pressure, is important to know in assessing cardiovascular risk but will not affect the prescription of simvastatin. Answer D is incorrect. A muscle biopsy is unnecessary and invasive. Answer B is incorrect. A creatinine kinase can be useful to check if an underlying myopathy is suspected. If raised, then simvastatin should not be prescribed. However, creatinine kinase is not a blood test that is required to be checked before starting a statin. Answer E is incorrect because simvastatin is not dosed according to weight.

10. C. Clarithromycin is an inhibitor of the cytochrome P450 enzyme. This enzyme breaks down warfarin and thus the combination of these two medications results in a potentially serious interaction. The presence of clarithromycin results in warfarin not being metabolized thus increases the plasma levels and consequently results in bleeding and a raised INR.

11. A. Refer to p. 48, Hints and Tips box. ACE inhibitors, β-blockers and nitrates with hydralazine and spironolactone have been found to have a proven mortality benefit in patients with heart failure.

Chapter 5 Kidney and urinary system

1. A. The distal convoluted tubule is the main site of potassium secretion because of the negative potential difference that moves sodium into parietal cells and potassium out of cells. Answer B is incorrect as the glomerulus is the site where plasma is filtered in general. Answer C is incorrect; juxtaglomerular apparatus is where renin is secreted. Answer D is incorrect; the loop of Henle is where approximately 25% of filtered sodium is reabsorbed. Answer E is incorrect; the proximal tubule is where two-thirds of the filtrate volume is reabsorbed, including bicarbonate (refer to pp. 70–72).

2. C. Thiazide diuretics can cause hyperuricaemia and therefore should be avoided in patients known to have gout. They can also cause hyponatraemia, hypokalaemia, hypermagnesaemia and hypercalcaemia (refer to p. 74).

3. D. Furosemide, a loop diuretic, causes the excretion of 25% of filtered sodium and can result in a profound diuresis. Furosemide is the mainstay of treatment in acute heart failure and is usually administered intravenously. Answer C is incorrect. Bumetanide, although a loop diuretic, that acts at the thick ascending segment of the loop of Henle, is usually reserved for patients who are resistant to furosemide. Answer B is incorrect. Indapamide is a thiazide diuretic more commonly used as an antihypertensive. Answer A & E are both potassium-sparing diuretics used in the management of CHF (refer to pp. 74–75).

4. D. Spironolactone is a potassium-sparing diuretic, known to cause hyperkalaemia because of its action at the late distal tubule and collecting duct (see Fig. 5.5). Spironolactone is a competitive antagonist at aldosterone receptors and reduces Na+ reabsorption and therefore K+ and H+ secretion. Answer A is incorrect. Amlodipine is a calcium-channel blocker and has little effect on potassium (see Chapter 4). Answer B is also incorrect because aspirin is an antiplatelet with minimal effect on potassium. Answer C is incorrect because furosemide is a loop diuretic and, in fact, lowers serum potassium levels through inhibition of the Na+/K+/2Cl– cotransporter. Answer E is incorrect because simvastatin is a cholesterol-lowering medication with little effect on potassium (see Chapter 4).

5. B. Doxazosin is an α-blocker. It increases the flow of urine by relaxing the smooth muscle around the urethra opening of the bladder. However, its vasodilator properties can result in postural hypotension (refer to p. 75). Answer A is incorrect. Bethanechol is a parasympathomimetic that increases detrusor muscle contraction and is not commonly used in the treatment of BPH. However, postural hypotension is not a common side effect associated with it, whereas bradycardia and intestinal colic are. Answer C is incorrect. Duloxetine is a serotonin noradrenaline reuptake inhibitor that is sometimes used in patients with stress incontinence and thus would not be prescribed in patients with BPH. Answer D is incorrect. Finasteride is an inhibitor of the enzyme 5α-reductase, and although used in the treatment of BPH, it is not thought to cause postural hypotension (refer to p. 75). Answer E is also incorrect. Oxybutynin is a muscarinic receptor antagonist used in the treatment of urge incontinence, not BPH (refer to p. 75).

6. C. Oxybutynin is an antimuscarinic and is used to relax the detrusor muscle of the bladder. It has anticholinergical properties and thus causes the following constellation of symptoms: dry mouth, constipation, blurred vision, urinary retention and nausea and vomiting. Answers A, B, D and E are therefore all incorrect (refer to p. 76).

7. D. Sildenafil is a selective inhibitor of phosphodiesterase type 5 and acts by enhancing the vasodilator effects of nitrous oxide. This results in maintenance of an erection if there is sexual stimulation. It is administered orally. Therefore answer E is incorrect. Alprostadil is a synthetic prostaglandin E1 analogue administered as a direct injection into the corpus cavernosum or applied to the urethra, it is not given orally and thus answer B is incorrect. Answers C & E are also incorrect because papaverine is a nonselective phosphodiesterase inhibitor, which is injected directly into the corpora cavernosa causing vasodilation and an erection (refer to pp. 75–77).

8. D. When patients are on diuretic medication, it is important to monitor their renal function and their electrolytes. Diuretics affect the function of the kidney and affect the excretion and reabsorption of potassium, sodium, calcium and magnesium. Answer A, blood pressure, is incorrect. Although it would be important to check the blood pressure while the patient is taking furosemide, especially if the patient becomes symptomatic, it is not the most important parameter to monitor. Remember that furosemide can lower the blood pressure because water follows sodium and is excreted into the urine in larger quantities, reducing the circulating volume. Answer C is incorrect because furosemide does not affect the full blood count and answer E is incorrect because

urinary sodium is not routinely measured when patients are on furosemide.

Chapter 6 Gastrointestinal system

1. B. A gastrinoma is a gastrin-secreting tumour found in the duodenum or pancreas, which causes multiple, refractory and recurrent peptic ulcers in the distal duodenum and proximal jejunum. These gastrin-secreting tumours and subsequent excessive HCl secretion characterize Zollinger-Ellison syndrome. Patients with Zollinger-Ellison syndrome often have severe diarrhoea because of the HCl causing hyperperistalsis and inhibition of the activity of lipase. The answer is B because multiple ulcers plus diarrhoea in a young man should highlight the possibility of gastrin secreting tumours.

Although he has risk factors for answers A, C, D and E, they are unlikely to have caused several ulcers throughout the gastrointestinal tract and diarrhoea (refer to p. 81).

2. C. Ranitidine is an H2 antagonist that works by inhibiting parietal cell secretion of hydrochloric acid. Ranitidine can cause nausea and diarrhoea and, in the long-term gynaecomastia, because of its modest affinity for androgen receptors. Answer A is incorrect because aluminium hydrochloride does not cause gynaecomastia, although is used as an antacid for dyspepsia (refer to p. 82). Answer B is incorrect because amoxicillin is an antibiotic that is not known to cause gynaecomastia. Answer D is incorrect because misoprostol, a synthetic prostaglandin analogue used as prophylaxis against NSAID induced ulceration, is more likely to cause diarrhoea and, in females, menstrual abnormalities (refer to p. 81). Answer E is incorrect; omeprazole (a PPI) causes gastrointestinal upset and headaches (refer to p. 81).

3. B. Cimetidine inhibits the P450 enzyme, reducing the metabolism of drugs such as warfarin, potentiating its pharmacological effect. It is likely that this patient was previously on a double dose PPI and then her GP added in a H2 receptor antagonist. Cimetidine is thought to be a more potent inhibitor of the P450 enzyme than ranitidine. This patient was likely to be overcoagulated, causing her to bleed. Answers A, C, D and E are not known to inhibit the P450 enzyme (refer to p. 81).

4. D. Metoclopramide is a prokinetic and improves gastric motility and is, therefore, the most useful antiemetic in patients with symptoms because of poor gastric emptying. Cyclizine (an H1-receptor antagonist) is useful in the treatment of motion sickness and vestibulocochlear disease (refer to pp. 82–83) and therefore answer A is incorrect. Answer B, dexamethasone is also incorrect. This is

typically used in the treatment of nausea and vomiting associated with cytotoxic therapy. Answer C is incorrect because levomepromazine is a dopamine antagonist used usually for nausea and vomiting in palliative care. Answer E, ondansetron, a 5-HT3 antagonist is not the preferred antiemetic in patients with gastroparesis.

5. D. Ondansetron has been recommended in guidelines as an effective antiemetic in chemotherapy induced nausea and vomiting. This is because it antagonizes 5-HT3 receptors in the chemoreceptor trigger zone, which is stimulated by cytotoxic toxins associated with chemotherapy (refer to p. 84). Answers A, B, C and E are incorrect because these antiemetics work slightly differently. Metoclopramide and domperidone are dopamine receptor antagonists, whereas cyclizine is a histamine-receptor antagonist. Prochlorperazine antagonizes dopamine, histamine and muscarinic receptors.

6. B. Chlorpromazine (an antiemetic) antagonizes several receptors including dopamine receptors. The reduction in dopamine in patients with Parkinson disease results in worsening symptoms and is therefore contraindicated. Answer A is incorrect; cimetidine is an H2-receptor antagonist that is used to reduce gastric acid secretion and is not typically used as an antiemetic. Answer C is incorrect; cyclizine is an H1—receptor antagonist that is not known to affect dopamine receptors and thus is not contraindicated in patients with Parkinson disease. Answer D is incorrect; dexamethasone, a glucocorticosteroid is used in the treatment of nausea and vomiting but has no known effect on Parkinson symptoms. Similarly, ondansetron is not known to cause problems in these patients (refer to pp. 84–88).

7. E. Oral Mesalazine–5-ASA is the treatment of choice for induction and maintenance of remission of mild to moderate ulcerative colitis (UC). Mesalazine is also thought to reduce the risk of colorectal cancer associated with UC (refer to p. 88). Answer A azathioprine is incorrect because this medication is used when patients are intolerant to corticosteroids or who require several courses of steroids. Azathioprine interferes with purine synthesis and depresses antibody-mediated immune reactions thus dampening down the inflammation. Answer B cyclosporine is also incorrect because it typically is prescribed in patients with severe refractory colitis. Answer C ispaghula husk is used in the treatment of proximal constipation associated with ulcerative colitis because it is a stool bulking laxative but is not used in maintaining remission. Answer D is incorrect because infliximab is a monoclonal antibody used in inducing remission in patients with moderate to severe UC whose disease has been resistant to steroids and/or the other immunosuppressive drugs.

8. E. Senna is a stimulant laxative whereas lactulose (answer B) is an osmotic laxative that increases the water content of the bowel. Answer A ispaghula husk is a bulk forming laxative (refer to pp. 85–86) and thus is incorrect. Answer C methylcellulose is thought to be a bulk-forming agent but is predominantly used in the management of obesity and is therefore incorrect. Answer D peppermint oil is incorrect. It is used as a smooth muscle relaxant and antispasmodic (refer to p. 85).

Chapter 7 Endocrine and reproductive

1. B. This question is related to the rare complication of bone marrow suppression and neutropenia associated with carbimazole. A full blood count will indicate whether there is a neutropenia, therefore answer B is the most important investigation to because the patient is presenting with a sore throat. Before prescribing carbimazole, it is imperative that the physician informs the patient to report any symptoms of infection, including a sore throat, so that drug-induced neutropenia can be identified and if present, carbimazole stopped. Although carbimazole can cause hepatitis, and checking the liver function test would be sensible, hepatitis is rare and the patient has presented with a sore throat, and thus answer B is more appropriate than answer D (refer to p. 93). Answer A and E would be useful to do but as indicated are not the most important investigation to do initially. There is no indication in the history that this patient is diabetic, so answer C is not the most important to check.

2. A. Amiodarone is class III antiarrhythmic (see Chapter 4) that blocks sodium and calcium channels. It is prescribed to patients with structural heart disease who require treatment for atrial fibrillation. Amiodarone is rich in iodine, which inhibits the conversion of T4 to T3 and inhibits hormone secretion. Amiodarone can cause either hyperthyroidism (symptoms this gentleman presents with) or hypothyroidism and thyroid function tests should be checked before prescribing it and 6 months thereafter (refer to Hints and Tips box on p. 94). Answer B is incorrect. Carbimazole is used in the treatment of hyperthyroidism but is not prescribed for the management of atrial fibrillation. Answer D is incorrect. Levothyroxine is used in the treatment of hypothyroidism. Answer E is incorrect. Although β-receptor antagonists are used to rate control patients with atrial fibrillation, it does not cause symptoms of hyperthyroidism. In fact, propranolol is prescribed to patients to relieve the tachycardia, tremor and nervousness associated

with hyperthyroidism. Answer C is incorrect because iodide is used in the treatment of thyrotoxicosis and is not used in the treatment of atrial fibrillation.

3. D. A β-blocker (e.g., atenolol) can mask the warning signs (e.g., tremor, racing heart) of hypoglycaemia. Patients taking gliclazide (a sulfonylurea) are at risk of hypoglycaemia because they stimulate endogenous insulin secretion through ATP-dependent sodium channel blockade in pancreatic β-cells (refer to p. 98), therefore the combination of gliclazide and a β-blocker should be prescribed with caution. Answer A is incorrect. As indicated, gliclazide can cause hypoglycaemia, particularly in the elderly and those with renal impairment. Answer B is incorrect. Alcohol can cause flushing if a patient is on gliclazide as well as increasing the risk of severe hypoglycaemia. Answer C is incorrect. Gliclazide causes weight gain (as do the other sulfonylureas). Answer E is incorrect. If a dose of gliclazide is missed, the patient should not take a double dose because the risk of hypoglycaemia is very high.

4. D. The case points towards type I diabetes as the most likely diagnosis. The patient, a child, is presenting with polyuria, polydipsia and weight loss with associated hyperglycaemia and glycosuria. The most appropriate management of type 1 diabetes is subcutaneous insulin (refer to p. 96), because patients with type I diabetes do not produce enough insulin as a result of autoimmune destruction of their pancreas, therefore answer D is correct. Answer A is incorrect. Acarbose is an α-glucosidase inhibitor used in the treatment of type 2 diabetes in combination with metformin and dietary control (refer to p. 98). Type 2 diabetes typically affects older patients who are overweight and inactive and is not the diagnosis in this case. Answer B is incorrect. Although it is important for all patients with diabetes to avoid foods with a high fat or sugar content, dietary modification is not sufficient treatment for the management of type I diabetes, and for patients who have the inability to secrete insulin and who are at risk of significant, uncontrolled hyperglycaemia that can lead to diabetic ketoacidosis and death. Answer C and E are both medications used in the treatment of type 2 diabetes and are therefore incorrect.

5. B. Pioglitazone can be used second-line or third-line in the treatment of type 2 diabetes but can take up to 3 months to have a maximum effect (refer to p. 98). Nevertheless, it can reduce the need for exogenous insulin by 30% so answer B is correct. Pioglitazone has been associated with an increased risk of bone fractures and bladder cancer and therefore answers C and D are incorrect. Pioglitazone causes weight gain and thus answer A is incorrect. Pioglitazone causes fluid retention

and is contraindicated in patients with heart failure, therefore answer E is incorrect. Metformin is the antidiabetic medication that is safe to give in heart failure (refer to pp. 97–98). Pioglitazone can cause liver failure and the prescriber should check liver function tests.

6. B. Dapagliflozin is an SGLT-2 inhibitor. It is used in combination with other antidiabetic medications in the treatment of type 2 diabetes. In addition to causing polyuria, hypotension and hypoglycaemia, one of its main side effects is urinary tract infections (e.g., penile discharge and dysuria) hence B is the correct answer. Acarbose is an α-glucosidase inhibitor and it causes flatulence and diarrhoea as side effects and thus answer A is incorrect. Linagliptin is a DPP4 inhibitor and its side effects include gastrointestinal upset, worsening heart failure and pancreatitis, hence answer C is incorrect. Liraglutide is a GLP-1 agonist that also causes gastrointestinal disturbances and pancreatitis. Pioglitazone causes weight gain, fluid retention and increases the risk of bladder cancer but does not typically cause urinary tract infections. Therefore answers D and E are incorrect (refer to pp. 98–100).

7. C. Fludrocortisone (answer C) is used as mineralocorticoid replacement in primary adrenal insufficiency. With regards to glucocorticoid replacement, hydrocortisone is used in patients with Addison disease (refer to p. 104). Answers B and D are incorrect. Dexamethasone and prednisolone are glucocorticoids, but they are typically used in the treatment of allergic and inflammatory diseases. They are not first-line replacement in adrenal insufficiency (refer to p. 104). Answer A is incorrect. Beclometasone is a very potent glucocorticoid drug with no mineralocorticoid that is used topically to treat allergic rhinitis and eczema (refer to p. 104). Answer E is incorrect. Triamcinolone is a glucocorticoid used for the treatment of arthritis.

8. C. Osteoporosis is a metabolic side effect of glucocorticosteroids long-term caused by the catabolism of protein matrix in bone. Answer A is incorrect. Glucocorticosteroids cause hyperglycaemia because of disturbed carbohydrate metabolism. Patients' blood glucose levels should be monitored when on steroids because they are at risk of diabetes mellitus. Answers B and D are incorrect. Glucocorticosteroids cause muscle wasting and thinning of the skin because of altered protein metabolism. Answer E is incorrect. Glucocorticoids cause fat redistribution and thus patients develop a characteristic moon face and central obesity (refer to p. 102).

9. C. The COCP contains both oestrogen and progestogen. It is an effective contraception but

must not be prescribed to patients with certain conditions. Patients with a migraine should not be prescribed the COCP, because of the risk of an ischaemic stroke, therefore answer C is the correct answer. Answer A is incorrect. Asthma is not a contraindication to the COCP. Answer B is incorrect. It is hypertension that is a contraindication to the COCP again because of the risk of a stroke. Answer D is incorrect. Having had a previous pregnancy is not a contraindication to the COCP. Liver disease is a contraindication to the COCP, not renal disease thus answer E is incorrect (refer to p. 107).

10. D. Phenytoin is a cytochrome p450 inducer and consequently, the metabolism of the progesterone-only pill is increased, reducing the contraceptive effect. Answer A (amiodarone), B (ciprofloxacin), C (erythromycin) and E (sodium valproate) are all cytochrome P450 inhibitors and subsequently the metabolism of the progesterone-only pill is reduced.

11. A. Bisphosphonates, of which alendronate is an example, are used first line for the prevention and treatment of osteoporosis. It is contraindicated in severe renal impairment. Atypical femoral fractures can develop if taking long-term bisphosphonate treatment. This complication can also occur in patients taking denosumab (refer to p. 111). Answer B is incorrect. Ergocalciferol is the inactive form of vitamin D which helps the gastrointestinal tract absorb calcium. It is used in the treatment of osteoporosis but is not known to cause atypical fractures. Answer C is incorrect. Raloxifene stimulates osteoblasts and inhibits osteoclasts and is used as third-line management of osteoporosis. It is contraindicated in patients who have had a previous venous thromboembolism but is not known to cause atypical fractures. Answer D is incorrect. Strontium is prescribed by specialists for the treatment of severe osteoporosis. Answer E is incorrect. Teriparatide is a recombinant parathyroid hormone, which when given in small doses stimulates osteoblast activity. It causes a headache and arthralgia but not atypical fractures (refer to p. 112).

12. B. Bendroflumethiazide, a thiazide diuretic used in the management of hypertension and is known to cause hyperglycaemia, particularly in at-risk patients. It is unclear how, but the current understanding is that thiazide diuretics induce hypokalaemia. The K+ deficiency is known to inhibit insulin secretion by the pancreas, thus blood sugar levels are not reduced as normal (refer to Chapter 5). Allopurinol, answer A, is used in the prophylaxis of gout and of uric acid stones but is not known to cause hyperglycaemia. Celecoxib (answer C) is an NSAID used in the management of inflammation associated with severe osteoarthritis. It can cause several side effects including bleeding, stomach ulcers and kidney

failure but it is not known to cause hyperglycaemia. Paracetamol (answer D) is used to manage pain and is not known to cause hyperglycaemia. Ramipril, answer E, is an angiotensin-converting enzyme inhibitor used in the treatment of hypertension but is not known to cause hyperglycaemia. Statins (used in the treatment of hypercholesterolaemia) and steroids (used in the treatment of inflammation) can also cause hyperglycaemia and blood glucose levels should be monitored in patients started on these medications.

Chapter 8 Central nervous system

1. A. Levodopa is usually given for symptom control in patients with newly diagnosed Parkinson disease. However, it is an immediate precursor of dopamine and penetrates the blood barrier. It is then carboxylated to dopamine by dopa decarboxylase and therefore answer D is incorrect (refer to p. 114). Carbidopa is the correct answer. This drug inhibits dopa decarboxylase in the periphery and cannot cross the blood-brain barrier. This inhibits the extracerebral conversion of L-dopa to dopamine. It is often combined with levodopa as co-careldopa and given to most patients to minimize adverse effects (refer to p. 115) and is an effective treatment for Parkinson disease. Answer B is incorrect. Domperidone is a dopamine agonist that blocks the stimulation of dopamine receptors in the periphery (refer to p. 115). Answer C is incorrect. Entacapone is a COMT inhibitor, which inhibits dopamine degradation in the CNS and does not affect dopa decarboxylase (refer to p. 116). Answer E is incorrect. Selegiline is a monoamine oxidase inhibitor. MAOB enzyme is normally responsible for the degradation of dopamine but this is inhibited by selegiline (refer to p. 7).

2. C. Benzodiazepines have several adverse effects; drowsiness, ataxia and reduced psychomotor performance are common. Therefore answer C is correct. Given this, patients taking benzodiazepines should take care when driving, so answer A is not the correct answer. Answer B is incorrect. Taking benzodiazepines with alcohol can potentiate the CNS depressants effects and can result in respiratory depression. Answer D is incorrect. If a patient takes a benzodiazepine only overdose, this can be reversed with flumazenil. Answer E is incorrect. Patients taking benzodiazepines for more than 4 to 6 weeks can become dependent and as such if stopped abruptly can result in a withdrawal syndrome, therefore patients should only be prescribed short courses or benzodiazepines should be withdrawn slowly (refer to pp. 118–119).

3. D. Propanolol is a beta-adrenoceptor blocker and can be very effective in alleviating the somatic manifestations of anxiety caused by marked

sympathetic arousal. Propranolol blocks excessive catecholamine release. However, they also cause bronchoconstriction and should be avoided in patients with asthma (refer to p. 120). Answer A is incorrect. Buspirone is a serotonergic (5-HT1A) agonist indicated for the short-term relief of generalized anxiety disorder. It is not particularly helpful in the somatic manifestations of performance related anxiety (refer to p. 120). Answer B is incorrect. Midazolam is a benzodiazepine. While short-acting benzodiazepines (e.g., diazepam) are useful in short-courses for treating anxiety, midazolam has a slower onset and longer half-life and is typically used in the cessation of status epilepticus or in anaesthesia (refer to p. 133). Answer C is incorrect. Pheobarbital is a barbiturate and acts to increase GABA-mediated inhibition on the GABAA receptor. Barbiturates can be used to reduce anxiety but are not commonly prescribed because of the significant adverse effects associated with them (e.g., respiratory failure) (refer to p. 133). Answer E is incorrect. Zolpidem is a newer-generation hypnotic that is typically used to manage insomnia rather than anxiety.

4. B. Citalopram is an example of an SSRI. SSRIs are usually first line for moderate to severe depression alongside psychological therapies. They block serotonin transporters, which inhibits serotonin reuptake into nerve terminals from the synaptic cleft. It would be important for the GP to warn the patient of increased anxiety and agitation during the early stages of treatment (refer to p. 122). Answer A is incorrect. Amitriptyline is a TCA. TCAs are used as second-line or third-line treatment of depression (refer to p. 122). Answer C is incorrect. Mirtazapine is an atypical antidepressant that has α2-adrenoceptor-blocking activity, which results in an increase in the amount of noradrenaline in the synaptic cleft (refer to p. 124). Answer D is incorrect. Moclobemide is an example of a reversible inhibitor of MAOA. MAO inhibitors block the action of enzymes that metabolize the monoamines and have antidepressant properties. They are particularly effective in patients with atypical or hysterical features. However, given their dietary and drug interactions, are reserved for refractory depression in most cases (refer to p. 124). Answer E is incorrect. Venlafaxine is an SNRI and is contraindicated in patients with hypertension. This is because SNRIs increase blood pressure. It is also prescribed as a second-line treatment if two SSRIs are unable to control the depressive symptoms (refer to p. 123).

5. E. Before prescribing lithium, a patient must have their renal function checked. Lithium is renally excreted and should not be given to patients with renal impairment because there is a significant risk of lithium toxicity. Answer E is correct. Thyroid function

tests should be performed before starting treatment and every 6 to 12 months because lithium can cause hypothyroidism. Answer A is incorrect. Although a full blood count is useful to have before starting any medication, it is not essential to check, unlike urea and electrolytes (U+Es) and thyroid function tests. Answer B is incorrect. Checking liver function tests is important when commencing any medication but because lithium is renally excreted, checking U+Es is more important. Answer C is incorrect. Lithium causes many drug interactions and side effects. It is imperative that lithium levels are checked at least every 3 months and during any intercurrent illness, that renal function and thyroid function are checked at baseline and 6 to 12 monthly. Answer D is incorrect. Although checking parathyroid hormone and calcium is worth doing, it is not essential to do before prescribing lithium. Note that before prescribing lithium it is important to also do an EKG and check a patient's weight because lithium can cause cardiac arrhythmias and weight gain (refer to p. 124).

6. B. Lithium is a commonly used mood stabilizer and although its mechanism is unclear, it is useful in the treatment of mania and bipolar disorder. However, lithium has a long half-life and a narrow therapeutic index. It is renally excreted and therefore should be used with caution in patients with renal impairment, and drugs that may affect kidney function should be avoided. Answer A. Amlodipine, a calcium channel antagonist, is an appropriate hypertensive because it is not known to cause a rise in plasma lithium concentrations. Answers B and C are incorrect. Bendroflumethiazide is a thiazide diuretic and furosemide is a loop diuretic. Diuretics promote renal sodium loss and affect reabsorption at renal tubules. Their pharmacological action can result in an increase in plasma lithium resulting in toxicity; vomiting, tremor, ataxia and drowsiness. Answers D and E are incorrect. Losartan, an angiotensin-receptor blocker, and ramipril, an angiotensin–converting enzyme (ACE) inhibitor reduce the glomerular filtration rate and enhance tubular reabsorption of lithium, thus increasing the risk of lithium toxicity. Therefore diuretics and ACE inhibitors should be avoided in patients taking lithium. If they have to be prescribed, careful monitoring of renal function and lithium levels should be undertaken. Note that NSAIDs also affect kidney function and increase the risk of toxicity (refer to p. 124 and Chapter 5).

7. D. Answer D is correct. Moclobemide is safe to give in patients with cardiovascular disease. MAO inhibitors, such as moclobemide, are useful in the treatment of depression or phobias with atypical or hysterical features. However, TCAs should be avoided in patients with cardiovascular disease given that they can cause conduction abnormalities. Answer A is

incorrect. Moclobemide should not be coprescribed with SSRIs (e.g., fluoxetine) because the combination can cause a potentially fatal serotonergic syndrome of hyperthermia, tremor, agitation, sweating and dilated pupils, which can result in cardiovascular collapse (refer to p. 122). Answer B is incorrect. TCAs (e.g., amitriptyline and imipramine) should be used cautiously in patients with epilepsy because they lower the seizure threshold. Moclobemide is not known to cause significant problems in patients with epilepsy (refer to p. 129). Answer C is incorrect. Moclobemide blocks the action of MAOA and MAOB enzyme, involved in the metabolism of the monoamines. MAO in the gut wall and liver normally breaks down ingested tyramine but when MAO is inhibited, tyramine causes the release of noradrenaline within the circulation, resulting in a potentially fatal rise in blood pressure. Cough mixture contains sympathomimetic amines and therefore should be avoided because of the significant risk of severe hypertension. Diets rich in cheese and game should be avoided for the same reasons (refer to p. 124). Answer E is incorrect. Moclobemide causes a dry mouth, blurred vision and postural hypotension as a result of the muscarinic and sympathetic blockade. TCAs cause weight gain in addition to blurred vision and dry mouth (refer to p. 124).

8. D. Answer D is correct because sodium valproate is often used as first line in the treatment of tonic-clonic seizures (as described in the question). It blocks use-dependent voltage-gated sodium channels while also increasing the GABA content of the brain when given over a prolonged period. Sodium valproate should not be given to patients with hepatic dysfunction (refer to p. 132). Answer A is incorrect. Ethosuximide inhibits T-type calcium channels and dampens down the thalamocortical oscillations that are critical in the generation of absence seizures. Ethosuximide can make tonic-clonic seizures worse (refer to p. 133). Answer B is incorrect. Lamotrigine, one of the newer anticonvulsants, inhibits the release of glutamate (refer to p. 133). Answer C is incorrect. Phenytoin does block use-dependent voltage-gated sodium channels but is no longer commonly used as first-line treatment of epilepsy given its poor side effect profile and narrow therapeutic window (refer to p. 132). Answer E is incorrect. Vigabatrin inhibits GABA degradation in the CNS through inhibition of GABA transaminase, the enzyme normally responsible for the metabolism of GABA within the neurone (refer to p. 44).

Chapter 9 Drug misuse

1. C. Cannabis causes an altered state of consciousness and users feel "high", euphoric and socially uninhibited. Answer A is incorrect.

Cannabis causes a tachycardia and dilated pupils. Answer B is incorrect. Cannabis stimulates appetite and users often get the "munchies". Answer D is incorrect. Cannabis is used to treat spasticity in multiple sclerosis and as an antiemetic in certain situations. Opioids are used clinically as analgesics. Cannabis is typically smoked or taken orally with food, it is not injected, and therefore answer E is incorrect. Negative experiences include anxiety, paranoid thoughts and self-consciousness. Long-term use of cannabis increases the risk of developing schizophrenia (refer to pp. 143–144).

2. E. Opioid withdrawal results in users feeling irritable, distressed and restless. Answer A is therefore incorrect. Answer B is incorrect as appetite is unchanged acutely. Autonomic cold turkey symptoms include fever, sweating and piloerection; therefore answer C is incorrect. Answer D is incorrect. Patients have dilated pupils when they are withdrawing. Patients who have opioid toxicity may have constricted pupils (refer to p. 143).

3. E. Varenicline is a partial agonist at nicotinic acetylcholine receptors and reduces the craving for nicotine. It is safe to give to patients with epilepsy. It causes abnormal dreams, headaches and flatulence (refer to p. 142). Answer A is incorrect. Bupropion, although it reduces nicotine craving through selective inhibition of the neuronal uptake of noradrenaline and dopamine, is contraindicated in patients with epilepsy because it can lower the seizure threshold (refer to p. 142). Answer B is incorrect. Disulfiram is used to help patients stay off drinking alcohol (refer to p. 142). Answer C is incorrect. Flumazenil is a benzodiazepine receptor antagonist. Answer D is incorrect. Ethanol is used as an antidote to methanol poisoning (refer to p. 142).

Chapter 10 Pain and anaesthesia

1. C. This gentleman is currently on step 1 of the WHO analgesic ladder; he is taking a nonopioid (paracetamol) and an adjuvant (ibuprofen). Given that his pain is persisting, his analgesia should involve step 2; a weak opioid (codeine), a nonopioid (paracetamol) and an adjuvant if it is working and there are no contraindications (ibuprofen), therefore answer C is correct. Answer A is incorrect; aspirin is not a weak opioid. Answer B is incorrect; morphine is a strong opioid that should be given when pain is increasing despite the analgesia given at step 2 or when it is very severe. Answer D is incorrect, given that the patient is at step 2 not step 3 on the WHO ladder. In addition, the ibuprofen should continue, given that there are no contraindications and it is an antiinflammatory that is useful for osteoarthritic pain. It is important for

patients with pain to take regular paracetamol as a form of analgesia and thus just ibuprofen and codeine is not enough (refer to Fig 10.1 on p. 145).

2. B. Mr Jones requires opioid analgesia given the severity of his pain and he requires it to act quickly. He also requires medication that is not, predominantly, excreted renally given his acute kidney injury as evidenced by the raised creatinine. Fentanyl is a selective μ receptor agonist that is mainly metabolized by the liver. It has a rapid onset of action (5 minutes) when absorbed buccally. It has an extensive first-pass metabolism so is not especially effective when given orally. Therefore, fentanyl lozenges are the best as required medication for Mr Jones' breakthrough pain, given his renal impairment (refer to p. 147). The other options listed are inappropriate because they accumulate in renal impairment. If the renal function was normal, diamorphine (answer A) is a helpful medication to use for breakthrough pain, given its rapid onset. Morphine sulphate and oxycodone (answer D and E) have a slightly longer onset of action and are less useful for pain that comes on quickly. Methadone (answer C) is used predominantly to help misusers wean themselves off morphine or diamorphine.

3. E. Flushing (answer E) is caused by the histamine release associated with opioid analgesia. Answer A is incorrect; opioids suppress a cough. Answer B is incorrect; opioids cause constipation (not diarrhoea) because of the stimulation of cholinergic activity in the gut wall ganglia, resulting in smooth wall spasm. Answer C is incorrect; opioids stimulate the parasympathetic third cranial nerve nucleus, which results in pupillary constriction. Patients with opioid toxicity present with "pinpoint" pupils. Answer D is incorrect; opioids cause a reduction in the sensitivity of the respiratory centre to carbon dioxide, leading to shallow and slow respiration. This can cause the serious adverse effect of respiratory depression. Opioids also cause pancreatic stasis, drowsiness, sedation and vomiting (refer to pp. 147–148).

4. A. Sumatriptan is a 5-HT1 receptor agonist and is thought to constrict the dilated arteries associated with migraines. Triptan medication can cause chest tightness and a tingling sensation. Answer B is incorrect. Pizotifen is a 5-HT1 receptor antagonist. However, it is used in the prophylaxis of a migraine because it can reduce the vascular inflammation associated with migraines (refer to p. 149). Answer C is incorrect. β-Receptor antagonists are used in the prophylaxis of a migraine, but this is not the action of sumatriptan. Answer D is incorrect. Nonsteroidal antiinflammatories (e.g., ibuprofen) are used as the treatment for acute migrainous attacks. Answer E is incorrect. Serotonin-noradrenaline reuptake inhibitor (e.g., amitriptyline) is a tricyclic antidepressant,

which is sometimes used in the prophylaxis of a migraine, but again is not the mechanism of action of sumatriptan (refer to p. 149).

5. B. Isoflurane is used in the maintenance of anaesthesia but has fewer effects upon the cardiorespiratory system (as compared with halothane) and therefore is an appropriate medication to use. However, isoflurane can be an irritant to the respiratory tract causing cough and laryngospasm. It can also precipitate myocardial ischaemia in patients with coronary disease (refer to p. 156). Answer A is incorrect. Although enflurane is an inhalational anaesthetic used in the maintenance of anaesthesia, it is contraindicated in patients with epilepsy and therefore should be avoided in this patient. Answer C is incorrect. Halothane is used as an inhalational maintenance anaesthetic; however, it has a narrow therapeutic window and there is a risk of cardiorespiratory depression in addition to severe hepatic necrosis (refer to p. 155). It has therefore largely been replaced by isoflurane or sevoflurane. Answer D is incorrect. Etomidate, given intravenously, is not used in the maintenance of anaesthesia but is given for rapid induction of general anaesthesia (refer to p. 154). Answer E is incorrect. Ketamine, given intravenously, can be used to maintain anaesthesia but given the high incidence of dysphoria and hallucinations in adults, it is not commonly used (refer to p. 154).

Chapter 11 Inflammation, allergic diseases and immunosuppression

1. D. Ibuprofen is an example of a NSAID. It should be avoided in patients with renal impairment and gastrointestinal ulceration because of its effects on platelets, gastric mucosa and renal vasculature (refer to Box 11.5). Therefore answers A and C are incorrect. In some patients with asthma, taking NSAIDs can induce bronchospasm and thus should be used with caution in this patient population. Therefore answer B is incorrect. NSAIDs can cause liver disorders, rarely and thus should be used cautiously in patients with liver failure. Ibuprofen and other NSAIDs are used for the treatment of joint inflammation, so answer D is correct (refer to Box 11.5).

2. E. Hydroxychloroquine is a DMARD and one of the antimalarial medications. The major adverse effect is retinal toxicity and thus patients should have their vision monitored regularly while taking hydroxychloroquine. Gold salts can cause diarrhoea, ulceration and bone marrow suppression; therefore, answer A is incorrect (refer to p. 163). Answer B is incorrect. Sulfasalazine has been reported as causing oligospermia (refer to p. 163). Answer C is incorrect. Steroids (e.g., prednisolone) cause thinning of the skin

(refer to p. 167). Answer D is incorrect. Penicillamine causes a transient loss of taste in addition to bone marrow suppression.

3. E. Adalimumab is a monoclonal antibody that binds TNF-α and suppresses the immune system. It can therefore lead to reactivation of old tuberculosis and thus a history of tuberculosis should be excluded before starting therapy. Adalimumab is also contraindicated in patients with heart failure and in females who are pregnant or breastfeeding. Answers A to D are not reasons to exclude the prescription of monoclonal antibodies.

4. E. Patients with psoriasis should be given emollients to use liberally and frequently to help hydrate the skin. First-line therapy for psoriasis includes topical therapies (corticosteroids, vitamin D analogues and dithranol with tar preparations). Second-line therapy includes phototherapy, psoralen and systemic agents such as cyclosporine and methotrexate (answer B is therefore incorrect). Third-line treatment is with TNF antagonists adalimumab and etanercept. Answer E is correct. Coal tar modifies keratinisation but adverse effects include skin irritation, acne-like eruption and photosensitivity (refer to p. 167). Answer A is incorrect. Clobetasone butyrate is a moderately potent topical steroid, a very potent steroid is clobetasol propionate (refer to Box 11.11). Answer C is incorrect. Dithranol and coal tar should not be used in patients with pustular psoriasis (refer to p. 167). Answer D is incorrect. Calcipotriol is a vitamin D analogue that inhibits epidermal proliferation and keratinocyte differentiation. Given its involvement in vitamin D metabolism, it should not be given to patients with disorders of calcium (refer to p. 167).

5. C. This scenario indicates an anaphylactic reaction to penicillin. Treatment involves intramuscular adrenaline (therefore answer E is incorrect) that acts at α2-receptors to cause vasoconstriction and β2-receptors to cause bronchodilation (therefore answer C is correct). Intravenous adrenaline may cause a patient's heart to stop because of a huge dose of adrenaline reaching the heart, resulting in a fast arrhythmia and should be avoided. Bronchoconstriction is caused by prostaglandins, not histamine, therefore answer A is incorrect (refer to Box 11.13). An anaphylactic reaction is mediated by IgE antibodies (not IgA) and is a type I hypersensitivity reaction (not type II). Therefore answer B is incorrect. Promethazine is an old, sedative H1-receptor antagonist and therefore answer D is incorrect (refer to p. 169).

Chapter 12 Infectious diseases

1. B. Gentamicin (an aminoglycoside) is a protein synthesis inhibitor, which is useful against gram-negative bacteria. It irreversibly binds the 30S portion of the bacterial ribosome, inhibiting the translation of mRNA to protein. Gentamicin is bactericidal and is used in the treatment of severe urine infections and bacterial endocarditis (refer to pp. 177–178). Tetracyclines (refer to p. 178), macrolides (refer to p. 179) and clindamycin (refer to p. 179) are also protein synthesis inhibitors.

Co-amoxiclav and meropenem (refer to p. 4) are cell wall synthesis inhibitors so answers A & C are incorrect. Metronidazole inhibits nucleic acid and DNA synthesis so answer D is incorrect (refer to p. 179). Metronidazole is used in the treatment of anaerobic bacteria (e.g., in patients with aspiration pneumonia or intraabdominal sepsis). Trimethoprim is an antifolate and affects the synthesis of purines and bacteria DNA, thus answer E is incorrect (refer to p. 177).

2. E. Vancomycin is a glycopeptide used in the treatment of severe C. difficile pseudomembranous colitis. It has been associated with ototoxicity, nephrotoxicity and red man syndrome, particularly at high plasma doses. It is therefore essential to check the level of the vancomycin when treating patients (refer to pp. 177–178). Gentamicin (an aminoglycoside) also causes nephrotoxicity and ototoxicity (refer to pp. 177–178). Levofloxacin (a quinolone) is known to cause gastrointestinal upset and tendon damage (refer to p. 177), and so answer B is incorrect. Metronidazole also causes gastrointestinal upset and alcohol should not be consumed while taking it (refer to p. 179), therefore answer C is incorrect. Erythromycin and trimethoprim are not known to cause ototoxicity and nephrotoxicity, therefore answers C, A, and D are incorrect. Erythromycin (a macrolide effective against most gram-positive bacteria) may cause liver damage and jaundice if used long term (refer to p. 179) and trimethoprim may cause a severe rash, but it is more likely to be Stevens-Johnson syndrome. It can also cause a transient rise in creatinine and an acute kidney injury (refer to p. 177).

3. A. This patient's history suggests a sexually transmitted infection, such as chlamydia. Azithromycin (a macrolide) can be given as a one-off dose for uncomplicated chlamydial infections of the genital tract. Macrolides reversibly bind to the 50S subunit of the bacterial ribosome and affect protein synthesis. They are also used as an effective alternative in penicillin-sensitive patients (refer to p. 179). Ciprofloxacin (a quinolone) is usually used in patients with pyelonephritis and they present more acutely unwell with flank and suprapubic pain, pyrexia and rigors. Answer B is therefore incorrect. Co-amoxiclav is usually prescribed in patients with lower respiratory tract infections (refer to p. 174) therefore answer C is incorrect. Meropenem (answer

D) is used as a second-line or third-line antibiotic and is not used in the treatment of chlamydia (refer to p. 177). Trimethoprim, although used in the treatment of UTIs, is not typically used in the treatment of chlamydia (refer to p. 177). Therefore answer E is incorrect. Doxycycline, however, is also used in the treatment of chlamydia (refer to p. 178).

4. B. Clarithromycin is a macrolide antibiotic used in the treatment of respiratory infections, particularly in patients allergic to penicillin. However, it is cytochrome p450 enzyme inhibitor and can, therefore reduce the effectiveness of warfarin. Macrolides can also cause cholestatic hepatitis. Monitoring of liver function tests and the INR should be considered in patients. Answers A and B are incorrect. Although amoxicillin and co-amoxiclav are used in the treatment of lower respiratory tract infections (LRTIs), it would not be sensible to give these antibiotics in a patient with an allergy to penicillin (refer to p. 174). Co-trimoxazole (answer D) is used in the treatment of respiratory infections but is used predominantly for the treatment of P. jiroveci pneumonia, most commonly seen in patients who are immunocompromized (refer to p. 192). Answer E is incorrect. Although levofloxacin is sometimes used in severe LRTIs, it is not known to affect the cytochrome p450 enzyme (refer to p. 177).

5. D. Answer A is incorrect because not treating the asymptomatic bacteriuria can result in cystitis or pyelonephritis for the mother or result in reduced intrauterine growth of the foetus and premature labour and neonatal delivery. Trimethoprim (answer B) is contraindicated in the first and second trimester of pregnancy because it is teratogenic (refer to p. 177). Doxycycline (answer C) is also incorrect because it is not a typically used antibiotic in the treatment of a urinary tract infection but importantly can cause impaired bone growth and dental hypoplasia, thus it is contraindicated in pregnant and breastfeeding women (refer to p. 178). Nitrofurantoin is the safest of the antibiotics listed for treatment of the asymptomatic bacteriuria (refer to pp. 179–180). However, it should be avoided in the third trimester because it can cause neonatal haemolysis. Ciprofloxacin (answer E) should be avoided because there is a theoretic risk of causing neonatal joint problems if taken during pregnancy.

6. E. Rifampicin inhibits DNA-dependent RNA polymerase causing a bactericidal effect in the treatment of tuberculosis. However, it is known to cause an orange discolouration of bodily fluids. In addition, patients taking rifampicin must be cautious when taking other medications because rifampicin is a cytochrome p450 enzyme inhibitor (refer to p. 18). Ethambutol is bacteriostatic and given orally. It causes a reversible optic neuritis and therefore answer A is the incorrect answer. Isoniazid is bactericidal

and can be hepatotoxic, cause agranulocytosis and a peripheral neuropathy. Therefore answer B is incorrect. Pyridoxine (answer D) is also incorrect because it is given to help reduce the risk of peripheral neuritis associated with isoniazid. Pyrazinamide is the final medication used to treat tuberculosis and it causes hepatotoxicity and is contraindicated in patients with gout because it is known to raise plasma urate levels. Therefore pyrazinamide, answer C, is incorrect (refer to p. 180).

7. C. Nevirapine is a nonnucleoside reverse transcriptase inhibitor, similar to efavirenz. Both these medications are given orally and can cause a rash, dizziness and headache. Nonnucleoside reverse transcriptase inhibitor also induce the cytochrome p450 enzyme (refer to p. 185). Lamivudine, didanosine and zidovudine are nucleoside reverse transcriptase inhibitors and therefore answers A, B and E are incorrect. Nucleoside reverse transcriptase inhibitors are given orally in the management of HIV infection and can cause bone marrow suppression, resulting in anaemia and neutropenia in addition to nausea, headaches and myalgia (refer to p. 184). Ritanovir is a protease inhibitor therefore answer D is incorrect. Protease inhibitors prevent the virus-specific protease of HIV cleaving the inert polyprotein product of translation into various structural and functional proteins and are used in the management of HIV infections in combinations with nucleoside reverse transcriptase inhibitor (refer to p. 184).

8. E. Rubella, measles, mumps and oral polio are vaccines containing live attenuated viruses. Diphtheria vaccine contains inactivated bacterial toxins, so answer A is incorrect. Hepatitis A and parenteral polio are vaccines made up of inactivated viruses and therefore answers B and D are incorrect. Hepatitis B vaccine is genetically engineered thus answer C is incorrect (refer to p. 194).

9. C. Mebendazole is used in the treatment of pinworm. It is an example of the benzimidazole family, which prevents the polymerisation of microtubules. They should not be given to pregnant women (refer to p. 193).

    Ivermectin is used in the treatment of tapeworm by causing tonic paralysis of the worm's peripheral muscle system. It is also used in the treatment of strongyloides infection, but not pinworm. Therefore answer A is incorrect (refer to p. 194). Levamisole is used in the treatment of A. lumbricoides round worm infection, thus answer B is incorrect. It stimulates nicotinic receptors at the neuromuscular junction and results in a spastic paralysis and expulsion of the worm (refer to p. 194). Niclosamide is also used in the treatment of tapeworm (refer to p. 192) and therefore answer D is incorrect. Praziquantel is the drug of choice for all schiztosome infections and not pinworms, therefore answer E is incorrect.

10. A. Chloroquine is a schizonticide and is considered safe to use in pregnant women. It does not affect hypnozoites and in most areas P. falciparum is resistant to chloroquine, necessitating combination chemoprophylaxis with antifolates (refer to p. 190). Mefloquine (answer C) is incorrect. It is not considered safe in pregnancy because it can cause foetal abnormalities. Mefloquine is also a schizonticide but has no effect on gametocytes of P. falciparum. Nevertheless, it is used as chemoprophylaxis (refer to p. 190). Quinine (the same family as mefloquine) is however safe in pregnancy and is the treatment of choice for falciparum malaria resistant to chloroquine. Dapsone and sulphonamide are both antifolates and affect all growing stages of the malarial parasite. However, because they are antifolates they should be avoided in pregnancy, therefore answers B and E are incorrect. Primaquine is effective against hypnozoites and gametocytes. It is useful in the radical cure of relapsing malarias and prevention of transmission of P. falciparum. However, it is contraindicated in pregnancy and thus answer D is incorrect (refer to p. 191).

Chapter 13 Cancer

1. C. Melphalan is an alkylating agent used to treat haematological malignancies (refer to p. 199). Cisplatin is a platinum compound that inhibits DNA synthesis; therefore answer A is incorrect. Dactinomycin is a cytotoxic antibiotic that interferes with RNA polymerase and therefore answer B is incorrect. Methotrexate is a folate antagonist, antimetabolite medication and therefore answer D is incorrect (refer to p. 199). Vinblastine is a vinca alkaloid that inhibits the polymerisation of microtubules (refer to p. 200) and therefore answer E is incorrect.

2. B. Cyclophosphamide causes haemorrhagic cystitis because a urinary metabolite of cyclophosphamide, acrolein causes urothelial toxicity. This can be reduced by high fluid intake concomitantly. Cyclophosphamide can also cause interstitial pulmonary fibrosis, anorexia, pancreatitis and at high doses, cardiotoxicity (refer to p. 199). Chlorambucil, used in the treatment of haematological malignancies, can cause bone marrow suppression and severe widespread rash but is not known to cause haemorrhagic cystitis, therefore answer A is incorrect. Doxorubicin causes generalized toxicity and dose-dependent cardiotoxicity but not haemorrhagic cystitis, therefore answer C is incorrect (refer to pp. 199–200). Melphalan is an alkylating agent, similar to cyclophosphamide but is not known to cause haemorrhagic cystitis, therefore

answer D is incorrect (refer to p. 199). Methotrexate is an antimetabolite, which competitively inhibits dihydrofolate reductase, inhibiting the synthesis of DNA. It causes myelosuppression rather than haemorrhagic cystitis, therefore answer E is incorrect (refer to p. 199).

3. C. Vincristine is a vinca alkaloid or mitotic inhibitor and this class of chemotherapy is known to cause neurological problems because tubulin polymerisation is relatively indiscriminate (refer to p. 9). Bleomycin is not known to cause neuropathy therefore answer A is incorrect. Bleomycin is used in the treatment of lymphoma but typically causes pulmonary fibrosis (refer to pp. 199–200). Methotrexate is not known to cause neuropathy, it more commonly causes myelosuppression, mucositis and pneumonitis thus answer B is incorrect (refer to p. 199). Mercaptopurine is converted into a fraudulent purine nucleotide that impairs DNA synthesis and is used as maintenance therapy for acute leukaemia and does not commonly cause neurotoxicity, therefore answer C is incorrect (refer to p. 199). Rituximab is used in the treatment of lymphoma, but it is not known to cause neuropathies thus answer D is incorrect. It commonly causes hypotension and fever during infusion and can worsen cardiovascular disease (refer to p. 203).

4. C. The BCR-ABL fusion gene is found in most patients with chronic myeloid leukaemia (CML) and in some patients with acute lymphoblastic leukaemia, found on chromosome 22 and is known as the Philadelphia chromosome. Imatinib is a BCR-ABL tyrosine kinase inhibitor, which targets the abnormal tyrosine kinase, created by the Philadelphia chromosome abnormality. Therefore imatinib is the most appropriate treatment in this scenario (refer to p. 201). Everolimus acts as an mTOR kinase inhibitor and is not known to treat CML, therefore answer A is incorrect (refer to p. 201). Hydroxyurea is used in the treatment of CML and polycythaemia rubra vera, but it acts through the inhibition of ribonucleotide reductase rather than on the BCR-ABL gene, therefore answer B is incorrect (refer to p. 201). Oxaliplatin is a platinum compound that inhibits DNA synthesis and is used in the treatment of lung, cervical, bladder and testicular cancers, therefore answer D is incorrect (refer to p. 200). Procarbazine is a methyl-hydrazine derivative with monoamine oxidase inhibitor actions and cytotoxicity. It inhibits DNA and RNA synthesis and is used in the treatment of Hodgkin lymphoma. It causes an adverse reaction with alcohol, therefore answer E is incorrect (refer to p. 201).

5. D. Rituximab lyses B lymphocyte by its effect on the CD20 protein expressed on the surface of white blood

cells. It is given via an infusion for the treatment of lymphoma. Cetuximab is licensed for the treatment of metastatic colorectal cancers overexpressing epidermal growth factor receptors, therefore answer A is incorrect. Patients who have EGFR mutations overexpressed lung cancers are treated with erlotinib which inhibits the intracellular phosphorylation of tyrosine kinase associated with the EGFR, therefore answer B is incorrect.

Nivolumab is an anti-PDL1 antibody that has been approved for the treatment of advanced melanoma, therefore answer C is incorrect. Patients with HER2 receptor-positive breast cancer are treated with trastuzumab, which targets the HER2 receptor and cells undergo arrest during the G1 phase of the cell cycle so there is a reduced proliferation of the malignant cells, therefore answer E is incorrect.

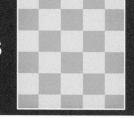

Chapter 1 Introduction to Pharmacology
Receptor interactions and pharmacokinetics

1. C. Activation of adenylyl cyclase. Continued activation of adenylyl cyclase of the cholera toxin results in secretion of large amounts of fluid.
2. A. Drug absorption. Drugs that are usually absorbed in the small intestine and enter the portal circulation where they are extensively metabolized, which results in less of the drug entering the systemic circulation. This is known as first pass metabolism. Lidocaine has a high degree of first past metabolism and therefore must be given via another route.
3. G. Competitive antagonist. Naloxone acts as a competitive antagonist at the opioid receptors and thus reduces the ability of the agonist, heroin, to activate the receptor.
4. Q. Phase 2 metabolic reaction. Paracetamol is conjugated with glucuronic acid and sulphate. When high doses of paracetamol are ingested, these pathways become saturated and the drug is metabolized by the mixed function oxidases resulting in the formation of the toxic metabolite N-acetyl-benzoquinone which is inactivated by glutathione. When glutathione is depleted, this toxic metabolite reacts with nucleophilic constituents in the cell leading to necrosis in the liver and kidneys. N-acetylcysteine can be administered because these increase liver glutathione formation and the conjugation reactions.
5. L. Continued inactivation of adenylyl cyclase.
6. I. Drug distribution. Highly lipid soluble drugs such as thiopental will accumulate in fat and their half-life will be much longer in obese patients than in thinner patients.
7. A. Drug absorption. Morphine is a weak base and is highly charged in the stomach, it is poorly and erratically absorbed from the stomach and therefore must be given as an injection or delayed release capsules.
8. P. Phase 1 metabolism. Phenytoin induces the hepatic P450 system, therefore increasing the metabolism of several drugs. Therefore levels may be subtherapeutic rendering them ineffective. This highlights the importance of knowing how drugs are metabolized.
9. O. Pharmacokinetic interaction. NSAIDS bring about this effect by reducing prostaglandin synthesis in the kidney, thus impairing blood flow and consequently decreased excretion of waste and sodium. Thus increasing blood volume and blood pressure because of the pharmacokinetic property of the drug on absorption, distribution, metabolism and excretion.
10. J. Drug excretion. Glomerular filtration, tubular resorption and tubular secretion all determine the extent to which a drug will be excreted by the kidneys which can be reduced in the elderly and in patients with kidney diseases.
11. D. Adherence. For some drugs to be effective, they must be taken at regular intervals to maintain "steady-state" plasma levels. This is particularly important for some antibiotics because the plasma levels need to be sufficient to kill bacteria.

Chapter 2 Peripheral nervous system
Medications – their actions and side effects

1. G. Lidocaine is a local anaesthetic that blocks sodium channels and thus nerve conduction by binding to the sixth transmembrane region of the fourth domain. Small nociceptive (painful) fibres are blocked preferentially because of the high surface to volume ratio. Local anaesthetics are therefore useful as movement and touch are not affected (refer to p. 20).
2. C. Botulinum toxin A can be given via local injection. It inhibits acetylcholine release by inactivating actin, which is necessary for exocytosis. It can cause motor paralysis thus relieving symptoms (refer to p. 22).
3. A. Atracurium is a nondepolarising neuromuscular blocking agent, which acts as a competitive antagonist by binding to the nicotinic acetylcholine receptor. The main side effect is hypotension, but bronchospasm may be a problem in patients with asthma because of histamine release from mast cells (refer to p. 22).
4. D. Clonidine is an α2-adrenoreceptor agonist used in the treatment of hypertensive migraine. It can cause drowsiness and hypotension (refer to Table 2.5).
5. L. Phenylephrine is an α1-adrenoreceptor agonist used in the treatment of nasal decongestion. It can cause hypertension and reflex bradycardia (refer to Table 2.5).
6. I. Neostigmine is an anticholinesterase and can be used to reverse nondepolarising blockers (e.g., atracurium) but not depolarising blockers. It works by inhibiting acetylcholinesterase and thus increases the amount of acetylcholine in the synaptic cleft, enhancing cholinergic transmission.

7. B. Atropine is a muscarinic antagonist which results in tachycardia and thus counteracts the bradycardic effects of depolarising neuromuscular blocking agents, which activate muscarinic receptors (refer to p. 12).

8. I & N. Pyridostigmine is used orally in the treatment of myasthenia gravis and has few parasympathetic actions. The correct answer is physostigmine, which is an anticholinesterase drug that crosses the blood–brain barrier and has selectivity for the postganglionic parasympathetic junction. It can reduce intraocular pressure and thus is used in the treatment of glaucoma. However, side effects include bradycardia, hypotension, excessive secretions and bronchoconstriction (refer to p. 24).

9. J. Phentolamine binds reversibly. Note that phenoxybenzamine is an irreversible antagonist at α-adrenoreceptors. They cause a fall in blood pressure caused by block of α-receptor–mediated vasoconstriction (refer to p. 26).

10. E. Carbidopa inhibits dopa decarboxylase and increases dopamine levels but does not affect noradrenaline synthesis (refer to p. 26).

11. P. Reserpine is a drug used in the treatment of schizophrenia and reduces the stores of noradrenaline presynaptically by preventing the accumulation of noradrenaline in vesicles. The displaced noradrenaline is immediately broken down by monoamine oxidase and is, therefore, unable to exert sympathetic effects (refer to p. 27).

12. K. Phenelzine (monoxidase inhibitor). They prevent the breakdown of leaked catecholamines so that noradrenaline that leaves the vesicle is protected and eventually leaks out from the nerve ending (refer to p. 27).

Chapter 3 Respiratory system

Respiratory system drugs and their side effects and contraindications

1. H. Salbutamol. An adverse effect of salbutamol is tremor (refer to p. 35).

2. D. Montelukast. These are common side effects of Montelukast (refer to p. 37).

3. C. Ipratropium. Benign prostatic hyperplasia and glaucoma are contraindications (refer to p. 37).

4. E. Naloxone. It is used to reverse the effects of opiates (refer to p. 41).

5. A. Aminophylline. It has a narrow therapeutic range and thus levels must be checked frequently (refer to p. 37).

Chapter 4 Cardiovascular system

Mechanism of action of antiarrhythmics

1. H. Lidocaine. Class Ib drugs are given for ventricular arrhythmias following a myocardial infarction (refer to p. 50).

2. B. Amiodarone. Class III drugs are potassium-channel blockers. Amiodarone also blocks sodium and calcium channels (refer to p. 51).

3. L. Verapamil. Class IV drugs that reduce the action potential duration through calcium antagonism (refer to p. 51).

4. E. Digoxin. A cardiac glycoside with antiarrhythmic properties. They are used in the treatment of atrial fibrillation and inhibit the membrane Na/K ATPase of myocytes (refer to p. 47).

5. J. Procainamide. A class Ia drug that is used in the treatment of ventricular arrhythmias (refer to p. 50).

6. F. Flecainide. A class 1c drug that blocks sodium channels similar to class Ia and Ib but shows no preference for refractory channels. It is used in the treatment of atrial fibrillation in patients with structurally normal hearts (refer to p. 50).

7. I. Metoprolol. A class II drug (a β-adrenoceptor antagonist). They increase the refractory period of the AV node and prevent recurrent attacks of supraventricular tachycardias (refer to pp. 50–51).

8. A. Adenosine. This antiarrhythmic is used to help with the diagnosis of supraventricular tachycardia (refer to p. 66).

Side effects and contraindications of cardiovascular medications

1. A. Adenosine (refer to p. 66)
2. M. Procainamide (refer to p. 50)
3. B. Amiodarone (refer to p. 51)
4. O. Verapamil (refer to p. 51)
5. K. Losartan (refer to p. 56)
6. I. Glyceryl trinitrate (refer to p. 52)
7. L. Metoprolol (refer to pp. 50–51)
8. E. Digoxin (refer to p. 47). The cardiac glycosides have a very narrow therapeutic window, and toxicity is therefore relatively common. Effects of cardiac glycosides are increased if plasma potassium decreases, because of reduced competition at the K+ binding side on the NA/K-ATPase. This is clinically important because many diuretics, which are often used to treat heart failure, decrease plasma potassium thereby increasing the risk of glycoside-induced dysrhythmias.
9. N. Spironolactone (refer to p. 48)
10. F. Enoxaparin (refer to p. 65)

Appropriate management

1. A. Adrenaline 1.10,000 intravenously must be given in a cardiac arrest situation. Adrenaline 1.1000 intramuscularly is given in anaphylaxis (refer to p. 59).

2. I. Fondaparinux. This low-molecular-weight heparin is used in the prevention of further clots following a myocardial infarction (refer to p. 65).

3. F. Digoxin. This cardiac glycoside is used in the treatment of atrial fibrillation. For rate control, ß-blockers are commonly prescribed but as this patient has asthma, these are contraindicated. Second-line rate control is then calcium-channel blockers, but given her allergy, this is inappropriate. Digoxin can be used as a treatment for rate control (refer to p. 47).

4. K. Phenoxybenzamine. This is an α-adrenoceptor antagonist which is used in the treatment of phaeochromocytoma-related hypertensive crises. Treatment with ß-blockers (e.g., bisoprolol) is dangerous because the tumour secreted sympathomimetics act unopposed on α-adrenoceptors, increasing both peripheral vascular resistance and blood pressure (refer to p. 58).

5. E. Dipyridamole. This medication inhibits phosphodiesterase enzymes involved in the inhibition of platelet aggregation. It is used in conjunction with aspirin in the prophylaxis of stroke in patients with transient ischaemic attacks (refer to p. 66).

6. G. Ezetimibe. This lipid-lowering medication is indicated when cholesterol remains high despite intensive dietary changes and treatment with statins at high doses. It inhibits the absorption of cholesterol from the duodenum (refer to p. 61). Fish oils are used in the treatment of severely raised triglycerides (refer to p. 61).

Chapter 5 Kidney and urinary system
Mechanism of action and adverse effects of medications

1. P. Sildenafil is contraindicated in patients taking nitrates because both medications cause vasodilation, which can result in severe hypotension (refer to pp. 76–77).

2. B. Amiloride blocks sodium reabsorption by the principal cells, thus reducing the potential difference across the cell, reducing K+ secretion. Whereas spironolactone (answer R) is a potassium-sparing diuretic, it acts through competitive antagonism at aldosterone receptors, reducing Na reabsorption and therefore K+ and H+ secretion (refer to p. 75).

3. L. Lithium is a mood stabilizer given to manage bipolar disorder. However, it can inhibit the action of ADH. ADH is released from the posterior pituitary gland resulting in the increased expression of aquaporins. This increases the amount of water passively reabsorbed thus concentrating the urine. In the presence of lithium, ADH does not exert its effects and thus patients excrete large amounts of dilute urine. Desmopressin (answer D) is an analogue of ADH and thus has the opposite effect to lithium (refer to Clinical Note on p. 71).

4. K. Indapamide is a thiazide diuretic. It inhibits the Na+/Cl– cotransporter. Similar to loop diuretics (answer H) it increases the secretion of K+ and H+ into the collecting ducts but, in contrast, thiazide diuretics decrease Ca2+ excretion by a mechanism possibly involving the stimulation of a Na+/Ca2+ exchange across the basolateral membrane (refer to p. 74).

5. R. Solifenacin is a muscarinic receptor antagonist used in the treatment of urge continence. Given its anticholinergical properties, it is contraindicated in patients with glaucoma (as is oxybutynin and tolterodine) (refer to p. 76).

6. M. Mannitol is an osmotic diuretic and causes a reduction in passive water reabsorption because of its presence within the tubule lumen. Osmotic diuretics, unlike thiazide and loop diuretics, are not used in the treatment of heart failure (refer to p. 75).

7. J. Ibuprofen is a nonsteroidal antiinflammatory (refer to the Clinical note on p. 70) that inhibits prostaglandin production by inhibiting cyclooxygenase. In patients in whom renal blood flow is dependent on vasodilator prostaglandins, ibuprofen can precipitate renal failure. Paracetamol (answer N) has little effect on the kidney and no effect on salt and water retention.

8. P. Sildenafil causes vasodilation because of its inhibition of phosphodiesterase-mediated degradation of cGMP and is used in the treatment of erectile dysfunction but can affect other vascular beds resulting in these symptoms (refer to p. 76). Although alprostadil (answer A) is used in the treatment of erectile dysfunction its main side effects include penile pain and priapism.

9. G. Eplerenone is a potassium-sparing diuretic that acts through competitive aldosterone antagonism whereas amiloride (answer B) works through sodium-channel blockade. The combination of potassium-sparing diuretics and an ACE inhibitor increases the risk of hyperkalaemia. ACE inhibitors cause hyperkalaemia because of their inhibition of the renin-angiotensin aldosterone system (see Chapter 4) whereas potassium-sparing diuretics reduce the secretion of potassium in the late distal tubule and collecting ducts (refer to p. 75).

10. I. Furosemide is a loop diuretic that inhibits the Na+/K+/2Cl– cotransporter. This increases the amount of sodium reaching the collecting duct and thereby increases K+ and H+ secretion. Calcium and magnesium reabsorption is also inhibited, owing to the decrease in potential difference across the cell normally generated from the recycling of potassium. Indapamide is incorrect because it is a thiazide diuretic. Similar to loop diuretics, thiazide diuretics increase the secretion of K+ and H+ into

the collecting ducts but, in contrast, they decrease Ca2+ excretion by a mechanism possibly involving the stimulation of a Na+/Ca2+ exchange across the basolateral membrane.

11. H. Finasteride is a 5α-reductase inhibitor that converts testosterone to the more potent androgen dihydrotestosterone. This inhibition leads to a reduction in prostate size, and improvement of urinary flow. Thus is used in the management of BPH.

12. N. Mirabegron is a selective β agonist that has been licensed recently for treatment of overactive bladder. Solifenacin, although used in patients with overactive bladder, is a muscarinic receptor antagonist. Duloxetine is a serotonin noradrenaline reuptake inhibitor (see Chapter 8) used as second-line treatment for stress incontinence.

Chapter 6 Gastrointestinal system

1. J. Enterochromaffin-like paracrine cells release histamine. Histamine then acts locally on the parietal cells where activation of the H2 receptor results in the stimulation of adenylyl cyclase and the subsequent secretion of acid. Answer T parietal cells is incorrect because they directly secrete acid and answer U peptic cells is incorrect because they secrete digestive enzymes (refer to p. 79).

2. Z. Ursodeoxycholic acid is used in the treatment of gallstones because it reduces cholesterol within bile (refer to p. 28). Cholestyramine (answer D) is incorrect because it acts as an anion exchange resin, binds acids in the gut and prevents their reabsorption as used in treatment of pruritic (refer to p. 89).

3. L. Ispaghula husk is a bulk-forming laxative that stimulates peristaltic activity. It is contraindicated if there is any intestinal obstruction (refer to p. 84). Docusate sodium (answer H) is a faecal softener and is therefore incorrect.

4. V. Pantoprazole is a PPI that irreversibly inhibits H+/K+ ATPase. They are used in the treatment of GORD, peptic ulcers and in combination to eradicate H. pylori. In some patients on multiple medications, PPIs can cause hyponatraemia (refer to p. 81).

5. Q. Metoclopramide. This can cause an oculogyric crisis and torticollis secondary to its dopamine receptor antagonism within the nigrostriatum of the brain, which causes an excess of cholinergic output resulting in the extrapyramidal symptoms. Domperidone (answer I), although a dopamine antagonist, does not penetrate the blood–brain barrier to the same extent as metoclopramide (refer to p. 83).

6. A. Aluminium hydroxide causes constipation and is antacid (refer to p. 82). Answer O magnesium salts cause diarrhoea and therefore is the incorrect answer.

7. P. Mebeverine is an antispasmodic that works to directly relax smooth muscle. Answer W propantheline is incorrect because, although it is used as an antispasmodic in the treatment of irritable bowel syndrome, it is a muscarinic-receptor antagonist (refer to p. 85).

8. Y. Terlipressin is often used in the treatment of oesophageal varices to prevent catastrophic varial haemorrhage (refer to p. 82).

9. C. Biscodyl is a stimulant laxative that takes 15 to 30 minutes to take effect. It is important only to prescribe this medications for short courses to prevent damage to the nerve plexuses within the gut (refer to p. 86).

10. S. Orlistat is licensed in the treatment of obesity but can cause flatulence and abdominal pain. Methycellulose (answer R) works by promoting early satiety to reduce food intake (refer to p. 88).

11. B. Azathioprine is an immunosuppressant used in the management of inflammatory bowel disease. It is metabolized to 6 mercaptopurine (refer to p. 88).

12. M. Lactulose is a semisynthetic disaccharide that produces an osmotic load, increasing the fluid content within the bowel, helping the passage of stool. It can cause flatulence and abdominal discomfort as well as electrolyte disturbance (refer to p. 86).

13. X. Sulfasalazine can cause infertility in males secondary to oligospermia (refer to p. 88).

Chapter 7 Endocrine and reproductive systems

Adverse effects of endocrine drugs

1. I. Octreotide is an analogue of somatostatin, which is used in the treatment of acromegaly as it ihibits growth hormone release. Cholelithiasis (gallstones) is a well-recognized complication (refer to p. 105).

2. D. Clomifene is an antioestrogen used in the treatment of infertility. Ovarian hyperstimulation is a rare complication (refer to p. 108). Tamoxifen (answer K) has antioestrogen effects but is not known to cause ovarian hyperstimulation.

3. A. Alendronate, a bisphosphonate, is used in the treatment of postmenopausal osteoporosis and can cause oesophagitis, ulcers and erosions. Prescribers must advise patients to swallow tablets with a full glass of water and to remain sat upright for at least 30 minutes afterwards. Denosumab (answer E) is used as second-line treatment of osteoporosis but is not known to cause this complication (refer to p. 110).

4. F. Iodide is used in the treatment of a thyrotoxic crisis and inhibits the conversion of T4 to T3. It should

not be given to pregnant or breastfeeding women because it can cause a goitre in infants (refer to p. 8). Carbimazole (answer C) is used in the treatment of hyperthyroidism but is not known to cause impotence, depression and insomnia. Levothyroxine (answer G) is used in the treatment of hypothyroidism.

Chapter 8 Central nervous system

Medications used in the treatment of Parkinson disease, dementia and the eye

1. G. Levodopa can cause cardiac arrhythmias arising from increased catecholamine stimulation following the excessive peripheral metabolism of L-dopa (refer to p. 114).
2. B. Cabergoline is a dopamine agonist effective in treating the motor features of Parkinson disease. Dopamine agonists are commonly prescribed in younger patients because they cause fewer motor fluctuations. However, patients should be warned about the risk of developing compulsive or disinhibited behaviours while taking cabergoline (refer to p. 116). Selegiline (option L) selectively inhibits the MAOB enzyme in the brain normally responsible for the degradation of dopamine and therefore is incorrect (refer to p. 116).
3. K. Procyclidine is an example of an anticholinergic. It acts as an antagonist at muscarinic receptors that mediate cholinergic excitation and is prescribed for patients with Parkinson disease who have a severe tremor (refer to p. 116).
4. H. Memantine selectively inhibits the excessive and pathological activation of NMDA receptors. Memantine can cause a headache, dizziness and constipation and is contraindicated in patients with a history of seizures. Donepezil (option D), although used in the management of mild to moderate Alzheimer dementia, is a cholinesterase inhibitor, which prevents the breakdown of ACh within the synaptic cleft, and therefore is the incorrect answer (refer to p. 117).
5. F. Latanoprost is prescribed in the treatment of open-angle glaucoma because it promotes outflow of aqueous fluid from the anterior chamber via an alternative drainage route (refer to p. 136). Timolol (option M), a beta-adrenoceptor antagonist is also used to reduce intraocular pressure within the eye but is not known to cause brown pigmentation of the iris (refer to p. 134).
6. J. Pilocarpine, a muscarinic antagonist, is used in the management of acute closed angle glaucoma because it causes constriction of the pupil, allowing aqueous fluid to drain from the anterior chamber into the trabecular meshwork. It is also used to reverse mydriasis at the end of an ophthalmic examination (refer to p. 136).

Medications used in the treatment of mood disorders and insomnia

1. G. Mirtazapine is an atypical antidepressant that results in an increased amount of noradrenaline in the synaptic cleft. A dangerous but rare side effect of mirtazapine is agranulocytosis (where the white blood cells become very low). If this occurs, then the medication must be stopped because of the risk of severe infection. Reboxetine (option I) is incorrect because it acts as a selective inhibitor of noradrenaline uptake (refer to p. 124).
2. A. Buspirone is a 5-HT1A agonist that is prescribed orally and given for the short-term relief of generalized anxiety disorder. Adverse effects include dizziness, headache and light-headedness. Sertraline and fluoxetine (option E & K) are incorrect because they are SSRIs (refer to p. 120).
3. J. Risperidone acts as an antagonist at both dopamine and 5-HT receptors. Neuroleptic medications cause a variety of adverse effects as a result of the disruption of dopaminergic pathways (refer to p. 127). The effects are more pronounced with typical neuroleptics but can occur with newer, atypical neuroleptics. (Options C & H are also correct).
4. C. Clozapine acts at dopamine receptors and is an effective medication for the treatment of schizophrenia but has several unpleasant side effects including hypersalivation, sedation, tachycardia and significant weight gain. It is therefore used in severe, longstanding schizophrenia (refer to p. 127).
5. B. Chlordiazepoxide is a benzodiazepine and potentiates the effect of GABA release and has inhibitory effects on postsynaptic cells within the CNS. Although zopiclone (option L), a newer-generation hypnotic, is thought to act on the GABAA receptor, it is not the same site as benzodiazepines, and zopiclone are used in the short-term treatment of insomnia, not acute alcohol withdrawal (refer to p. 119).
6. F. Melatonin acts at the MT1 receptor and improves sleep onset and quality in patients aged over 55 years and in children with autism (refer to p. 121). Zopiclone (option L) is used in the treatment of insomnia but it acts on the GABAA receptor and therefore is the incorrect answer.
7. H. Olanzapine has low affinity for the D2 receptor and high affinity for D1 and D4 receptors as does clozapine. However, olanzapine is usually first line whereas clozapine (option C) is used in refractory cases of schizophrenia and therefore is incorrect (refer to p. 127).
8. D. Flumenazil is a benzodiazepine antagonist and can be given to patients suspected of taking a benzodiazepine overdose. Patients with severe social anxiety may be prescribed short-courses of benzodiazepines (refer to p. 127).

Medications used in the treatment of epilepsy

1. A. Carbamazepine or G. Phenytoin. Both are commonly used anticonvulsants that induce the hepatic cytochrome P450 oxidase enzyme resulting in the increased metabolism of warfarin. This also results in reduced amounts of warfarin, limiting its anticoagulant effects. Female patients on carbamazepine or phenytoin should be warned that oral contraception might be less effective (refer to p. 132).

2. C. Diazepam is a short-acting benzodiazepine that potentiates chloride currents through the GABAA channel complex and is commonly used in the management of status epilepticus. A potentially harmful side effect is respiratory depression (refer to p. 133). Clonazepam (option B) is a longer-acting benzodiazepine and is not commonly used in the management of status epilepticus.

3. A. Carbamazepine is a commonly prescribed anticonvulsant for generalized tonic-clonic seizures. Be aware that it is a hepatic enzyme inducer and interacts with many medications (e.g., warfarin) (refer to p. 125).

4. D. Ethosuximide is useful in treatment of absence seizures, which are caused by oscillatory neuronal activity between the thalamus and cerebral cortex (refer to p. 133). Vigabatrin (option I) should not be given to patients with absence seizures and is typically only prescribed for patients with difficulty to control epilepsy by specialists only.

5. E. Lamotrigine inhibits glutamate release and is taken orally. Adverse effects include rash, fever, hepatic impairment and malaise (refer to p. 133).

Chapter 9 Drug misuse
Drugs of misuse

1. J. LSD, an example of a psychomimetic, can also cause hallucinations and delusions, some are pleasant, and others are frightening. bad trips. In chronic toxicity, flashbacks may occur long after the trip (refer to p. 144).

2. C. Delta-9-tetrahydrocannabinol (THC). Hashish (option G) is the extracted resin of the cannabis plant (refer to p. 144).

3. A. Clonidine is an α2-adrenoceptor agonist that reduces nausea, vomiting and diarrhoea associated with opioid withdrawal. Methadone (option K) is incorrect because it is a long acting opiate. Methadone is used to help reduce the intensity of opioid withdrawal, through substitution (refer to p. 143).

4. N. Naloxone is an opioid antagonist used in acute toxicity of an opiate overdose. Bronchospasm and flushing are caused by a histamine release

(refer to p. 17). Flumazenil (option F) is incorrect because it is a benzodiazepine receptor antagonist. Benzodiazepine toxicity causes hypotension and confusion (refer to p. 143).

5. D. Diazepam is a benzodiazepine that acts by potentiating the inhibition of GABA transmission. Benzodiazepines are widely abused drugs because they induce a dream-like effect. Withdrawal includes rebound anxiety and insomnia (refer to p. 142). Ethanol (option E) also potentiates inhibitory GABA transmission but is not prescribed, therefore is incorrect.

6. F. Ethanol can cause Wernicke encephalopathy which presents as a classic triad of confusion, ataxia and ophthalmoplegia. Long-term alcohol abuse can result in thiamine deficiency and subsequently, Korsakoff syndrome can develop. This causes amnesia and confabulation (refer to p. 142).

7. E- Disulfiram, an aldehyde dehydrogenase inhibitor given to patients trying to achieve alcohol cessation (refer to p. 142).

8. I. Ketamine causes thickening of the bladder and urinary tract and can cause severe bladder dysfunction. Ketamine and MDMA (option K) are taken because they cause feelings of relaxation and pleasant out of body experiences. NMDA causes patients to overhydrate and have hyponatraemia, therefore is not the correct answer (refer to p. 141).

9. B. Cocaine is usually snorted or smoked and causes euphoria. Adverse effects include paranoid psychosis and tissue damage to the nostrils and at sites of injection (refer to p. 4). Amphetamines also cause the release of monoamines and inhibit monoamine reuptake (refer to p. 140).

Chapter 10 Pain and anaesthesia
Analgesia and anaesthesia

1. J. Lidocaine is a local anaesthetic that is directly injected into the skin and underlying tissue. This allows local surgery to be performed while the person is awake.

2. O. Nitric oxide diffuses into air containing closed spaces and accumulates in gaseous cavities. This increases the pressure within the lungs and will worsen a pneumothorax and will significantly compromise breathing. It is useful in the maintenance of anaesthesia or as analgesia (e.g., labour). Although halothane (option N) is an inhaled anaesthetic it is not as associated with this complication as nitric oxide.

3. C. μ-Receptors. These receptors are also responsible for the major adverse effect of opioids, respiratory depression. δ Receptors (option A) is incorrect. These do contribute to analgesia but are

thought to be more important in the periphery (refer to p. 145).

4. E. Amitriptyline. The pain described in this statement suggests neuralgic pain, discomfort in the distribution of a particular nerve. Amitriptyline, a tricyclic antidepressant, is used in the management of neuralgic pain. Carbamazepine and gabapentin are also useful for the treatment of neuropathic pain (refer to p. 150). Morphine (option L), although a strong opioid, is not effective in the treatment of nerve-related pain.

5. B. κ Receptors. These receptors may also cause sedation but do not contribute to physical dependence. σ Receptors are not selective opioid receptors, but they may account for the dysphoria produced by some opioids (refer to p. 154).

6. K. Midazolam, a benzodiazepine, reduces anxiety and can also lessen the amount of general anaesthetic required to achieve and to maintain unconsciousness. Atropine (option F) is incorrect because it is a muscarinic antagonist given to help reduce bronchial secretions and counteract the bradycardia caused by some inhalation agents (refer to p. 153). These two medications, alongside analgesia and antiemetics, are given at the induction of general anaesthesia.

7. G. Etomidate can also cause pain on injection. Thiopental (option P) is incorrect, even though it is an induction agent it typically causes bradycardia and respiratory depression (refer to p. 154).

8. N. Naltrexone has a half-life of 10 hours, whereas the shorter acting opioid receptor antagonist, naloxone has a 2- to 4-hour half-life (refer to p. 149).

9. D. Adrenaline causes vasoconstriction of the blood vessels around the site of the LA injection preventing the spread of the LA. Adrenaline should not be used at extremities (e.g., end of digits) because of the risk of ischaemia.

10. I. Ketamine, a dissociative anaesthetic, is commonly used as a general anaesthetic in children but given the high incidence of dysphoria and hallucinations in adults, it is less frequently used (refer to p. 154).

11. N. Halothane is an inhaled anaesthetic used as a maintenance agent. It has the potential to induce hepatotoxicity and hepatic necrosis and has been replaced largely by newer volatile anaesthetic (e.g., isoflurane). Nitric oxide (option O) is incorrect. This has low blood solubility and produces rapid induction and recovery because relatively small amounts are required to saturate the blood. Nitric oxide must always be given with oxygen (refer to 10.11 and p. 155).

Chapter 11 Inflammation, allergic diseases and immunosuppression
Medications used in the treatment of inflammation and immunosuppression

1. R. Thromboxane A2 is involved in platelet aggregation and vasoconstriction. Prostaglandin (option Q) is incorrect because they produce increased vasodilation, vascular permeability and oedema in an inflammatory reaction. Prostacyclin (option P) is incorrect because they inhibit platelet aggregation and cause vasodilation (refer to box 11.2).

2. N. Methotrexate has cytotoxic and immunosuppressant activity and acts as a competitive inhibitor of dihydrofolate reductase, which is important for DNA synthesis. Although it is a common first choice drug for the treatment of rheumatoid arthritis, a full blood count and liver function test should be checked regularly because it can cause bone marrow suppression and liver cirrhosis. Patients should be coprescribed folic acid (refer to p. 8). Patients on methotrexate can also develop interstitial pulmonary fibrosis and may present with progressive shortness of breath. Penicillamine (option O) is a DMARD but it is not a folic acid antagonist. It chelates metal and is sometimes used in the treatment of Wilson disease that causes excess copper deposition (refer to p. 163).

3. G. COX-1 is expressed on platelets, gastric mucosa and renal vasculature. It is also involved in physiological cell signalling. Inhibition of COX-1 causes the majority of adverse effects associated with NSAIDs. COX-2 (option H) provides the analgesic and antiinflammatory effects of NSAIDs when inhibited (refer to p. 159).

4. A. Aspirin irreversibly blocks the formation of thromboxane A2 and is therefore used in the primary and secondary prevention of cardiovascular disease. It also irreversibly inhibits cyclooxygenase. It can cause tinnitus in toxic doses. Celecoxib (option E) is incorrect because it is a COX-2 specific inhibitor. This drug is associated with an increased incidence of cardiovascular effects (e.g., myocardial infarction) (refer to p. 159).

5. J. Etanercept contains the ligand-binding component of the human TNF receptor. It is used to treat severe rheumatoid arthritis when DMARDs have not provided an adequate response. Infliximab is a monoclonal antibody that binds TNF-α preventing its interaction with cell surface receptors. Neither infliximab or etanercept should be given to patients with live vaccines (refer to p. 164).

6. K. Febuxostat reduces uric acid synthesis and is used in the prophylactic treatment of gout. Allopurinol works in the same way. These medications can cause dyspepsia, headaches and a rash. They should not be given during an acute attack (refer to p. 165). Colchicine (option F) is incorrect. It inhibits the migration of leucocytes into the inflamed joint because colchicine inhibits microtubular function and mitotic spindle formation. It causes nausea, vomiting and diarrhoea but is commonly used in the treatment of an acute gout attack (refer to p. 165).

7. I. Efudix (5 Fluorouracil) is used topically for the treatment of basal cell carcinomas and other areas of skin damage (e.g., actinic keratosis). Benzoyl peroxide (option C) is incorrect because it is an antibacterial/keratolytic used in the treatment of acne vulgaris (refer to Table 11.8).

8. L. H1-receptor antagonists are used to counteract the actions of histamine that arise during an allergic reaction. Histamine at H1-receptors causes capillary and venous dilation, increased vascular permeability and contraction of smooth muscle. H2-receptor (option M) is incorrect because they are involved in the regulation of gastric acid secretion (refer to Table 11.11).

9. D. Cyclosporine reversibly suppresses both cell-mediated and antibody-specific immune responses. It has a selective inhibitory effect on T cells and is used for the prevention of graft and transplant rejection. Although it does not cause bone marrow suppression, it is very nephrotoxic and can cause kidney failure and hypertension (refer to pp. 170–172).

10. B. Azathioprine is a prodrug that has cytotoxic action on dividing cells, used to prevent graft and transplant rejection as well as treatment for autoimmune conditions when corticosteroid therapy is inadequate. Guidance in the United Kingdom is that patients commencing azathioprine have their thiopurine methyltransferase (TPMT) enzyme measured because if a patient has no or low TPMT activity, then they are at risk of developing the severe side effects associated with azathioprine (e.g., bone marrow suppression, infections, alopecia and gastrointestinal disturbances) (refer to p. 172).

Chapter 12 Infectious diseases

Medications used in the treatment of inflammation and immunosuppression

1. Q. Tazocin is used in the treatment of neutropenic sepsis (refer to p. 174). It is part of the penicillin family and inhibits cell wall synthesis and is bactericidal.

2. J. Flucloxacillin is used in the treatment of skin infections (refer to p. 174). Benzylpenicillin (answer C) is incorrect because it is often inactivated by β-lactamase.

3. D. Ceftriaxone. This antibiotic is part of the cephalosporin family and is good against gram negatives (refer to p. 176).

4. H. Doxycycline. This tetracycline antibiotic can depress bone growth and cause permanent discolouration of teeth. It also causes gastrointestinal reflux and photosensitivity. Doxycycline is typically used in the treatment of acne and atypical chest infections (refer to p. 178).

5. R. Trimethoprim. This antifolate antibiotic causes bilirubin displacement and affects the synthesis of purine and bacterial DNA. Nitrofurantoin (answer K) is incorrect. It can be given safely in the treatment of UTIs up until the third trimester, however, it should be avoided in the third trimester of pregnancy given the risk of neonatal haemolysis.

6. E. Ciprofloxacin is a quinolone that inhibits prokaryotic DNA gyrase and works effectively against gram-negative organisms. Ciprofloxacin is effective in the treatment of pyelonephritis and levofloxacin is used for respiratory infections (refer to p. 177).

7. F. Clindamycin is a lincosamide used in the treatment of severe cellulitis (refer to p. 179).

8. M. Metronidazole is a medication that is both an antiprotozoal and has good anaerobic cover. It is additionally used in the treatment of intraabdominal sepsis (refer to p. 179).

9. S. Zanamivir is delivered via inhalation and is used in the treatment of influenza A and B virus within 48 hours after onset of symptoms (refer to p. 182). Amantadine (answer B) is incorrect. Amantadine blocks a primitive ion channel in the viral membrane (named M2) preventing fusion of a virion to host cell membranes and inhibits the release of newly synthesized viruses from the host cell. It is not a neuraminidase inhibitor and is only used in the treatment of influenza A.

10. A. Acyclovir is used in the treatment of HSV and VZV infections. Side effects include encephalopathy and renal impairment. Ganciclovir (answer K) is used in the treatment of CMV infection because it is resistant to acyclovir; the CMV genome does not encode thymidine kinase (refer to p. 183).

11. T. Zidovudine is a nucleoside reverse transcriptase inhibitor used in the treatment of HIV. Enfuvirtide (answer I) works by preventing fusion of the HIV virus with the host cell (refer to p. 184).

12. L. Indinavir is a protease inhibitor. Answer N (nevirapine) is a nonnucleoside reverse transcriptase

inhibitor which inactivates reverse transcriptase and is thus incorrect (refer to p. 185).

13. P. Nystatin binds to ergosterol in the fungal cell membrane resulting in death and treatment of candida.

Chapter 13 Cancer

Medications used in the treatment of cancer

1. I. Fluorouracil is converted into a fraudulent pyrimidine nucleotide, fluorodeoxyuridine monophosphate, that inhibits thymidylate synthetase, impairing DNA synthesis. It is used in the treatment of superficial basal cell carcinoma and gastrointestinal tract cancers (refer to p. 199). Methotrexate competitively antagonizes dihydrofolate reductase and prevents the regeneration of intermediates (tetrahydrofolate) essential for the synthesis of purine and thymidylate, therefore answer L is incorrect (refer to p. 199).

2. G. Doxorubicin is used in the treatment of acute leukaemia and lymphoma. It can be given intrathecally to treat bladder cancer. It produces a dose-dependent cardiotoxicity because of irreversible free radical damage to the myocardium (refer to p. 200). Bleomycin acts on DNA fragments and may cause pulmonary fibrosis, but has virtually no myelosuppression, therefore answer C is incorrect.

3. D. Cisplatin is a platinum compound used in the treatment of lung, cervical, bladder and testicular cancer. It acts by inhibiting DNA synthesis and transcription. However, platinum compounds (e.g., carboplatin and oxaliplatin) cause significant nausea and vomiting, often requiring concomitant 5-HT3 antagonist antiemetics (e.g., ondansetron) and can cause nephrotoxicity and ototoxicity (refer to p. 200).

4. E. Crisantaspase breaks down circulating asparagine and is used as a form of chemotherapy in acute lymphoblastic leukemia. It causes severe toxicity to the liver and pancreas as well as CNS depression (refer to p. 201).

5. M. Prednisolone is an adrenocortical steroid that inhibits the growth of some cancers but is also used in the treatment of oedema associated with cancer and can be used in palliative settings (refer to p. 201).

6. O. Tamoxifen acts as a competitive inhibitor at oestrogen receptors. Side effects include nausea, flushing and bone pain. Tamoxifen also increases the risk of endometrial cancer (refer to p. 202).

7. F. Degarelix is a GnRH antagonist that reversibly binds to GnRH receptors in the pituitary gland, blocking the release of LH and FSH, suppressing the release of testosterone from the testes and is used in the treatment of prostate cancer. Bicalutamide is an androgen antagonist that acts at androgen receptors thus suppressing testosterone production, therefore answer B is incorrect (refer to p. 202).

8. J. Gardasil is one of the cervical cancer vaccines given to girls aged 12 to 13 years (refer to p. 202). Sipuleucel T is an example of autologous cellular immunotherapy and is used in the treatment of metastatic prostate cancer, therefore answer N is incorrect (refer to p. 202).

9. H. Filgastrin is an example of recombinant human granulocyte colony stimulating factor used to raise white blood cell counts after cytotoxic chemotherapy (refer to p. 202). Aldesleukin is a cytokine, specifically an IL-2 used in the treatment of metastatic renal cell carcinoma, therefore answer A is incorrect (refer to p. 202).

10. K. Gonadorelin stimulates the production of oestrogen and testosterone in a nonphysiological manner, resulting in the disruption of endogenous hormonal feedback systems, reducing the amount of testosterone production. It is used in the treatment of prostate cancer (refer to p. 202).

Index

Note: Page numbers followed by *f* indicate figures, *t* indicate tables and *b* indicate boxes.

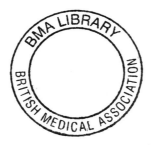